OXFORD MEDICAL PUBLICATIONS

Regional Anaesthesia, Stimulation, and Ultrasound Techniques

T0177676

Oxford Specialist Handbooks published and forthcoming

Oxford Specialist Handbooks in Anaesthesia
Regional Anaesthesia, Stimulation, and Ultrasound Techniques

Edited by

Dr Paul Warman
Consultant Anaesthetist
Leeds General Infirmary
Leeds Teaching Hospitals
NHS Trust
Leeds
and
Honorary Senior Lecturer
University of Leeds
Leeds

Dr David Conn
Consultant Anaesthetist
Royal Devon and Exeter Hospital
Royal Devon and Exeter NHS
Foundation Trust
Exeter
and
Honorary University Fellow
University of Exeter Medical
School

Dr Barry Nicholls
Consultant in Anaesthesia and
Pain Management
Musgrove Park Hospital
Taunton and Somerset NHS
Foundation Trust
Taunton

Mr David Wilkinson
Physicians' Assistant
(Anaesthesia)
Royal Devon and Exeter
Hospital
Royal Devon and Exeter NHS
Foundation Trust
Exeter

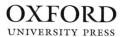

OXFORD
UNIVERSITY PRESS

OXFORD
UNIVERSITY PRESS

Great Clarendon Street, Oxford, OX2 6DP,
United Kingdom

Oxford University Press is a department of the University of Oxford.
It furthers the University's objective of excellence in research, scholarship,
and education by publishing worldwide. Oxford is a registered trade mark of
Oxford University Press in the UK and in certain other countries

Published in the United States of America by Oxford University Press
198 Madison Avenue, New York, NY 10016, United States of America

British Library Cataloguing in Publication Data
Data available

Library of Congress Control Number: 2014930094

ISBN 978–0–19–955984–8

Printed in Great Britain by
Ashford Colour Press Ltd, Gosport, Hampshire

Oxford University Press makes no representation, express or implied, that the drug
dosages in this book are correct. Readers must therefore always check the product
information and clinical procedures with the most up-to-date published product
information and data sheets provided by the manufacturers and the most recent
codes of conduct and safety regulations. The authors and the publishers do not
accept responsibility or legal liability for any errors in the text or for the misuse or
misapplication of material in this work. Except where otherwise stated, drug dosages
and recommendations are for the non-pregnant adult who is not
breast-feeding

Links to third party websites are provided by Oxford in good faith and
for information only. Oxford disclaims any responsibility for the materials
contained in any third party website referenced in this work.

Foreword

For a (large) pocket-sized handbook, this new addition to the Oxford Handbook series contains an impressive range and depth of information about regional anaesthesia, a sub-specialty of anaesthesia, which has truly come of age in recent years.

The current popularity of regional anaesthesia can be attributed to three main factors: advances in nerve location technology, especially the application of ultrasound guidance; recognition of the central importance of anatomy in achieving safe and successful results; and a better understanding of the potential benefits and limitations of regional anaesthesia in the management of surgical anaesthesia, postoperative analgesia, and other causes of acute pain. The very experienced editors of this practical and informative book are well placed to attract an impressive array of authors and to ensure that these three fundamental principles are used as a consistent framework throughout the book. The result is a very readable approach to all the techniques described, literally from head to toe. The expertise, enthusiasm, and common sense of all the contributors are clearly communicated throughout the text, enhanced by the excellent diagrams and ultrasound pictures.

It would be unusual to agree with the details of every technique, as described, in an instructional textbook. While I might take a different view on some of the nuances of practice, I can commend the book as a comprehensive and authoritative guide for the novice. It will also stimulate the more experienced practitioners to question their own practice and encourage debate to continue the evolution of regional anaesthesia for the benefit of the next generation.

It is a privilege to be asked to write a foreword for such an instructive book, if only because it has allowed me to update my knowledge base prior to its general release. More importantly it allows me to pay tribute to the many contributors who, during their working lifetimes, have worked hard to ensure that regional anaesthesia has found its proper place in modern anaesthetic practice.

Barrie Fischer
Dr H B J Fischer
Worcestershire, UK

Preface

The purpose of this handbook is to provide clinicians with an easy access to the art and science of regional anaesthetic techniques. We believe we have provided the reader with a practical guide, in the familiar format of the Oxford Handbook series, combined with aspects of a larger reference text, in a handy pocket-sized book. We have deliberately included both landmark or peripheral nerve stimulator-guided techniques and ultrasound techniques to provide a complete clinical guide. Anatomy features strongly throughout the chapters as it remains the cornerstone of good clinical regional anaesthesia, whether using an ultrasound or a peripheral nerve stimulator, and indeed the legendary Alon P. Winnie remarked 'Regional anesthesia is simply an exercise in applied anatomy'.[1]

The first section covers a wide range of topics on the background of regional anaesthesia. There is an amusing and enlightening chapter on the history of regional anaesthesia. There are chapters covering the basic science of physiology of pain, pharmacology of drugs, physics and use of ultrasound, and peripheral nerve stimulators. Whilst maintaining a strong science base, we have tried to make these chapters as clinically relevant as possible and have useful clinical tips on the practice of regional anaesthesia and frequent summaries of published evidence. There are also sections to deal with risks and complications of regional anaesthesia. Included in this section are some more advanced techniques of wound and nerve catheters and paediatric regional anaesthesia.

The remainder of the book provides detailed descriptions of almost all conceivable regional anaesthetic techniques over the whole of the body. The obvious upper and lower limb blocks are there, with descriptions of all common approaches. Unlike some pocket guides we have included head and neck blocks and ophthalmic regional anaesthesia. We have also covered trunk blocks, those of both the chest, including the increasingly popular paravertebral blocks, and of the abdominal wall; such as TAP and rectus sheath blocks. Each chapter provides a representation of the complexity of the block, the indications, contraindications, and complications. There is an overview of the anatomy with frequent diagrams to illustrate. The step-by-step 'hands on' guides of the blocks are again complemented with diagrams to aid understanding and to help the practice of block performance and of course ultrasound images of the appropriate anatomy. There are frequent helpful clinical tips and hints throughout.

Although familiar to many, we have included a section describing central neuraxial techniques. Although the basics of the practical techniques are covered, there is perhaps more of a focus on the use of these techniques in certain situations and there is a chapter to describe and illustrate the emerging skill of spinal ultrasonography in regional anaesthesia.

There are many contributors to the text of the book; all are clinical anaesthetists with an enthusiasm and passion for regional anaesthesia. Many of them will be familiar names from the 'aristocracy' of regional anaesthesia in this country, teaching and preaching on national and international stages over many years of dedication. Our thanks to them all for their expert contributions and their forbearance on bringing this book to publication.

The text and images have been checked, but we apologies in advance for any errors (or differing points of view) and would welcome your feedback, comments, and corrections. Whilst we hope that this handbook provides an invaluable guide and reference, it is not a substitute for the proper study, training, practice, and mentorship to attain proficiency in the safe and effective delivery of regional anaesthesia to your patients.

Paul Warman
David Conn
Barry Nicholls
David Wilkinson

Reference

1. Winnie AP, Håkansson L (eds) (1993). *Plexus Anesthesia. Vol 1* (3rd edn). Philadelphia: WB Saunders.

viii

Acknowledgements and dedications

I would like to acknowledge the kind assistance of the Anatomy Department at the University of Leeds. My thanks to Barry Nicholls and David Conn for their teaching, guidance, and friendship. I dedicate this book to my wife, Claire, who makes everything possible and to my children Harry and Barnaby who make everything worthwhile. —PW

For the support and training shown to me by teachers and friends Dr Edmund J Charlton and Dr Angus Pridie. —BN

To Sherdil Nath, Angus Pridie, and Barry Nicholls, who are the reason I practise regional anaesthesia. Also to Clare, who keeps me sane. —DC

For IAW and AMR. —DW

Contents

Part 5 **Lower Limb**

Part 6 **Neuraxial**

Contributors

Dr Nigel M. Bedforth
(Chapter 3)
Consultant Anaesthetist
Honorary Associate Professor
Queen's Medical Centre
Nottingham University Hospitals
NHS Trust
Nottingham, UK

Dr Claire Blandford
(Chapter 7)
Consultant Anaesthetist
Torbay Hospital
South Devon Healthcare NHS
Foundation Trust
Torquay, UK

Dr Mark Blunt
(Chapters 47, 48, 49)
Consultant in Critical Care and
Anaesthesia
Queen Elizabeth NHS Foundation
Trust
King's Lynn
Norfolk, UK

Dr George Bostock
(Chapter 1)
Specialist Registrar in Anaesthesia
Imperial College Healthcare NHS
Trust
London, UK

Dr Matthew Checketts
(Chapters 9, 14)
Consultant Anaesthetist
Ninewells Hospital
Tayside NHS Trust
Dundee, UK

Dr Christina Cleary
(Chapters 32, 33, 34, 35)
Senior Registrar Anaesthetist
Galway University Hospital
Galway, Ireland

Dr David Conn
(Chapters 10, 11, 19, 21, 23–29)
Consultant Anaesthetist
Royal Devon and Exeter NHS
Foundation Trust
Exeter, UK

Dr Matthew Grayling
(Chapters 36–46)
Consultant Anaesthetist
Christchurch Public Hospital
Christchurch, New Zealand

Dr James Griffin
(Chapter 7)
(Posthumous)
Consultant Anaesthetist
Torbay Hospital
South Devon Healthcare NHS
Foundation Trust
Torquay, UK

Dr Sumit Gulati
(Chapter 18)
Consultant in Pain Medicine and
Anaesthesia
The Walton Centre and Aintree
University Hospital
Liverpool, UK

Dr William Harrop-Griffiths
(Chapter 1)
Consultant Anaesthetist
St Mary's Hospital
Imperial College Healthcare NHS
Trust
London, UK

Dr Sunil Jamadarkhana
(Chapter 20)
Consultant in Anaesthesia and
Intensive Care Medicine
Lister Hospital, East and North
Hertfordshire NHS Trust
Stevenage, UK

Dr Deepa Jadhav
(Chapter 3)
Consultant Anaesthetist
Department of Anaesthesia
Frimley Park Hospital
Portsmouth Road
Frimley
Surrey, UK

Mr Richard Kerr
(Chapter 17)
Associate Specialist in Oral and
Maxillofacial Surgery
Royal Devon & Exeter Foundation
NHS Trust
Exeter, UK

Dr John McDonnell
(Chapters 32, 33, 34, 35)
Consultant Anaesthetist
University Hospital Galway
Galway, Ireland

Dr Andrew McEwen
(Chapter 2)
Consultant Anaesthetist
Torbay Hospital
South Devon Healthcare NHS
Foundation Trust
Torquay, UK

Dr Hamish McLure
(Chapter 16)
Consultant Anaesthetist
St James's University Hospital
Leeds Teaching Hospitals NHS
Trust
Leeds, UK

Dr Barry Nicholls
(Chapters 36–46)
Consultant in Anaesthesia and Pain
Management
Musgrove Park Hospital
Taunton and Somerset NHS
Foundation Trust
Taunton, UK

Dr Matthew Oldman
(Chapters 21, 23–29)
Consultant Anaesthetist
Derriford Hospital
Plymouth Hospitals NHS Trust
Plymouth, UK

Mr David Pagliero
(Chapter 17)
Associate Specialist in Oral and
Maxillofacial Surgery
Royal Devon & Exeter Foundation
NHS Trust
Exeter, UK

Dr David Pappin
(Chapter 50)
Locum Consultant Anaesthetist
Torbay Hospital
South Devon Healthcare NHS
Foundation Trust
Torquay, UK

Dr John Picard
(Chapter 4)
Consultant Anaesthetist
Imperial College Healthcare NHS
Trust
London, UK

Dr Steven Roberts
(Chapter 13)
Consultant Paediatric
Anaesthetist
Alder Hey Children's Hospital
Liverpool, UK

Dr Graham Simpson
(Chapter 11)
Fellow in Pain Management
Royal Devon & Exeter Foundation
NHS Trust
Exeter, UK

Dr James Stimpson
(Chapters 8, 47, 48, 49)
Consultant Anaesthetist
Queen Elizabeth NHS Foundation
Hospital
Kings Lynn, UK

Dr David Tew
(Chapter 5)
Consultant Anaesthetist
Addenbrooke's Hospital
Cambridge University Hospital
NHS Foundation Trust
Cambridge, UK

Dr Sean Q.M. Tighe
(Chapters 30, 31)
President RA-UK
Consultant Anaesthetist
Countess of Chester Hospital
NHS Foundation Trust
Chester, UK

Dr Paul Warman
(Chapters 6, 15, 18, 22)
Consultant Anaesthetist
Leeds General Infirmary
Leeds Teaching Hospitals NHS
Trust
Leeds, UK
and
Honorary Senior Lecturer
University of Leeds
Leeds, UK

Dr Morné Wolmarans
(Chapter 8)
Consultant Anaesthetist
Norfolk and Norwich University
Hospital
Norfolk and Norwich University
Hospitals NHS Foundation Trust
Norwich, UK

Symbols and Abbreviations

	US technique: easy
	US technique: medium
	US technique: difficult
	PNS/landmark technique: easy
	PNS/landmark technique: medium
	PNS/landmark technique: difficult
⮑	cross reference
~	approximately
±	plus/minus
↑	increased
↓	decreased
1°	primary
2°	secondary
AAGBI	Association of Anaesthetists of Great Britain and Ireland
Ach	acetylcholine
APTT	activated partial thromboplastin time
ASIS	anterior superior iliac spine
ASRA	American Society of Regional Anesthesia and Pain Medicine
CGRP	calcitonin gene-related peptide
CNB	central neuraxial block
CNS	central nervous system
COX	cyclo-oxygenase
CPR	cardiopulmonary resuscitation
CSA	continuous spinal anaesthesia
CSE	combined spinal epidural
CSF	cerebrospinal fluid
CTL	costotransverse ligament
CUSUM	cumulative sum
CVS	cardiovascular system

CWI	continuous wound infusion
DCS	dorsal column stimulation
ECG	electrocardiogram
EDRA	European Diploma in Regional Anaesthesia and Pain Therapy
ESRA	European Society of Regional Anaesthesia and Pain Therapy
FCU	flexor carpi ulnaris
FDP	flexor digitorum profundus
FDS	flexor digitorum superficialis
FOI	fibreoptic intubation
GA	general anaesthetic
GABA	gamma-aminobutyric acid
GI	gastrointestinal
GSN	greater sciatic notch
GT	greater trochanter
HTM	high-threshold mechanoreceptor
INI	intraneural injection
IP	in-plane
IT	ischial tuberosity
IU	international units
IV	intravenous
LA	local anaesthetic
LAST	local anaesthetic systemic toxicity
LC	locus coeruleus
LCNTH	lateral cutaneous nerve of the thigh
LMWH	low-molecular-weight heparin
LPB	lumbar plexus block
LT	low-threshold
MLAC	minimum local anaesthetic concentration
MRI	magnetic resonance imaging
NICE	National Institute for Health and Care Excellence
NMDA	N-methyl-D-aspartate
NO	nitric oxide
NRM	nucleus raphe magnus
NS	nociceptive-specific
NSTT	neospinothalamic tract
ODP	operating department practitioner
OOP	out-of-plane
PABA	para-amino benzoic acid
PAG	periaqueductal grey
PBA	peribulbar anaesthesia
PCA	patient-controlled analgesia

PDPH	postdural puncture headache
PIM	posterior intercostal membrane
PMN	polymodal mechanoheat nociceptor
PNB	peripheral nerve block
PNC	peripheral nerve catheter
PNS	peripheral nerve stimulator/stimulation
PONV	postoperative nausea and vomiting
psi	pounds per square inch
PSIS	posterior superior iliac spine
PSTT	paleospinothalamic tract
PT	pubic tubercle
PVB	paravertebral block
PVS	paravertebral space
RA-UK	Regional Anaesthesia-United Kingdom
RBA	retrobulbar anaesthetic
RBH	retrobulbar haemorrhage
RCT	randomized controlled trial
RLN	recurrent laryngeal nerve
RVM	rostral ventromedial medulla
SC	subcutaneous
SCGM	sacrococcygeal membrane
SCM	sternocleidomastoid
SH	sacral hiatus
SLN	superior laryngeal nerve
SP	spinal process
STB	sub-Tenon's block
STT	spinothalamic tract
SVR	systemic vascular resistance
TAP	transversus abdominis plane
TENS	transcutaneous electrical nerve stimulation
TGC	time gain compensation
TP	transverse process
UGRA	ultrasound-guided regional anaesthesia
UH	unfractionated heparin
US	ultrasound
VCH	vertebral canal haematoma
VIB	vertical infraclavicular block
VIP	vasoactive intestinal polypeptide
WDR	wide-dynamic-range
WHO	World Health Organization

Part 1

General Considerations

Chapter 1

A brief history of regional anaesthesia

A brief history of regional anaesthesia

Introduction

A chapter of this size cannot describe every detail of the history of regional anaesthesia; this would be beyond the scope and remit of this short introduction to the fascinating past of our subspecialty. Instead we focus on some of the more interesting, compelling, or entertaining moments within the last few centuries that acted as nodes or turning points along the winding path that regional anaesthesia has followed.

Regional anaesthesia—the first few centuries

One of the native plants of South America is an unassuming bush with dull green leaves and red berries that was given the name *Erythroxylon coca* by Western botanists after the invasion and conquest of the Incan peoples by the Spanish conquistadors. For centuries before the arrival of the Spanish in the early 16th century, the native Indians had chewed coca leaves, presumably for their ability to give the chewer extra energy and a diminished appetite. We know this because traces of cocaine have been found in mummified bodies up to 3,000 years old. The Spanish invaders were aware of the propensity of their new subjects to chewing the leaves, and presumably that chewing the plant made your lips go numb, but there was no hint that there might be medicinal uses for the drugs therein until the writings of Father Bernabe Cobo in 1653. His 43-volume magnus opus entitled *Historia del Nuevo Mundo* contains this passage:

> 'And this happened to me once, that I repaired to a barber to have a tooth pulled, that had worked loose and ached, and the barber told me how he would be sorry to pull it because it was sound and healthy. A monk friend of mine who happened to be there and overhearing, advised me to chew for a few days on coca. As I did, indeed, soon to find my toothache gone.'

It is a disappointment that although any one of thousands of Spanish visitors to South America in the 17th and 18th centuries could have made the mental leap required to realize that a plant that takes pain away and makes the lips go numb might have some uses beyond giving the natives an extra spring in their step, none did. It is not for 2 centuries after this that the story is picked up by a German professor and his Austrian assistant.

Cocaine—its early years in Europe

Friedrich Wöhler was the Professor of Chemistry at the University of Göttingen in 1857. A remarkable man, he was the first to synthesize urea and calcium carbide, and discovered aluminium, silicon, yttrium, beryllium, and titanium. He also asked a young scientist named Carl Scherzer to pick up a few bales of *Erythroxylon coca* while he was circumnavigating the world between 1857 and 1859 on the Austrian frigate *Novara*. Wöhler gave the material to one of his students called Albert Niemann, who isolated the active drug in the plant and gave it the name cocaine. He even noted that cocaine made his lips go numb, but he was also unable to make the mental leap to realize the potential medicinal use of cocaine. Niemann died shortly after naming the drug, and his work was continued by Wilhelm Lossen, who determined cocaine's molecular formula in 1865 ($C_{17}H_{21}NO_4$). Lossen, too, noted that cocaine made his lips go numb but he too failed to make the required mental leap. The actual structure of cocaine was eventually determined by Richard Willstätter in his doctoral thesis of 1894, a discovery that allowed Einhorn to produce the first synthetic cocaine derivative (procaine) in 1905.

Cocaine and its many uses

A number of scientists and entrepreneurs became interested in cocaine and its effects. An Italian chemist called Paolo Mantegazza devised his own purification process in 1859 and conducted a series of experiments with the drugs, initially on animals and then on himself. Sadly, he suffered the consequences of so many cocaine experimenters from that day to this: he developed an unhealthy appetite for the drug. An excerpt from his writings makes this clear:

'I sneered at the poor mortals condemned to live in this valley of tears while I, carried on the wings of two leaves of coca, went flying through the spaces of 77,438 words, each more splendid than the one before. An hour later, I was sufficiently calm to write these words in a steady hand: God is unjust because he made man incapable of sustaining the effect of coca all life long. I would rather have a life span of ten years with coca than one of 10,000,000,000,000,000,000,000,000 centuries without coca'.

While Mantegazza did not seek to make money out of the stimulant and euphoric effects of cocaine, this was not true for Angelo Mariani, who built a greenhouse in the garden of his house in a small town in France and grew coca plants, macerating the leaves and mixing the resultant juices with red wine to produce a delicious and invigorating beverage that he called Vin Mariani. This became a very popular beverage indeed, and its popularity even spread as far as the Vatican, where Pope Leo XIII, who reigned from 1878 to 1903, was so enamoured of it that he awarded it a Papal Gold Medal. Not wishing to be left behind, an American pharmacist named John Pemberton spotted the opportunities in producing cocaine-laced drinks and devised his own version of Vin Mariani. Denied the use of wine for admixture by local prohibition laws, he flavoured the drink with cola nuts and produced a drink that is enjoyed to this day: Coca Cola.

Thomas, Basil, Carl, Sigmund, and William

The first person to identify the potential use of cocaine as a local anaesthetic was Thomas Moreno Y Maiz, a Peruvian surgeon who, in 1868, noticed that injected cocaine caused insensitivity in 'rats, guinea pigs and, above all, frogs'. However, he failed to translate this observation to clinical use in humans. This historic first almost certainly went to Vassily (Basil) von Anrep, who recommended cocaine as a surgical anaesthetic in a little-read paper in 1880 and was probably the first person to use the drug clinically. However, in the same way that Crawford Long used ether before Thomas Morton but did not get the accolade he arguably deserved, he did not advertise or promote its use sufficiently to earn the epithet 'the father of regional anaesthesia'. This fell to a young ophthalmic surgery intern at the Vienna General Hospital in 1884, named Carl Koller.

A colleague of his, one Sigmund Freud, had been researching the effects of cocaine and published a review article in 1884 entitled 'Über Coca'. The article mentioned the alkaloid's local anaesthetic effects on mucous

membranes, and it is possible that Freud was about to conduct some
experiments on this use of cocaine when he left the hospital to spend
time with his fiancée Martha Bernays. As love—or perhaps lust—drew
Freud away from his study of cocaine, his colleague Koller placed a little
of the powder on his tongue and noted, as so many had in the centuries
before, that it made his lips go numb. He then made the mental leap that
had been waiting for centuries to be made. After a brief series of experiments on nearby laboratory animals, he performed his first operation
under local anaesthesia on 11 September 1884. This was proclaimed to
a meeting in Heidelberg on 15 September, but not by Koller himself as he
could not afford the travel. A review of the conference was published in a
New York journal in October 1884, the same month in which Koller published his first paper on the anaesthetic use of cocaine in the Viennese
Weekly Medical Journal. The word of Koller's discovery spread throughout
the Western world like wildfire, and the first true nerve block—that of
the mandibular nerve—was performed by an American surgeon, William
Stewart Halsted, in December 1884. It was Halsted who performed first
ever brachial plexus block in 1885. After cocaine infiltration of the skin and
subcutaneous tissues, Halsted dissected out what was probably the upper
trunk of the plexus and injected a small amount of cocaine directly into it.
An excellent block resulted with no ensuing damage to the nerve in spite of
the evidently intraneural injection. Interestingly, Halsted suffered the same
fate as Mantegazza, becoming addicted to cocaine, which he may well have
taken to wean himself off his pre-existing morphine habit. In spite of being
doubly addicted, he managed to conduct a highly successful career as the
first Professor of Surgery at Johns Hopkins Hospital in Baltimore, although
it was noted at the time that he was moody, elusive, sarcastic, and prone to
leaving operations half way through.

Early neuraxial blocks

James Leonard Corning was a New York neurologist who, in 1885, armed
with a pioneering spirit and a syringe of cocaine, performed a single spinal injection on a dog. He noted the now predictable effects on the dog
and its inability to move its legs, and determined to perform a similar injection on a human being as some form of therapy. He soon found a suitable patient, a man who had been referred to him suffering from 'addiction
to masturbation' and 'spinal weakness and seminal incontinence'. Corning
performed what was probably an accidental epidural injection of cocaine,
and afterwards assessed the unfortunate victim's skin sensation with a
wire brush. He noted that after 20 minutes, application of the brush to
the penis and scrotum caused neither pain nor reflex contraction, which
makes one wonder what it must have been like for the patient before
the analgesia had developed, and whether the treatment was successful.
I suspect that it might have been.

Formal descriptions of spinal anaesthesia come from the great German
trauma surgeon Karl August Gustav Bier. Bier and his laboratory assistant, August Hildebrandt, combined the now established practice of using
cocaine as a local anaesthetic for infiltration and peripheral nerve blocks
and the work of his colleague Heinrich Quincke, (of needle tip fame) who
was performing spinal injections in an attempt to treat tuberculosis, and

developed spinal anaesthesia. The two experimented on each other on 24 August 1898, and the tale is worth relating briefly. Hildebrandt was not a surgeon and his ham-fisted attempts to push the large needle through Bier's dura proved very painful. The syringe of cocaine and needle did not fit well together and a large volume of Bier's cerebrospinal fluid leaked out and he started to suffer a headache shortly after the procedure. Also, presumably due to the poor needle–syringe connection, Hildebrandt's attempt to inject 5mL of cocaine 1% did not result in anaesthesia. It was now Bier's turn to perform a spinal anaesthetic on Hildebrandt and with the trained hands of a talented surgeon, Bier performed a near painless dural puncture and successfully injected all the cocaine with minimal leakage. After 5 minutes, it was time to test the block. Bier pinched Hildebrandt with his fingernails, hit his legs with a hammer, stubbed out a burning cigar on him, pulled out his pubic hair, and then firmly squeezed his testicles. It was most likely a disappointment to Bier that Hildebrandt felt none of this. However, it was undoubtedly a great moment for the future of regional anaesthesia. The two celebrated their success that evening by smoking cigars and drinking wine. The thumping headaches that they suffered the next day were presumed to be hangovers, although it is more likely that they were two of the earliest post-dural puncture headaches on record.

The pioneers and educators

The end of the 19th century and the early years of the 20th century saw the flowering of regional anaesthesia and the development of almost all of the useful nerve blocks that are still in use today, in one form or another and with one eponymous name or another. Many names of the early pioneers are worth mentioning, but space does not allow us to mention all of them.

Louis Gaston Labat was born in the Seychelles in 1876. Working with French surgeon Victor Pauchet, he was a co-author of the 3rd edition of Pauchet's seminal work *L'Anésthesie Régionale*, which was published in 1921. Labat moved to the United States in 1920 and published his own book in 1922: *Regional Anesthesia: its technique and clinical application*. This tome bore a remarkable resemblance to the book that Labat had produced with Pauchet. Labat was a hugely successful physician who was in large part responsible for the popularization of regional anaesthesia in the United States, and was one of the founding fathers of the first incarnation of the American Society of Regional Anesthesia (ASRA), which lasted from 1923 to 1940. Indeed, it is said that his colleagues pressed him to allow it to be called the 'Labat Society'. It is perhaps with uncharacteristic modesty that he declined this suggestion.

Woolley and Roe

No commentary on the history of regional anaesthesia, particularly one published in the UK, is complete without mention of the sad story of Albert Woolley and Cecil Roe. On 13 October 1947, Dr JM Graham performed spinal anaesthesia on these men. Both suffered permanent spastic paraparesis that blighted the remainder of their lives.

The ensuing case did not get to court until 1953. The plaintiffs alleged that some toxic substance had been introduced into their spinal canal either because of a manufacturing fault in the production of the ampoules of nupercaine or because of the way that the needles and ampoules were sterilized.

The late 1940s were the early years of autoclaving, which was not then universal. The needles and syringes had been boiled in water and then rinsed in distilled water. The ampoules had been soaked in a coloured phenol solution.

The main witness for the defence was Professor Robert Macintosh, author of a leading textbook on spinal anaesthesia and the inaugural Nuffield Professor of Anaesthetics at Oxford University. In the course of the case, the opinion that he developed, and the one that the judge found compelling, was that phenol had entered the ampoule to contaminate its contents through microscopic cracks that were invisible to the human eye, and in sufficient quantities to cause nerve damage but not in sufficient quantities to cause visible discolouration of the contents. The judge therefore found for the defence and neither Woolley nor Roe received compensation.

A contemporary report of the trial is well worth a read, as is a 1990 re-analysis of the case by Hutter (see ➲ Further reading, p. 10). He draws a different conclusion to that reached by Macintosh and the trial judge by suggesting the effects were due to residual mineral acid (used for descaling) in the sterilizers on that Monday morning. The pathological changes seen in the two patients were compatible with the intrathecal injection of a mineral acid.

Whatever the cause of Woolley and Roe's paraparesis, the effects upon regional anaesthesia in general and spinal anaesthesia in particular were negative, dramatic, and long lasting. They greatly added to concerns about the safety of spinal anaesthesia raised by a 1950 article written by Foster Kennedy and colleagues entitled: 'The grave spinal cord paralyses caused by spinal anesthesia' and fuelled a fear of regional anaesthesia in general. These reports cast a grey pall over spinal anaesthesia, and may well have delayed its enthusiastic introduction into obstetric anaesthesia.

ASRA—birth, death, and rebirth

As mentioned earlier, the original ASRA, founded by Labat and his colleagues in 1923, faded away and finally died in 1940. There were several reasons for this, but a recent article on the original society notes that the senior members of the society were actively involved in the creation of the American Society of Anesthetists (later the American Society of Anesthesiologists, ASA) in 1936, of the American Board of Anesthesiology (ABA) in 1938, and the journal *Anesthesiology* in 1940. The rebirth of ASRA had to wait until 1975, when the 'founding fathers' as they are called by ASRA today restarted the society. The founding fathers comprise Alon P Winnie, L Donald Bridenbaugh Jr, Harold Carron, P Prithvi Raj, and Jordan Katz. A year later, the first issue of the journal *Regional Anesthesia* appeared under the editorship of Harold Carron. Both the society, in its second incarnation as the American Society of Regional Anesthesia and Pain Medicine, and the journal, in its first, live on in ever ruder health. The title of the journal has now changed to *Regional Anesthesia and Pain Medicine* and rightly holds the position of the world's leading regional anaesthesia journal under the editorship of Marc A Huntoon.

ESRA—birth and survival

Regional anaesthesia in the UK had been kept alive in the post-Woolley and Roe doldrums years by the formidable knowledge, skills, and efforts of Alfred Lee, John Gillies, Robert Macintosh, Charles Massey Dawkins, Andrew Doughty, and, perhaps most notably, Bruce Scott. It was Scott who, after having worked with Ben Covino in the USA, was the prime mover in the creation of the European Society of Regional Anaesthesia. Along with Albert van Steenberge, he formed the society, which held its first meeting in 1982 in Edinburgh. The society, now called the European Society of Regional Anaesthesia and Pain Therapy, or ESRA for short, shows no sign of fading in spite of the usual European internecine shenanigans and occasional impromptu reorganizations.

The future of British regional anaesthesia

Regional anaesthesia in the UK has grown and developed since its resurgence in the early 1980s. While some have developed the science of regional anaesthesia (I might mention Wildsmith, Rubin, Charlton, and Armitage), others were content to be capable clinicians and enthusiastic teachers (I suppose I have to mention Fischer). They have all played their part in the promotion and development of the subspecialty, and have brought it to its current state of being a leading—arguably *the* leading—subspecialty in UK anaesthesia under the umbrella of Regional Anaesthesia UK (RA-UK). If readers wish to spot the leaders and stars of the subspecialty in the future, they could do worse than look at the list of contributors to this book.

Further reading

Cope RW (1954). The Woolley and Roe case. *Anesthesia*, **9**(4), 249–70.

Cote AV, Vachon CA, Horlocker TT, et al. (2003). From Victor Pauchet to Gaston Labat: the transformation of regional anesthesia from a surgeon's practice to a physician anesthesiologist. *Anesth Analg*, **96**(4), 1193–200.

Hutter CDD (1990). The Woolley and Roe case: a reassessment. *Anesthesia*, **45**(10), 859–64.

Mandabach MG, Wright AJ (2006). The American Society of Regional Anesthesia: a concise history of the original group—its birth, growth, and eventual dissolution. *Reg Anesth Pain Med*, **31**(1), 53–65.

McLeod GA, McCartney CGL, Wildsmith JAW (eds) (2012). *Principles and Practice of Regional Anaesthesia* (4th edn). Oxford: Oxford University Press.

Yentis SM, Vlassakov KV (1999). Vassily von Anrep, forgotten pioneer of regional anesthesia. *Anesthesiology*, **90**(3), 890–5.

The physiology of acute pain

Types of pain

'An unpleasant sensory or emotional experience associated with actual or potential tissue damage, or expressed in terms of such damage' (International Association for the Study of Pain, 1986).

Classification by duration

Acute pain

A physiological response to a harmful stimulus that provides survival benefit, e.g. rapid withdrawal from a burning object or resting and immobilizing an injured limb to promote healing. Sometimes termed 'physiological pain', it results from local tissue damage and is often associated with stimulation of the sympathetic nervous system. By definition, acute pain subsides within 3 months.

Chronic pain

This has no survival value or protective function. It extends beyond the period of normal healing and generally does not involve sympathetic nervous stimulation. Instead, it may be associated with negative symptoms such as impaired sleep, fatigue, loss of appetite, and depression. It is indicative of sustained pathophysiology such as inflammation or nerve injury (hence it is sometimes termed 'pathological pain').

Classification by aetiology

Nociceptive pain

Caused by noxious stimuli. Somatic pain originates in skin, muscle, and skeletal structures. Visceral pain originates in internal organs.

Neuropathic pain

Caused by a 1° dysfunction in the nervous system. Usually associated with chronic pain states, although acute neuropathic pain is also recognized after surgery and trauma.

Classification by primary afferent

First pain

Sharp, pricking, 'bright' pain, easily localized. Receptors are high threshold mechanoreceptors and impulses are carried by myelinated Aδ fibres.

Second pain

Dull, aching, diffuse, poorly localized pain. Receptors are widespread polymodal nociceptors and signals are transmitted via unmyelinated C fibres, e.g. visceral pain. It may last beyond the termination of the noxious stimulus.

Nociception

From the Latin 'noci' meaning harm or injury.

Describes the body's detection of noxious stimuli which are damaging to normal tissues and may be: mechanical (e.g. pressure, surgical incision), thermal (e.g. burn, cold injury), or chemical (toxins, ischaemia, infection).

There are 4 basic processes involved in nociception:

- Transduction
- Transmission
- Perception
- Modulation.

Transduction

Nociceptors are receptors which respond to noxious stimuli, or stimuli which would become noxious if prolonged. They are the free, naked endings of nerves and are found throughout the body.

If stimulated above their threshold values, Na^+ and Ca^{2+} ion channels open and action potentials are formed which travel via the nerve axon to the central nervous system (CNS) to form the conscious awareness of pain. Thus nociceptors transduce noxious information into an electrical signal which is transmitted to the CNS.

Several types have been described:

High-threshold mechanoreceptors (HTMs)

Respond to mechanical deformation, pinch, or pinprick.

Polymodal mechanoheat nociceptors (PMNs)

Respond to a variety of noxious stimuli including pressure, extremes of temperature (<18°C and >42°C), and chemical mediators (alogens). These may be exogenous (e.g. capsaicin) or endogenous and may be released by damaged cells following noxious stimulation.

Endogenous alogens include:

- Bradykinin
- Serotonin
- Substance P
- Histamine
- H^+, K^+
- Prostaglandins
- Leukotrienes
- Cytokines
- Acetylcholine (ACh).

PMNs are the most widespread nociceptor. In contrast to most other sensory receptors they fail to adapt to stimulation and keep firing until the stimulus is removed. They also display sensitization whereby repeated stimulation causes an increase in response (hyperalgesia). This is of protective benefit to the individual, e.g. it ensures an injured limb is not forgotten about and is rested and immobilized.

Silent nociceptors

Respond only in the presence of inflammation.

Subtypes

Various receptor subtypes have been isolated:
• Vanilloid receptors: sensitive to temperatures >43°C and expressed on C fibres. Capsaicin and H^+ decrease their threshold.
• ASIC (acid-sensing ion-channel) receptors: respond to H^+. Some types are also mechanoreceptors.
• Purinergic receptors: stimulated by adenosine and its metabolites.

Transmission

In simple terms, the transmission of pain impulses has 3 components:
• A 1st-order neuron that transmits pain signals from peripheral nociceptors to the dorsal horn.
• A 2nd-order neuron that synapses with the 1st-order neuron, crosses the midline, and ascends to the thalamus in the spinothalamic tracts.
• A 3rd-order neuron that projects from the thalamus to the postcentral gyrus via the internal capsule.

There are 2 types of 1st-order neurons: thinly myelinated Aδ fibres which conduct 'fast pain', and smaller, unmyelinated C fibres which conduct 'slow pain'.

Their cell bodies lie either in the dorsal root ganglia or the trigeminal ganglion. 70% of them enter the cord via the dorsal root whilst the rest double back to enter via the ventral or 'motor' root.

The characteristics of these nerve fibres are summarized in Table 2.1.

Table 2.1 Characteristics of Aδ and C 1° afferents

Fibre type	Diameter (μm)	Velocity (m/s)	Myelin?	Receptors	Stimuli	Pain quality
Aδ	1–6	5–30	Y	HTMs	Mechanical Thermal	Well-localized Sharp, pricking 'fast' or 'first' pain
C	<1.5	0.5–2	N	PMNs	Mechanical Thermal Chemical	Diffuse Dull, aching 'slow' or 'second' pain

The spinal cord

Consists of grey and white matter which contain cell bodies and nerve axons respectively. In 1952 Rexed divided the grey matter into 10 laminae or layers based on its histological appearance.

The dorsal horn

Contains laminae 1 to 6. 1° sensory afferents synapse with 2nd-order neurons here.

The dorsal horn has an important role in the modulation of pain transmission and this occurs through spinal and supraspinal mechanisms involving 1° afferents, interneurons, and descending fibres. For this reason the dorsal horn has been called a 'gate' where pain impulses can be 'gated' or modified.

Although they have discrete functions there are numerous connections between laminae. Nociceptive Aδ and C fibres terminate superficially in laminae 1 and 2 respectively. Aβ fibres which carry light touch and vibration, predominantly innervate the deeper laminae 3–6. They may also synapse with C fibres in lamina 2 and because of this, lamina 2 (the substantia gelatinosa) is an important site of pain modulation. Some afferent fibres ascend several spinal segments cranially or caudally in the posterolateral tract of Lissauer before synapsing with 2nd-order neurons.

The dorsal horn contains 3 types of interneurons which synapse with 1° afferents:

- Nociceptive-specific (NS) cells respond only to noxious stimuli and are found superficially mainly in lamina 1 where they synapse with Aδ and C fibres.
- Wide-dynamic-range (WDR) cells receive inputs from all 3 sensory fibres (Aβ, Aδ, and C) and therefore respond to the full range of sensory stimuli (touch, vibration, temperature, pinprick, and chemical). They are found mainly in lamina 5 and respond in a graded fashion (as opposed to all or none) according to the stimulus intensity. WDR cells also exhibit an important property known as 'wind up' where repetitive C-fibre stimulation leads to a successive increase in response.
- Low-threshold (LT) cells are innervated solely by Aβ fibres and therefore respond only to innocuous stimuli (touch and vibration). These cells are found deeper still, mainly in laminae 7 and 8.

The response of the NS and WDR cells is also influenced by excitatory glutamatergic and inhibitory gamma-aminobutyric acid (GABA)interneurons.

Ascending tracts

Noxious stimuli are transmitted in the spinothalamic tracts (STTs) which are divided into lateral and medial portions:

Neospinothalamic (lateral) tract (NSTT)

2nd-order neurons receive inputs from Aδ fibres (mainly laminae 1 and 5), cross through the anterior commissure to the contralateral side, and enter the lateral white matter columns. The NSTT carries discriminative aspects of pain, such as location (i.e. 'first pain'), intensity, and duration. For this reason it has been described as the sensory discriminative pathway of pain.

Axons are arranged somatotopically so that caudal areas are located more laterally to rostral areas. Most fibres ascend to the ventral posterolateral nucleus of the thalamus and from here 3rd-order neurons continue to other basal areas of the brain as well as the somatosensory cortex. Some fibres synapse with motor units allowing initiation of reflex arcs.

Paleospinothalamic (medial) tract (PSTT)

Phylogenetically more ancient and receives inputs from cells deeper in the dorsal horn, mainly lamina 5. These cells have themselves received inputs via 1 or more interneurons from C fibre terminations in the substantia gelatinosa. Fibres also cross through the anterior commissure to the contralateral side, but then ascend in the medial white matter columns.

The PSTT has little somatotopic organization and is involved mainly in the emotional experience of pain. 10% of its fibres project to the medial nucleus of the thalamus, the rest to 1 of 3 areas:
- The reticular formation
- The tectal area of the mesencephalon
- The periaqueductal grey (PAG) matter.

The reticular formation is a poorly differentiated area containing a diffuse network of cells and fibres. It is located in the central brainstem and projects via the reticular activating system to the hypothalamus, thalamus, and cortex. Therefore, via activation of this system pain can maintain the cortex in an alert, aroused state.

The hypothalamic projections of the reticular formation may explain the autonomic components of the pain response, whilst the emotional and affective components may be explained by projections to the frontal cortex, particularly the anterior cingulate gyrus in the limbic system.

The dual-tract system of pain pathways provides the body with immediate information on the location and intensity of an injury (NSTT) as well as giving a slow, unpleasant reminder that tissue damage has occurred (PSTT).

Perception

The thalamus is a key area for processing of pain signals. 3rd-order neurons project to the 1° and 2° somatosensory cortices, the insula, the cingulate gyrus, the limbic system, and prefrontal cortex.

The perception of pain is the conscious awareness—typically unpleasant—that pain is occurring in an area of the body. Localization of pain takes place in the somatosensory cortex but no discrete centre exists where perception occurs—almost the whole brain is involved. Thus the pain experience is heavily modified by cognitive, behavioural, social and cultural factors, conditioning, and past experiences.

The (IASP) define pain as 'associated with actual or potential tissue damage'. The key word here is 'potential'—stimuli can be interpreted as painful irrespective of whether tissue damage is actually occurring. The pain is real but it is a perception rather than a sensation like vision or hearing.

Modulation

This involves alteration in transmission of impulses and can be either excitatory or inhibitory. It occurs because the nervous system is not 'hard wired' and may adapt and change according to its environment. This is termed 'plasticity' or 'neuroplasticity' and is evident at all levels from nociceptor to cortex.

Facilitation leads to ↑ pain perception typically resulting in hyperalgesia (an ↑ response to a painful stimulus) and allodynia (a painful response to a normally non-painful stimulus). These are often features of chronic pain but can occur acutely. For example, consider the common scenario of putting on a shirt when you have a sunburnt back (allodynia).

Inhibition is also possible and in evolutionary terms this is essential for survival. For example, it allows a person to ignore pain from an injured limb and flee to safety.

In 1965, Ronald Melzack and Patrick Wall put forward the 'gate control theory of pain' to account for the influence that psychological and physiological variables have on pain transmission. Their theory stated that perception of pain is not just the result of nociceptor stimulation (Descartes' one-way alarm system). Instead, nociceptive signals pass from periphery to brain through a 'gate' in the spinal cord, the opening or closing of which is influenced by other neural pathways. Pain signals can therefore be inhibited ('gated') altering the perception of pain.

In fact, pain signal transmission can be modulated in 3 different ways:
- Peripheral modulation
- Dorsal horn modulation
- Supraspinal modulation.

Peripheral modulation

Inhibition

Nociceptors can be desensitized but at present little is known about this.

Facilitation

Repeated stimulation of peripheral nociceptors may cause sensitization. This occurs via the release of chemical mediators from damaged tissues such as histamine, bradykinin, prostaglandins, and leukotrienes. The result is a decrease in stimulation threshold and response latency, with an increase in frequency of response, i.e. 1° hyperalgesia.

In addition to individual nociceptor sensitization, the total number of nociceptors transmitting pain impulses may be ↑. This reflects the fact that normally a large proportion (roughly 30–50%) lie in a 'dormant state' and are not activated until tissue damage occurs.

Nociceptors can also have effects on other nociceptors. This occurs via the antidromic (retrograde) release of neuropeptides such as substance P and calcitonin gene-related peptide (CGRP) from 1° afferent C-fibres. These substances produce local inflammation (also termed 'neurogenic' inflammation) and sensitize other nociceptors. This results in 2° hyperalgesia (an ↑ response in normal or undamaged tissue).

Dorsal horn modulation

Inhibition

Stimulation of Aβ fibres can act via inhibitory circuits in the superficial layers of the dorsal horn to inhibit C fibre afferents and 'close the gate'. From a practical point of view this is the reason that the following are useful analgesic techniques:
- Transcutaneous electrical nerve stimulation (TENS)
- Dorsal column stimulation (DCS)
- Acupuncture
- Rubbing the skin locally.

Facilitation

The mechanisms for facilitation are:
- Wind up
- Receptive field expansion.

Wind up

As mentioned earlier, WDR cells exhibit an important property known as 'wind up', also referred to as hypersensitivity or hyperexcitability. This occurs with repetitive, high-frequency stimulation by C fibres and leads to an increase in amplification and number of action potentials elicited per stimulus. There are numerous chemical mediators involved including substance P, CGRP, vasoactive intestinal polypeptide (VIP), glutamate, and aspartate.

The underlying mechanism is release of glutamate from the sensitized C fibres. This occurs mainly via presynaptic neuronal voltage-gated-N-calcium channels. The glutamate interacts with postsynaptic N-methyl-D-aspartate (NMDA) receptors causing an influx of calcium into the WDR cell and stimulation of nitric oxide synthase to produce nitric oxide (NO).

Substance P is involved via its action on neurokinin 1 (NK1) receptors which phosphorylate the NMDA receptors and remove the Mg^{2+} ions which normally physiologically block them. Once formed, the NO diffuses out of the cell to enhance the expression of presynaptic voltage-gated-N-calcium channels thus resulting in wind up.

Ongoing bombardment of WDR cells also results in an increase in the number of postsynaptic NMDA receptors on the WDR cells and this appears to be the mechanism responsible for opioid tolerance. Over time, structural reorganization of the dorsal horn, involving degeneration of C fibre afferents into lamina 2 and sprouting of Aβ afferents into lamina 2 (rather than laminae 3 and 4), results in chronic pain symptoms such as allodynia.

With continual afferent input, death of inhibitory interneurons may also occur further resulting in excessive responses to nociceptive signals.

NMDA antagonists such as ketamine would appear to be ideal analgesic drugs for preventing wind up and central sensitization. However, in practice adequate analgesic dosing is limited by their side effect profile. They are therefore generally used in low doses in combination with other drugs.

Receptive field expansion

There is evidence that expansion of receptive fields occurs after tissue injury. The resultant overlap leads to activation of an ↑ number of dorsal horn cells.

Supraspinal modulation
Inhibition

Descending pathways from higher centres modulate nociceptive transmission by:

• Direct action on dorsal horn cells
• Inhibition of excitatory dorsal horn neurons
• Excitation of inhibitory neurons.

Descending inhibition involves the release of a wide range of neurotransmitters including the endogenous opioids (met-enkephalin, dynorphin, beta-endorphin, leu-enkephalin).

The key neurotransmitters, however, are serotonin and noradrenaline and these are utilized respectively by the 2 main descending pathways. The first originates in the PAG matter, the second in the locus coeruleus (LC). These anatomical pathways are sometimes called 'antinociceptive' and clinically they are made use of in cognitive behavioural therapy.

Originating in the PAG

The PAG receives inputs from the thalamus, hypothalamus, and cortex as well as collaterals from the STT. It is the main descending inhibitory control over the 'gate' mechanism in the dorsal horn. In rats it has been shown that electrical stimulation in the PAG can produce sufficient surgical analgesia for abdominal surgery. In human subjects, electrical stimulation also produces profound analgesia. Subjects remain alert and responsive to non-noxious stimuli. Furthermore, injection of morphine in the PAG produces more profound analgesia than at any other site in the body.

The PAG projects to the nucleus raphe magnus (NRM) in the upper medulla where connections are serotoninergic. From here axons continue to the substantia gelatinosa via the dorsolateral funiculus (reticulospinal pathway). The synapses here are enkephalinergic. The majority (about 70%) are presynaptic so most of the pain signal is blocked before it reaches the dorsal horn. Furthermore, activation of α_2 receptors on interneurons by dynorphin causes the release of GABA which hyperpolarizes the dorsal horn cells and further blocks pain transmission.

The presence of opioid receptors in the dorsal horn may account for the effect of intrathecal opiates, whilst the α_2 receptors explain the analgesic effects of α_2 receptor agonists such as clonidine.

Originating in the locus coeruleus

This noradrenaline-based descending pathway originates in the LC in the pons and pass via the NRM to the dorsal horn. Noradrenaline mediates its action via α_2 receptors and this may be one reason that noradrenaline reuptake inhibitors (e.g. amitriptyline) are effective analgesics.

Facilitation

Over time following nerve injury, there is evidence that substantial cortical and subcortical remodelling can occur in the brain.

Descending facilitatory pathways exist which travel down from the rostral ventromedial medulla (RVM) in the brainstem to the dorsal horn and can increase pain perception.

The fact that the brain can facilitate or inhibit pain transmission via its descending pathways may explain why attitudes (coping versus catastrophizing) can have such an impact on the level of pain perceived.

Other features of acute pain

Visceral pain

This arises from the viscera and compared with somatic pain, has several different features:

- Poorly localized
- Often radiates or is referred
- Colicky
- Associated with autonomic features and nausea
- Initiated by different noxious stimuli, e.g. distension, ischaemia, inflammation, or smooth muscle spasm.

The differences are because visceral sensory modality receptors differ from those in the skin: there are no proprioceptors, and few temperature and touch receptors. Nociceptors are more sparsely distributed and almost all innervation is via C fibres.

If the cause of the visceral pain also affects surrounding parietal structures (peritoneum, pleura, or pericardium) then the pain will also be sharp and well localized as these areas are extensively innervated by Aδ fibres. For example, early appendicitis causes diffuse central abdominal pain until the parietal peritoneum is involved at which point the pain becomes localized to the right iliac fossa.

Visceral afferents travel with autonomic neurons to reach the CNS via sympathetic and parasympathetic pathways. They synapse in the dorsal horn and from here transmission continues in the same tracts that carry somatic information. There is no distinct ascending pathway that carries visceral sensations alone.

Visceral and somatic afferents may converge on the same WDR cell in the dorsal horn. Because of the shared onward pathway, visceral afferent activity can thus be interpreted as arising from the converging somatic afferent. This gives rise to the phenomenon of referred pain. When visceral pain has both local and referred components it sometimes appears to spread from the local to the referred site and is said to 'radiate'.

Some afferents make collateral connections with postganglionic sympathetic neurons in sympathetic ganglia such as the inferior mesenteric ganglion. Such connections are involved in the reflex sympathetic control of the viscera.

Visceral pain may also initiate reflex contraction of nearby skeletal muscle as a protective mechanism, e.g. abdominal 'guarding'. In contrast to somatic pain which usually initiates a withdrawal reaction, visceral pain often results in tonic muscle spasm.

Referred pain

When visceral pain is referred, it is usually to the dermatomal segment from where the visceral organ originated in the embryo—sometimes termed the 'dermatomal rule'. It occurs because organs which migrate during embryological development take their nerve supply with them. In other words, segmental embryological innervation persists throughout growth.

For example, embryologically the heart originates in the neck and upper thorax so that its visceral pain fibres pass upwards and enter the dorsal horn of the spinal cord between segments C3 to T5. Here the fibres may converge on the same WDR cell with somatic afferents innervating dermatomes C3 to T5. Hence visceral pain from the heart can also be referred to any of these dermatomes giving rise to arm, neck, and jaw pain, for example.

Somatic and visceral afferents converge in the ipsilateral dorsal horn in laminae 1–6, but in lamina 7 afferents converge bilaterally. For this reason pain can also be referred to the contralateral side of the body.

Reflex responses and sympathetic nervous system involvement

As already discussed, nociception may initiate reflex motor responses via monosynaptic pathways in the spinal cord.

In a similar way, both visceral and somatic pain may also initiate reflex sympathetic responses. Mechanisms include collateral connections of afferents with postganglionic sympathetic neurons, the convergence of visceral and somatic afferent fibres in the dorsal horn, as well as the projection of ascending pathways to the hypothalamus. Pain may therefore cause sympathetic stimulation and the release of catecholamines from the adrenal medulla.

This results in typical features of sympathetic stimulation: tachycardia, hypertension, sweating, tachypnoea, delayed gastric emptying, and hyperglycaemia from gluconeogenesis. The emotional responses often include anxiety, catastrophizing, and fear.

Important neurotransmitters involved in nociception

Crucial neurotransmitters and their involvement in nociception are described in Table 2.2.

Table 2.2 Crucial neurotransmitters and their involvement in nociception

Excitatory	
Glutamate	Widespread NT—utilized by vast majority of 1° afferents in dorsal horn (Aδ or C fibres). Various receptors subtypes: • AMPA: rapid transmission of acute or low-frequency noxious inputs • Kainate: similar to AMPA • NMDA: slower, long-term responses such as modulation. Activated with repetitive, high-frequency stimulation of C fibres (wind up) • Metabotropic: G-protein linked. Least clearly understood
Tachykinins	Include substance P, neurokinin A and B. Act at NK1, NK2, and NK3 receptors respectively. Substance P is widespread in the DRG. 80% of projection neurons in lamina 1 express NK1
NO	Synthesized from L-arginine by NO synthase. Involved in peripheral and central sensitization

Inhibitory	
GABA	• Widespread in the brain and spinal cord. Over 40% of inhibition is GABAergic. At least 2 distinct receptor subtypes: • GABA$_A$: ligand gated Cl⁻ channel. Activation causes hyperpolarization. Agonists include benzodiazepines (allosteric modulation) • GABA$_B$: G-protein linked. Agonists include baclofen • Interneurons in laminae I, II, and III are GABA-rich, and mediate gate control
Glycine	Increases membrane Cl⁻ conductance causing hyperpolarization. Probably also involved in inhibitory pathways in the RAS
Cannabinoids	CB1 receptors present in peripheral and central neurons. G protein coupled

Descending pain regulation	
Noradrenaline	NT in the SNS, ascending RAS, and hypothalamus. Descending pain modulation via alpha-2 stimulatory effects
Serotonin	Inhibitory NT in the brainstem, descending spinal pathways, hypothalamic, cortical, limbic, and extrapyramidal systems

DRG = dorsal root ganglion; GABA = gamma-aminobutyric acid; NK = neurokinin; NMDA = N-methyl-D-aspartate; NO = nitric oxide; NT = neurotransmitter; RAS = reticular activating system; SNS = sympathetic nervous system

Further reading

Barrett KE, Barman SM, Boitano S (2010). *Ganong's Review of Medical Physiology*, 23rd edn. New York: McGraw-Hill.

D'Mello R, Dickenson AH (2008). Spinal cord mechanisms of pain. *Br J Anaesth*, **101**(1), 8–16.

Guyton A, Hall E (2006). *Textbook of Medical Physiology*, 11th edn. Philadelphia, PA: Elsevier Saunders.

Hunt S, Koltzenburg M (2005). *The Neurobiology of Pain*. Oxford: Oxford University Press.

Stannard CF, Booth S (2004). *Churchill's Pocket Book of Pain*, 2nd edn. Edinburgh: Elsevier Churchill Livingstone.

Venugopal K, Swamy M (2008). *Physiology of Pain*. Available at the World Federation of Societies of Anaesthesiologists website: ✆ http://www.anaesthesiologists.org

Local anaesthetics and additives

Structure and function

Local anaesthetics (LAs) are used clinically to produce a loss of sensation by reversibly inhibiting excitation and conduction in peripheral nerves.

LAs have a common structure consisting of:

- a lipophilic aromatic ring
- a hydrophilic amine
- a 'link' molecule which is either an ester or amide bond.

It is the variations within these chemical components that determine the clinical properties of different LAs. LAs are usually classified by their chemical structure (principally the 'link molecule') into either esters or amides (Fig. 3.1). Most LAs are weak bases and are presented in an acidic solution (usually their hydrochloride salt) and the LA molecules are therefore ionized, water-soluble, and stable in solution.

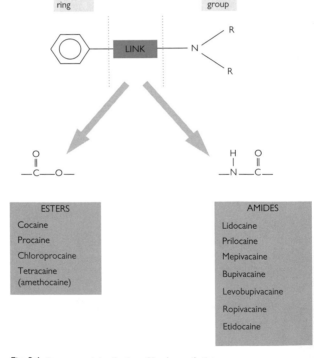

Fig. 3.1 Structure and classification of local anaesthetics.

Mechanism of action

LAs disrupt conduction of impulses along nerve axons by inhibiting the action of sodium channels required for cellular depolarization. In addition, LAs interact with other ionopores and G protein-regulated channels suggesting a more complex mechanism of action.

Unionized LA molecules traverse the lipid bilayer to enter nerve cells. A proportion of the drug then returns to its ionized state (dependant on pKa and intracellular pH) and may then bind to activated sodium channels preventing cellular depolarization (see Fig. 3.2).

LAs display phasic block, i.e. when a nerve undergoes depolarization the sodium channels are activated and open allowing direct entry of ionized drug molecules into the cell. This leads to a faster onset of action of LAs in stimulated nerves.

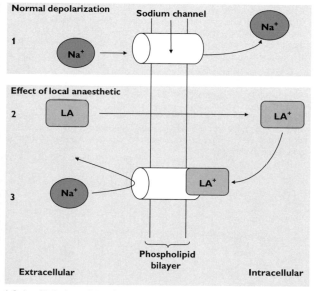

1. Sodium (Na$^+$) enters cell via sodium channels.
2. Unionized local anaesthetic (LA) crosses lipid bilayer to enter the cell where it is promptly ionized.
3. Ionized LA blocks the sodium channel from the internal surface, preventing sodium entry and depolarization. LA also inhibits conduction by acting on potassium and calcium channels and G protein-mediated receptors.

Fig. 3.2 Mechanism of action of local anaesthetics.

Isomerism and local anaesthetics

Stereoisomers are molecules with the same chemical formula and bond structure but different 3-dimensional, spatial arrangements. Optical stereoisomers occur when 4 different chemical groups are bound to a carbon or quaternary nitrogen atom known as a chiral centre. Two isomers are produced which are mirror images of each other and cannot be superimposed on each other, similar to your hands (see Fig. 3.3).

A mixture containing equal amounts of both isomers is called a racemic mixture; bupivacaine and prilocaine are racemic mixtures. Each optical isomer is known as an enantiomer and shares the same physico-chemical properties, but differs in its interaction with target receptor sites. This unique feature of stereoisomers has led to the development of single enantiomer preparations with an improved toxicity profile.

Enantiomers are described by several methods:
- A prefix is added depending on the direction the enantiomer rotates polarized light; *dextro* (right) or *levo* (left).
- The 'sequence rule notation'; the substituent group with the smallest atomic number is 'positioned' behind the plane of the page, if the atomic number of the remaining groups ascend clockwise it is called R (*rectus*, right) or anti-clockwise S (*sinister*, left).

Levobupivacaine and ropivacaine are enantiopure LAs in widespread clinical use. Levobupivacaine (the S-enantiomer of bupivacaine), has a superior cardiotoxicity profile compared to the racemic mixture, due to a faster dissociation of the LA from cardiac sodium channels.

Ropivacaine (also the S-enantiomer) when compared to racemic bupivacaine displays reduced cardiac and CNS toxicity, and when cardiotoxicity does occur it may be easier to treat due to a reduced affinity for cardiac sodium channels.

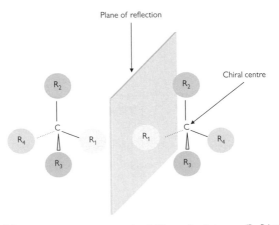

Fig. 3.3 Optical stereoisomers occur when 4 different chemical groups (R_1–R_4) are attached to a chiral centre; 2 enantiomers are formed which are mirror images of each other and interact with biological receptors differently.

Pharmacokinetics

Uptake

Factors that increase the uptake of LA into the plasma include:
- Patient factors:
  - ↑ cardiac output (determines perfusion of organs)
  - ↓ hepatic function (affects protein binding and metabolism).
- Drug properties:
  - low protein binding
  - vasodilatory effects: prilocaine > lidocaine > bupivacaine > ropivacaine > cocaine.
- Site:
  - intercostal > epidural > plexus/nerve > subcutaneous.

Distribution

Following uptake of LA into the plasma, initial distribution is to the highly perfused organs: brain, kidneys, and heart and then to the less vascular muscle, skin, and fat.

Placental transfer of local anaesthetic

The phenomenon of 'ion trapping' of LA occurs in pregnancy when LA molecules become ionized in the more acidic environment of the fetal circulation and are therefore unable to return to the maternal circulation via the placenta. This mainly affects amide LAs, as esters undergo rapid metabolism in the maternal circulation. Protein binding of LAs in the maternal plasma also reduces the quantity of free drug available to cross the placenta.

Metabolism and excretion

Esters are metabolized in the body by plasma cholinesterase and other non-specific esterases, except cocaine which is metabolized in the liver by ester hydrolysis and demethylation. Metabolites of ester LAs are excreted by the kidneys. A breakdown product of ester LAs is para-amino benzoic acid (PABA), which is implicated in the high incidence of allergic reactions to these agents.

Amides undergo phase I and II metabolism in the liver via the cytochrome p450 system. Allergic responses are rarely associated with these agents. Metabolism of amides is slower than esters, leading to a longer half-life and greater potential to accumulate if given as an infusion or repeated doses. The amide bond is stronger than the ester, allowing amide LAs to be stored for longer and even withstand autoclaving.

Prilocaine (an amide) is further metabolized in the lungs to produce o-toluidine which in high doses can induce methaemoglobinaemia.

Pharmacodynamics

The clinical properties of LAs are determined by their physicochemical characteristics. For a summary of the physicochemical characteristics of LAs see Table 3.1.

Onset of action

The onset of action is dependent on the relative concentrations of unionized (lipophilic) and ionized (hydrophilic) LA molecules. Onset time is quicker in LAs where the proportion of unionized molecules is greater (see Fig. 3.2).

The proportion of ionized to unionized drug depends on the local pH and the drug pKa (the equilibrium pH at which the unionized and ionized concentrations of LA are equal). Since the pKa of most LAs is higher than 7.4 and they are weak bases, they exist mainly in the ionized form *in vivo*; however, the proportion of unionized drug depends on the individual pKa of the agent.

For example, let us compare bupivacaine to lidocaine. Bupivacaine has a higher pKa than lidocaine; and is therefore a stronger base and more highly ionized at body pH. 85% of bupivacaine molecules are ionized at pH 7.4 compared to 72% of lidocaine, thus explaining the faster onset of action of lidocaine.

This concept explains why LAs are less effective near infected tissues; the acidic environment of the tissues causes an ↑ proportion of ionized drug which is unable to cross the cell membrane.

Duration of action

The duration of action of LAs is directly related to protein binding, agents which exhibit greater protein binding have a longer duration of action, e.g. bupivacaine. This follows since LAs act by binding to the protein-containing sodium channel.

Vascularity of the site of injection and the vasodilatory properties of the LA also influence duration of action. For example, lidocaine causes localized vasodilatation which leads to ↑ uptake of the drug away from the site reducing the duration of action.

Potency

Potency refers to the quantity of drug required to produce a desired effect. The potency of LAs *in vitro* is determined by lipid solubility. Highly lipid-soluble LAs can enter the cell easily to act on sodium channels, and therefore a smaller quantity of drug is required. However, other factors influence this relationship *in vivo*, e.g. vascularity of the area and the vasodilatory properties of the drug.

Bupivacaine is more potent than lidocaine (see Table 3.2), because it is more lipophilic. This is reflected by the concentrations of the drugs available. Lidocaine is commonly presented as 1% or 2% solutions whereas bupivacaine is available as equipotent 0.25% or 0.5% preparations.

Table 3.1 Summary of the physicochemical characteristics of local anaesthetics

Drug feature	Principal physical property responsible
Onset of action	pKa
Duration of action	Protein binding
Potency	Lipid solubility

Table 3.2 Properties of some local anaesthetics

Drug	Onset	Duration	pKa	% unionized at pH 7.4	Relative lipid solubility
Procaine	Slow	Short	8.9	3	1
Amethocaine	Slow	Long	8.5	7	200
Lidocaine	Fast	Medium	7.9	28	150
Prilocaine	Fast	Medium	7.7	33	50
Mepivacaine	Slow	Medium	7.6	40	50
Ropivacaine	Medium	Long	8.1	15	400
Bupivacaine	Medium	Long	8.1	15	1000

Drug	Relative potency	% protein bound	$t\frac{1}{2}$ min	Maximum recommended dose	Toxic plasma concentration micrograms/mL
Procaine	1	6			
Amethocaine	8	75			
Lidocaine	2	65	100	3 (6)[a]	>5
Prilocaine	2	55	100	6 (8)[a]	>5
Mepivacaine	2	77	115		>5
Ropivacaine	6	94	120	3	>4
Bupivacaine	8	95	160	2	>1.5

[a] Dose with epinephrine

Local anaesthetic adjuncts

Various drugs have been added to LAs in an attempt to improve the quality, duration, or onset of the resulting regional blockade.

Vasoconstrictors

Vasoconstrictors reduce uptake of LA from the target site and promote diffusion across the cell membrane, leading to a faster onset and ↑ duration of action. Specific effects depend on individual LAs; the duration of action of bupivacaine is not significantly prolonged or hastened by vasoconstrictors since it is already highly lipophilic. However, vasoconstrictors have a pronounced effect on the action of lidocaine which is less lipid soluble and a potent vasodilator when compared to other LAs.

Vasoconstrictors may also reduce the peak plasma concentration of LAs. The most commonly used vasoconstrictor is epinephrine. Pre-prepared solutions of lidocaine with epinephrine are available; however, the lower pH of these formulations may delay onset time of effect (by increasing the proportion of ionized drug).

Never add vasoconstrictors to LA when injecting near to an end artery, e.g. digits or penis, as this may cause irreversible, ischaemic damage. Many practitioners will also avoid vasoconstrictor containing LA solutions around the sciatic nerve due to a perceived poor blood supply.

Clonidine

Clonidine is primarily an α_2-agonist; a dose of 1–2 micrograms/kg intensifies and prolongs sensory and motor blockade in both central and peripheral nerve blocks. Side effects include sedation and hypotension.

Glucose

Glucose (usually 80mg/mL) is added to LAs to produce a hyperbaric solution for spinal anaesthesia. Baricity is the ratio of the density of a LA solution to the density of the cerebrospinal fluid (CSF), at a given temperature. Together with patient positioning, this provides more reliable spread of LA in the intrathecal space compared with isobaric solutions.

Ketamine

Ketamine inhibits transmission via central pain pathways by antagonizing NMDA receptors. It also has activity at opioid receptors and may have an intrinsic LA effect. Preservative-free ketamine is used in epidural analgesia, in particular caudal epidural analgesia in children (0.5mg/kg) to prolong the duration of postoperative analgesia. The main side effect is dysphoria.

Opioids

Opioids are added to LAs in neuraxial blocks to prolong the duration of analgesia. Pain transmission is inhibited by cellular hyperpolarization. Fentanyl and diamorphine are highly lipid soluble and have a short onset of action, with diamorphine having a more prolonged effect. Morphine is less lipid soluble which leads to a slower onset time and prolonged analgesia (due to a persistently higher CSF concentration). The side effects of intrathecal opioids include: nausea, vomiting, pruritus, delayed micturition, and the risk of late respiratory depression with longer-acting agents. Late respiratory depression has been associated with high intrathecal doses in combination with large boluses of sedative drugs administered by other routes.

Intra-articular injection of preservative-free morphine (1–5mg) with LA improves analgesia compared to LA alone for up to 24 hours after arthroscopy and anterior cruciate ligament repair.

Little evidence exists for the efficacy of opioids added to peripheral blocks.

Sodium bicarbonate

Addition of sodium bicarbonate increases the pH of the solution thereby increasing the proportion of unionized LA molecules, which hastens the onset of action. Excessive bicarbonate can lead to precipitation of the unionized insoluble LA.

Carbon dioxide

Carbon dioxide added to LA solution *in vitro* diffuses across into the axoplasm and acidifies the cell interior leading to 'diffusion trapping' of ionized LA molecules and a consequent faster onset of action. Whether this phenomenon actually hastens onset of action *in vivo* is unclear, since rapid buffering occurs within the cell.

Dexamethasone

There is no evidence that dexamethasone is more effective as an analgesic when added to the local anaesthetic solution than when given intravenously.

Future developments

The ideal LA to provide postoperative analgesia would be long acting and provide analgesia with minimal motor block. Two approaches are currently under research:
- Novel compounds.
- New drug delivery systems, such as a polymer or liposomal preparations which release the drug slowly, prolonging duration of action.

Tonicaine is a charged derivative of lidocaine and has shown a prolonged duration of action after subcutaneous infiltration in animals.

Sameridine is a LA which is also an opioid receptors agonist and may provide additional postoperative analgesia.

2-Chloroprocaine is an ester linked LA agent, which was introduced into clinical practice >50 years ago. Due to its favourable pharmacokinetic profile this agent has now been formulated for intrathecal use as a short-acting agent. It has recently received a licence for use in the UK.

Butyl amino-benzoate was originally discovered in 1923, but a new formulation has produced a poorly soluble agent with a low pKa which appears selective for Aδ and C nerve fibres. It appears to produce minimal motor impairment and may spare bowel and bladder function while providing a long duration of action.

Clinical notes

Adding epinephrine to local anaesthetic

Typically, epinephrine is added in a concentration of 1:200,000 or 5 micrograms per mL, up to a maximum absolute dose of 200 micrograms (total of 40 mL 1:200,000 solution delivered).

To prepare this concentration, use a 1mL syringe to draw up an ampoule of 1:1000 epinephrine (i.e. 1mg/mL epinephrine). Add 0.1 mL epinephrine to each 20mL LA.

Choice of local anaesthetic

- For a rapid onset of action and short duration, lidocaine or prilocaine are ideal.
- To provide postoperative analgesia, choose a long-acting amide such as levobupivacaine or ropivacaine. (Or consider the use of a continuous infusion.)
- Always consider recommended maximum dose of your chosen agent.

Further reading

Calvey TN, Williams NE (2001). Local anaesthetics. In *Principles and Practice of Pharmacology for Anaesthetists* (4th edn), pp. 148–69. Oxford: Blackwell Science.

Columb MO, MacLennan K (2007). Local anaesthetic agents. *Anaesth Intensive Care Med*, **8**(4), 159–62.

Gupta A, Bodin L, Holmström B, *et al.* (2001). A systematic review of the peripheral analgesic effects of intra-articular morphine. *Anesth Analg*, **93**(3), 761–7.

McCartney CJL, Duggan E, Apatu E (2007). Should we add clonidine to local anesthetic for peripheral nerve blockade? A qualitative systematic review of the literature. *Reg Anesth Pain Med*, **32**(4), 330–8.

Whiteside JB, Wildsmith JAW (2001). Developments in local anaesthetic drugs. *Br J Anaesth*, **87**(1), 27–35.

Local anaesthetic toxicity

Background

Introduction

It is accepted that pain is a bad thing. Systemic analgesics are only partially effective and have side effects, so clinicians in many different fields aim to reduce pain by interrupting nociception with LAs. Generally patients, clinicians, and hospital managers are delighted by the marvellous power of well-placed LA. Nerve blocks, plexus blocks, epidurals, intravenous (IV) regional anaesthetic (Bier's block), haematoma blocks, and even infiltration can expose patients to large doses of LAs and very occasionally free plasma concentrations rise too far in a patient, who then develops local anaesthetic systemic toxicity (LAST). Toxicity is estimated to occur between 1 in 1000 and 1 in 10,000 blocks.

Causes

- Drug overdose (exceeding maximum doses).
- Inadvertent intravascular injection:
  - needle tip in blood vessel
  - epidural vein cannulation
  - connection of LA infusions to IV cannula.
- Rapid absorption of bolus dose.
- Cumulative effect of infusions or repeated doses.
- Susceptible patients (metabolic mitochondrial defects, pre-existing cardiac conduction blocks) may be at higher risk of toxicity.

Pathophysiology

Clinical presentation

The central nervous system (CNS) and cardiovascular system (CVS) are principally affected by systemic toxicity (Table 4.1).

The pattern of toxicity is broadly similar for all LAs but variations exist in the relative severity and timing of CNS and CVS symptoms. Bupivacaine toxicity, for example, presents with earlier and more severe CVS sequelae than lidocaine. In addition it is not necessary, or indeed likely, that patients will exhibit all of the signs and symptoms described in Table 4.1 in a progressive manner and LAST should be considered with presentation of any of the signs and symptoms listed. The clinical scenario may also influence the observed pattern of symptoms:

- Doses of benzodiazepines (given as anxiolytics before regional blockade), sedation, or general anaesthesia may raise the seizure threshold.
- Tonic clonic seizures may not be noticed with the use of muscle relaxants.

Similarly the signs and symptoms can easily be attributed to other causes (which can make accurate estimates of the incidence of LAST difficult):

- The combination of surgery and anaesthesia offers many routes to cardiovascular collapse.
- In obstetric patients, seizure is often first attributed to eclampsia.
- CVS collapse from anaphylaxis.
- Hypotension (and CVS collapse) from neuraxial blocks.

Table 4.1 Signs and symptoms of LAST

CNS signs and symptoms	Increasing plasma concentration	CVS signs and symptoms
Perioral tingling		
Tinnitus		
Light headedness		
Slurred speech		Myocardial depression
Muscle twitching		Conduction defects
Loss of consciousness		
Convulsions		Dysrhythmias
Coma		
Respiratory arrest	↓	Cardiac arrest

Mechanism

Classically LAs were thought to act by binding and inhibiting voltage-gated sodium channels, dampening action potential propagation along nerves. In fact, widely used LAs are all amphipathic (they have hydrophobic and hydrophilic moieties) so they are apt to bind both hydrophilic proteins (dissolved in cytosol) and hydrophobic proteins (dissolved in the lipid bilayer of the cell or organelle wall). More specifically, LAs have been shown to bind voltage-gated potassium and calcium channels as well as sodium channels and also inhibit intracellular signal transduction after G protein activation.

These different actions can be correlated with the detail of the cardiovascular collapse during intoxication. Inhibition of voltage-gated calcium channels slows cardiac automaticity (bradycardia) and conduction (conduction block). Inhibition of voltage-gated sodium and potassium channels slows action potential propagation and repolarization, promoting re-entrant tachycardia before asystole supervenes.

LA can also damage muscle with direct injection, but as skeletal muscle is self-regenerating, this rarely causes a problem.

Pharmacokinetics

LA injected around a nerve or into the epidural space diffuses down a concentration gradient into the bloodstream. For a given dose of LA, the peak plasma concentration is more than double after an epidural, compared to subcutaneous infiltration, with a brachial plexus block's effect in between.

Once intravascular, a substantial proportion of LA molecules bind the carrier acid-glycoprotein before metabolism and excretion. The more dynamic a patient's circulation, the faster a given dose of LA will appear in the circulation and so the higher the peak plasma concentration. And the lower the concentration of acid-glycoprotein, the higher the plasma concentration of unbound LA molecules (which cause toxicity).

Treatment

Cardiorespiratory arrest from LAST had proven difficult to treat prior to the recent introduction of lipid emulsion. Whilst this has been used successfully in both animal models and human cases, there still exist debate about the optimal timing and dosing regimens. Most centres in the UK now have lipid emulsion readily available in clinical areas to treat LAST and would follow the Association of Anaesthetists of Great Britain and Ireland (AAGBI) guidelines. See Fig. 4.1.

As well as the use of lipid emulsion the guidelines also highlight the importance of immediate management (stop injection, call for help, secure airway, ventilation with 100% O_2, and seizure control) and following the standard treatment of cardiopulmonary arrest (CPR, arrhythmia treatment).

Controversies with treatment of LAST

Timing of lipid emulsion

The current AAGBI guidelines (2010) say to give IV lipid emulsion in patients in circulatory arrest, but to *consider* it in patients without circulatory arrest. The first proponents of treatment with lipid emulsion were anxious to avoid doing harm with a relatively novel therapy. Lipid emulsion was therefore recommended for patients already in refractory cardiac arrest—that is, those in whom further harm was virtually impossible. Since then other clinicians have reported using lipid treatment successfully in cardiac collapse before frank cardiac arrest. It has also been used with apparent success to treat acute, isolated, neurological changes attributed to LA intoxication. So the threshold for treatment with lipid is currently unclear, but it is sensible not to *wait* for full circulatory arrest to occur before giving lipid emulsion.

Dosing of lipid emulsion

Dosing studies in humans will be unlikely to occur (let alone randomized, controlled trails) due to the rare, catastrophic, and unpredictable nature of LAST. The AAGBI recommends a bolus (1.5mL/kg of 20% lipid emulsion) followed by an infusion (at 15mL/kg/hour). Differences of opinion about the relative merits of bolus and infusions stems from how the lipid emulsion is thought to work (see ➔ Mechanism of action of IV lipid emulsion, p. 42). If it is seen only as a circulating 'lipid sink', then giving only a bolus is appropriate. If, alternatively, the lipid has some metabolic effect, then adding an infusion would be rational. However, to date, patients that have received large doses of lipid emulsion have not reported any side effects.

Role of other drugs during resuscitation

Over the last years, the role of epinephrine in advanced cardiac life support protocols has diminished; in some animal models of severe LA intoxication epinephrine does more harm than good, apparently predisposing subjects to ventricular ectopy and pulmonary oedema. So it is conceivable that if lipid emulsion works quickly to restore effective cardiac output, adding large doses of epinephrine will only do harm.

The proper role of amiodarone is unclear. Many anaesthetists are familiar with amiodarone, and may wish to use it acutely. But it inhibits very largely the same channels as LAs. So amiodarone may compound the intoxication rather than treat it.

Some clinicians argue for the use of muscle relaxation in patients with obvious tonic–clonic seizures, to reduce the inevitable metabolic acidosis from such violent muscular activity which may make resuscitation more difficult. Others have argued that relaxants make detection of seizure more difficult. Prompt treatment of the seizures with benzodiazepines, thiopental, or propofol is probably the best course of action.

Mechanism of action of IV lipid emulsion

It remains uncertain how IV lipid emulsion works during LA toxicity. A full discussion is beyond the scope of this book, but in brief:

Lipid emulsion may act as a 'lipid sink', binding free LA molecules and thus reducing plasma concentration below toxic levels. The use of lipid emulsion to successfully treat overdoses of other lipophilic drugs supports this mechanism of action.

Some animal work and the original case leading to the use of lipid emulsion in LAST, suggest a biochemical mechanism of action. One of the toxic effects on the heart of bupivacaine (in particular) is to inhibit the transportation of lipid substrates (for metabolism) into the cardiac myocytes. High-dose lipid emulsion may improve intracellular substrate availability to maintain metabolism. This may be purely due to diffusion down a large concentration gradient.

AAGBI Safety Guideline

Management of Severe Local Anaesthetic Toxicity

1 Recognition	**Signs of severe toxicity:** • Sudden alteration in mental status, severe agitation or loss of consciousness, with or without tonic-clonic convulsions • Cardiovascular collapse: sinus bradycardia, conduction blocks, asystole and ventricular tachyarrhythmias may all occur • Local anaesthetic (LA) toxicity may occur some time after an initial injection	
2 Immediate management	• Stop injecting the LA • Call for help • Maintain the airway and, if necessary, secure it with a tracheal tube • Give 100% oxygen and ensure adequate lung ventilation (hyperventilation may help by increasing plasma pH in the presence of metabolic acidosis) • Confirm or establish intravenous access • Control seizures: give a benzodiazepine, thiopental or propofol in small incremental doses • Assess cardiovascular status throughout • Consider drawing blood for analysis, but do not delay definitive treatment to do this	
3 Treatment	**IN CIRCULATORY ARREST** • Start cardiopulmonary resuscitation (CPR) using standard protocols • Manage arrhythmias using the same protocols, recognising that arrhythmias may be very refractory to treatment • Consider the use of cardiopulmonary bypass if available **GIVE INTRAVENOUS LIPID EMULSION** (following the regimen overleaf) • Continue CPR throughout treatment with lipid emulsion • Recovery from LA-induced cardiac arrest may take >1 h • Propofol is not a suitable substitute for lipid emulsion • Lidocaine should not be used as an anti-arrhythmic therapy	**WITHOUT CIRCULATORY ARREST** Use conventional therapies to treat: • hypotension, • bradycardia, • tachyarrhythmia **CONSIDER INTRAVENOUS LIPID EMULSION** (following the regimen overleaf) • Propofol is not a suitable substitute for lipid emulsion • Lidocaine should not be used as an anti-arrhythmic therapy

4 Follow-up	• Arrange safe transfer to a clinical area with appropriate equipment and suitable staff until sustained recovery is achieved
	• Exclude pancreatitis by regular clinical review, including daily amylase or lipase assays for two days
	• Report cases as follows:
	    in the United Kingdom to the National Patient Safety Agency
	    (via www.npsa.nhs.uk)
	    in the Republic of Ireland to the Irish Medicines Board (via www.imh ie)
	If Lipid has been given, please also report its use to the international registry at www.lipidregistry.org. Details may also be posted at www.lipidrescue.org	

Your nearest bag of Lipid Emulsion is kept ....

This guideline is not a standard of medical care. The ultimate judgement with regard to a particular clinical procedure or treatment plan must be made by the clinician in the light of the clinical data presented and the diagnostic and treatment options available.

© The Association of Anaesthetists of Great Britain & Ireland 2010

Fig. 4.1 AAGBI guidelines for the management of severe local anaesthetic toxicity (with kind permission).

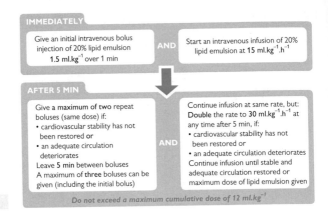

IMMEDIATELY

Give an initial intravenous bolus injection of 20% lipid emulsion **1.5 ml.kg⁻¹** over 1 min

AND

Start an intravenous infusion of 20% lipid emulsion at **15 ml.kg⁻¹.h⁻¹**

AFTER 5 MIN

Give a **maximum of two** repeat boluses (same dose) if:
• cardiovascular stability has not been restored or
• an adequate circulation deteriorates
Leave **5 min** between boluses
A maximum of **three** boluses can be given (including the initial bolus)

AND

Continue infusion at same rate, but:
Double the rate to **30 ml.kg⁻¹.h⁻¹** at any time after 5 min, if:
• cardiovascular stability has not been restored or
• an adequate circulation deteriorates
Continue infusion until stable and adequate circulation restored or maximum dose of lipid emulsion given

Do not exceed a maximum cumulative dose of 12 ml.kg⁻¹

An approximate dose regimen for a 70-kg patient would be as follows:

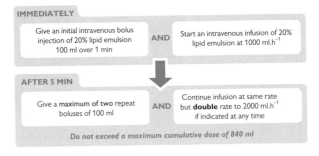

IMMEDIATELY

Give an initial intravenous bolus injection of 20% lipid emulsion 100 ml over 1 min

AND

Start an intravenous infusion of 20% lipid emulsion at 1000 ml.h⁻¹

AFTER 5 MIN

Give a **maximum of two** repeat boluses of 100 ml

AND

Continue infusion at same rate but **double** rate to 2000 ml.h⁻¹ if indicated at any time

Do not exceed a maximum cumulative dose of 840 ml

This AAGBI Safety Guideline was produced by a Working Party that comprised:
Grant Cave, Will Harrop-Griffiths (Chair), Martyn Harvey, Tim Meek, John Picard, Tim Short and Guy Weinberg.
This Safety Guideline is endorsed by the Australian and New Zealand College of Anaesthetists (ANZCA)

Fig. 4.1 (*Continued*)

Prevention

No single reform will prevent systemic intoxication by LAs, but there are means to control the risk.

Excessive doses

Thoughtless adherence to ostensibly safe dosages breeds complacency. Instead, doses should be tailored to the patient (see Table 4.2) and perhaps moderated where absorption will be fast. Epinephrine added to racemic bupivacaine slows absorption and so reduces the peak plasma concentration after peripheral nerve blocks.

Injection of a single-shot dose over a minute or so reduces the peak plasma concentration to which the heart is exposed.

Inadvertent intravascular injection

Intermittent aspiration during injection of a single-shot dose is obviously essential, but it is fallible. (Almost all case reports of LA overdose describe assiduous aspiration.) The Raj test (failure of loss of nerve stimulator-induced twitches on injection of 1mL of LA indicates potential IV injection) though its sensitivity is not known.

The use of ultrasound-guided regional anaesthesia should reduce the risk of intravascular injection but it has still been reported.

Addition of a 'marker' low concentration of epinephrine (say 1:400,000) to the LA injectate may reveal inadvertent intravascular injection before the entire intended dose is delivered. But anyone may become tachycardic with a needle stuck in them!

There have been plans to make all regional anaesthetic hardware non-interchangable/incompatible with IV luer connections. Whilst some examples are now available, the date of mandatory introduction keeps being pushed back. Whilst this may reduce risks, it will not eliminate the chance of injecting LA through an IV device.

Summary

In short, hoping to prevent all patients from developing toxic plasma concentrations of LA is probably futile. It is at least as important to ensure that toxicity is quickly detected and treated. Here the traditional advice stands: patients receiving potentially cardiotoxic doses of LA should be monitored as they receive the LA, and over the hour or so thereafter. The drugs, equipment, and trained personnel necessary to deliver advanced life support should be immediately available to them.

Table 4.2 Patient factors to consider when calculating maximum dose of local anaesthetic

Patient group	Effect on local anaesthesia toxicity	Recommendation
Elderly	↓ renal clearance, ↓ neural conduction	↓ dose by 10–20% in over 70s
Neonates	↓ α_1-acid glycoprotein (plasma protein which binds amides)	In newborns <4 months, ↓ large dose by 15%
Renal impairment	↑ α_1-acid glycoprotein Hyperdynamic circulation in uraemic patients	↓ large doses by 10–20%
Hepatic impairment	Altered fluid distribution Concurrent renal/cardiac disease in severe impairment	No dose change in mild disease ↓ dose 10–50% in severe liver dysfunction
Cardiac failure	Altered clearance & ↑ drug delivery to brain due to low cardiac output	No change in mild/moderate disease Severe heart failure, ↓ dose, especially infusions. Care if using epinephrine
Pregnancy	↑ sensitivity to neural blockade Progesterone ↑ cardiotoxicity from bupivacaine/ropivacaine ↓ protein binding. ↑ cardiac output enhances absorption of drug. Epidural venous engorgement and uterine compression ↑ epidural and intrathecal spread of drug	↓ dose

Further reading

Foxall G, McCahon R, Lamb J, *et al.* (2007). Levobupivacaine-induced seizures and cardiovascular collapse treated with Intralipid. *Anaesthesia*, **62**(5), 516–18.

Picard J, Meek T (2006). Lipid emulsion to treat overdose of local anaesthetic: the gift of the glob. *Anaesthesia*, **61**(2), 107–9.

LipidRescue™ Resuscitation … for drug toxicity website: ♒ http://www.lipidrescue.org.

Rosenblatt MA, Abel M, Fischer GW, *et al.* (2006). Successful use of a 20% lipid emulsion to resuscitate a patient after a presumed bupivacaine-related cardiac arrest. *Anesthesiology*, **105**(1), 217–18.

Spence AG (2007). Lipid reversal of central nervous system symptoms of bupivacaine toxicity. *Anesthesiology*, **107**(3), 516–17.

Peripheral nerve location using nerve stimulators

Background

The first peripheral nerve blocks (PNBs) were performed under direct vision by surgeons at the time of surgery. Once established as a useful method for providing surgical anaesthesia and postoperative pain relief, PNBs were performed 'blind' using surface landmarks to guide percutaneous approaches with paraesthesia as the endpoint prior to injection. During the 1960s, principles of electrical peripheral nerve stimulation (often using homemade devices) were evolved during attempts to localize peripheral nerves, exploiting the motor responses available from mixed (sensory and motor) peripheral nerves. These pioneering anaesthetists demonstrated the effectiveness of peripheral nerve stimulators (PNSs) as method of nerve location and paved the way for large-scale commercial development of the portable, battery-operated, micro-processor controlled devices that we recognize today.

Electrical principles

Mammalian nerve cell membranes have a negative resting intracellular potential and if this potential is reduced to a certain critical level (threshold) then an action potential is unleashed. The usual intrinsic triggers for this process are activation of voltage-gated sodium channels (from an arriving impulse), mechanical deformation of receptors, or specific ligand binding. PNSs attempt to deliver enough electrical energy to motor nerves to provide an extrinsic (non-physiological) trigger sufficient to reduce the resting potential to the threshold level.

This energy is delivered in the form of a monophasic square wave impulse with a 'strength' (current) of up to a couple of milliamps and a duration of less than a millisecond. Many combinations of strength and duration will provide enough energy to reach threshold and therefore elicit and action potential. A graphical plot of these variations in impulse morphology is known as a strength versus duration curve (Fig. 5.1) which is the key to understanding how PNSs work.

The rheobase is the minimum *current* (milliamps) capable of eliciting an action potential (at infinite duration). The chronaxie is the *duration* (milliseconds) required to elicit an action potential when using twice the rheobase current. The most efficient way to simulate mammalian nerves is to use impulse durations close to the chronaxie of the target nerves, typically around 0.1msec for motor fibres (and around 1msec for sensory fibres). Therefore as a general rule *0.1msec* should be selected (some older PNSs are internally set to this) when trying to elicit motor responses. An impulse duration of 0.1msec can be assumed for the remainder of the chapter. The

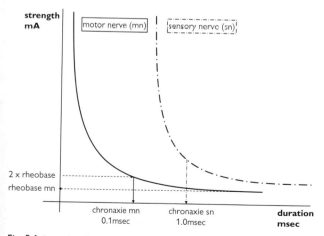

Fig. 5.1 Strength vs duration curves for mammalian motor and sensory nerves showing that stimulation at twice rheobase current for enough time (chronaxie) elicits an action potential.

longer chronaxie of sensory nerves (arising from their lack of myelination) make them more difficult to stimulate and allows some separation of motor (twitches) and sensory (pain) responses during the performance of awake blocks.

Polarity

If a negative needle is used to stimulate neural responses then less current will be required (than if a positive needle is used) due to the negative resting potential of the neurons and the way in which electrons flow through the nerve with stimulation by a cathode. Modern PNSs are automatically configured with a negative needle but it should be noted that some older machines may allow a positive needle to be selected.

Distance versus energy

For any given level of energy emitted from the tip of a stimulating needle, the distance between the target nerve and the needle tip is critical in eliciting any motor responses. The amount of energy delivered to a target (nerve membrane) from a point emitting source (needle tip) varies as an inverse square law (Coulomb's law). If this distance is doubled, 4 times as much energy will be required to produce the same effect.

In practical terms this means that a nerve stimulating needle is very 'short sighted' (no responses will be observed until you are very close to the nerve—say within 5–8mm at commonly used initial search settings) but gives *very accurate distance information on final approach* to the nerve (the amount of energy required for a response drops off rapidly as the nerve is approached—the closer you are, the better it gets). Modern regional anaesthesia needles are insulated, maximizing current density at the tip and ensuring the distance/energy relationship reflects the position of the tip of the needle. Research has shown that with a current of 1mA, motor response is first observed when the needle is 5.5mm (±1.5mm) from the target nerve.

Return electrode

Modern PNSs powered by 9V batteries use internal transformers to increase the internal voltage (to well over 60V) across a very high internal resistance to ensure constant current delivery to the patient (in spite of variations in patient–stimulator interactions such as high skin impedance at the return electrode). This means that the exact location of the return electrode is less critical than it once was so any sensible (e.g. avoiding current across pacemakers) convenient location is acceptable.

Clinical use

If a PNS is used to identify a peripheral nerve it needs to be done in a safe and effective manner. Safe implies that the procedure is carried out without damaging the target nerve and effective means that a suitably high proportion of attempted blocks are successful.

Setting up

Most modern PNSs have sophisticated internal diagnostics to detect faults and also allow the display to indicate most of the important electrical parameters. Before using this equipment the operator should be satisfied that the battery has sufficient energy, all cables and connections are functioning and placed properly, and that where possible the machine displays current actually flowing to the patient (strength and duration). The display should be visible to the operator who should communicate clearly with any assistant.

Either the needle should be moving or the current should be changing but never both at the same time (an operator moving the needle in or out while an assistant changes delivered current at the same time is a recipe for trouble).

Muscle relaxants are contraindicated (obviously).

When blocking awake patients, *careful* control of needle speed and chosen current will ensure that the procedure is not unpleasant.

The initial injection (first few mL) should be done particularly slowly and carefully to give the best feedback about any potential problems (intraneural or intravascular injection).

Avoiding intraneural injection (INI)

There are 5 safety rules to observe when performing a peripheral nerve block using a PNS in order to avoid INI.
1. Threshold current greater than 0.2mA (provided the impulse duration is set to 0.1msec);
2. Twitches should disappear immediately on starting injection;
3. The injection should be easy with low resistance (less than 25psi—the operator should only use one thumb to inject (gently));
4. Watch the patient (awake or asleep) for pain or abnormal movements;
5. If the going gets weird—JUST STOP.

Threshold current

Whenever a motor response (twitch) is seen, the minimum current required for eliciting the twitch should be checked *before* injection of LA (by reducing the current until the twitch is just abolished). A twitch continuing at a current of 0.2mA or less, suggests that the needle tip is extremely close to the target nerve, and may be intraneural. The needle tip should therefore be repositioned prior to injection of LA.

Most modern PNSs have this limitation stated in the product literature although the experimental evidence for this threshold to be used in practice is tenuous. In animal models, needles placed *into* nerves, under direct vision, have threshold stimulation below 0.2mA in only 33% of cases, but above 0.5mA in 44%. However care needs to be taken interpreting threshold data from experiments using exposed nerves as the surrounding tissues (that have been removed) can act as a volume conductor causing current channelling to occur which can reduce the threshold current.

Twitch disappears on injection

As soon as injection is started the observed twitches should stop immediately. Failure of the twitches to disappear should prompt the operator to STOP the injection, as this implies possible intraneural placement of the needle tip.

The original theories as to why the responses should stop were based on experiments where twitches were obtained and then either air, saline, or LA was injected. In all 3 cases the twitch stopped, implying that mechanical displacement of the nerve (critically increasing the distance between the stimulating needle and target nerve) was responsible for the cessation of response. It was noted that the response stopped too quickly for it to be due to pharmacological action of the local anaesthetic.

However, what is less widely reported from this study is that if stimulation is continued for several minutes then twitches will return: but after air and saline this return will take 10–15 seconds (as they are dispersed in the tissues) whereas following LA it takes 90 seconds for twitches to return at a much weaker level (due to LA beginning to act on the epineurium). This may have implications for multiple stimulation techniques, which will be discussed later.

Modern theory has modified this idea to embrace an electrophysiological explanation following experiments showing that solutions which conduct electrical energy are the significant factor in abolishing the twitch. Conductive solutions (LA and saline) *will* stop the twitch while non-conductive solutions *will not* stop the twitch (5% glucose actually enhances the twitch). These authors conclude that a tiny amount of conductive injectate emerging from the needle tip has the effect of 'increasing the size' of the tip and will reduce the perineural electric field thus abolishing the twitch. These findings are supported by a recent study using mathematical modelling techniques and have 3 clinical consequences. It may be helpful to use 5% glucose when placing stimulating catheters as this injectate will not interfere with stimulation responses. A 'trigger happy' assistant who prematurely injects so much as a drop of LA before the needle tip is where you want it, could impair your ability to locate a nerve accurately. Blood is also highly conductive, so significant amounts of blood in the region of the needle tip may diminish or abolish the expected twitches.

Resistance to injection

Animal studies of deliberate intraneural injection have shown that not all injections result in permanent nerve damage but that high initial injection pressures (>25psi) are most likely to be associated with permanent damage.

Traditional teaching has held that high resistance to injection is likely to indicate intraneural injection and may lead to permanent nerve damage. Recent data from ultrasound studies show that intraneural injection happens more commonly than previously thought but does not necessarily lead to permanent nerve damage (albeit at volumes of 2–3mL). This may be due to subepineurial injection with no fascicular damage.

Hadzic demonstrated the importance of high injection pressures being a major determinant of neurological damage. He exposed sciatic nerves in anaesthetized dogs and under microscopic guidance placed a needle tip either perineurally or intraneurally prior to injection (4mL of 2% lidocaine over 1 minute through a long-bevel, 25G needle). All perineural injections were associated with low injection pressures (<4psi) and no damage. Intraneural injection pressures fell into 2 groups (moderate pressures of 11psi or less and high *initial* injection pressures in excess of 25psi). Animals having moderate pressure intraneural injections did not suffer any neural damage whereas animals in the high-pressure group showed persistent motor deficits (after 7 days) and histological evidence of destroyed neural architecture (these high intraneural injection pressures were believed to represent intrafascicular injections although this was not formally demonstrated in the study). It should be noted that high initial pressures were followed by a sudden drop in pressure to the moderate level (believed to represent fascicular rupture and subsequent subepineural injection). Thus it is the *initial* injection pressure which is most informative. Commercial devices are now available to allow measurement of line pressure during LA injection. Why high pressure injection should be associated with nerve damage is beyond this chapter but mechanical disruption, LA toxicity, and ischaemia have all been implicated.

Once a needle is placed into a nerve, little can be done about the damage that it may have already caused (evidence suggest that short bevelled needles are actually unlikely to cause harm), but it by *avoiding injecting* when high resistance/pressure is felt, that further damage can be avoided.

Observe the patient (awake or asleep)
During positioning of the needle and injection of LA the patient should be watched closely for any reports or signs of distress. Severe lancinating pain, dysaesthesia, or shooting pains should all lead to the positioning/injection being stopped immediately. Some patients will report a low-intensity dull ache during LA injection which is due to 'pressure paraesthesia' and can be regarded as a normal response. Careful questioning is required to tell the difference. Paraesthesia rarely causes trouble; dysaesthesias commonly lead to longer-term problems (some studies documenting permanent nerve damage comment on the significance of dysaesthesia during needle placement or injection as an associated finding).

If LA is injected when the patient is sedated or anaesthetized they should be carefully observed for any signs of painful stimulation when the injection is started (laryngospasm, limb movement—localizing or non-specific— sudden tachypnoea); injection should be *stopped* if any of these are present.

'If the going gets weird—STOP'
If you are just not seeing what you expect to see during the performance of a block...**STOP**. Consider the reasons for things not adding up and check everything again before deciding whether to modify your technique or abandon it altogether. Better a failed block than a damaging one. This rule is best applied sooner rather than later. Inspection of case reports detailing damaging blocks often reveals a failure to apply one or more of the 'rules' in ➲ Avoiding intraneural injection (INI), p. 53. There are many reasons for things to become weird and you won't always get to the bottom of it.

Successful blocks

'Eliciting a relevant twitch at a suitably low current ensures the needle is close enough to the nerve to produce a successful block' is sadly too simplistic a concept and the clinical reality is more complicated.

All studies involving the use of nerve stimulators for nerve location report failure rates of anything up to 50% although a range of 5–20% would be representative and some claim rates of <2%. There are many reasons for this failure rate (related to variations in anatomy, electrophysiology, and operators) but all a nerve stimulator tells you is that the needle tip is close to the target nerve—it tells you little about what barriers (to diffusion) lie between the needle and the nerve or where the injectate is spreading. The bevel of a needle (giving a good-looking twitch) may not be within the fascial plane containing the nerve. Similarly the topography of individual motor and sensory fascicles within the same mixed nerve may lead to the block of one modality above the other.

A number of studies have attempted to correlate twitch threshold with either block success or needle position (proximity to the nerve) and the outcome has been mixed to say the least.

Threshold correlation with block success

There is some evidence that threshold does correlate with success (0.8mA:median, 0.6mA:radial, and 0.7mA:ulnar nerves for mid humeral blocks) and that higher currents predicted failure. In patients undergoing sciatic block threshold (0.4mA) was more important than the type of motor response in predicting success. Even this data make it difficult to draw meaningful conclusion.

Threshold correlation with needle position

Studies looking at this question have used paraesthesia or ultrasound guidance to 'confirm' that the needle is next to the nerve before turning on a PNS to determine the threshold current. A striking finding in these studies is the wide range of thresholds required to elicit a motor response after alleged nerve contact. A significant number of subjects (around 25%) needed well in excess of 0.5mA to elicit a motor response (and some >1mA). A recurrent and somewhat surprising finding is that in many cases where the needle is next to the nerve (paraesthesia elicited or visualized using ultrasound) *no* twitches are seen with an appropriate current despite the subsequent block being successful. A motor response (at or below 0.5mA) has been shown to be only 74.5% sensitive for detection of needle to nerve contact as seen on ultrasound (and paraesthesia was only reported in 38.2% of these patients). Injection of dye around animal nerves and subsequent histological analysis found no difference in spread around the nerves between high (0.99mA/0.2msec) and low (0.33mA/0.2msec) threshold currents.

Ideal endpoints

Accepting a threshold of ~0.5mA should produce reasonably reliable blocks (89% of patients with a motor response at 0.5mA (or less) developed a sensory block) but deliberately seeking thresholds below 0.4 mA may provide faster onset with no overall increase in success rate and that this may come at the price of an ↑ risk of nerve damage. The author aims to see a stable response at 0.5mA (with appropriate cues as the needle passes through the tissues) but often encounters (unsought) thresholds between 0.3mA and 0.5mA: injection proceeds in accordance with rules 1–5 (➜ Avoiding intraneural injection (INI), p. 53).

However, there are many other considerations in the production of a successful block. The feel of the needle in the tissues is a valuable guide to many experienced anaesthetists (fascial clicks). The stability of the twitch (a weak twitch that disappears with the slightest alteration in pressure on the needle shaft often precedes a failed block even though the correct muscle group is responding at what appears to be a suitable threshold). The way in which the needle approaches the nerve (strengthening up a weak twitch by 'levering' the needle tip towards the nerve) may precede a failed block because it is merely pushing tissues aside to reduce the needle to nerve distance allowing a good twitch but as injection proceeds these tissues remain as a barrier to stop the LA reaching the target nerve. It may be better to use the direction of leverage as a guide to the direction in which the needle should pass on the next attempt at location as you attempt to penetrate these tissue barriers.

It seems increasingly likely that patients with existing neurological impairment (previously diagnosed or undiagnosed subclinical disease) may require higher thresholds to elicit motor responses. This means that stimulation may not be possible at commonly used thresholds (≤0.5mA) without a higher chance of intraneural needle placement and subsequent intraneural injection. Diabetic patients in particular require careful thought in the application of PNB (in a hyperglycaemic animal model, low threshold stimulation (0.5mA/0.2msec) uniformly resulted in intraneural injection). It may be wise or necessary to consider accepting higher thresholds in these patients.

The double crush phenomenon has been evoked to explain why previously injured nerves (needle damage, neuropathy, slipped discs, chemotherapy) are more likely to suffer serious damage following a second injury attributed to a PNB.

Several types of PNB may require multi-stimulation and separate injection of several nerves in close proximity (axillary or infraclavicular approach to brachial plexus, popliteal fossa) to provide an effective block. This may mean that some LA diffuses from one target nerve to the surface of another during the performance of the block (such that PNS-guided location of the 2nd and/or 3rd nerves could become more difficult). If all nerves behave as expected during the course of a multi-stimulation technique then there is no problem (proceed as normal). If subsequent nerves behave as if they are more difficult to locate at expected thresholds then the cautious operator has the choice to prudently accept a higher threshold or employ 'rule 5' and abandon ship. Prolonged attempts to doggedly elicit expected thresholds (come what may) during multi-stimulation techniques may be unwise.

These and other factors have previously been referred to as the 'art' of regional anaesthetic blocking—we may be scientific but we need to be artful as well. Indeed, the lessons from ultrasound are that nerves are extremely mobile when approached by needles (difficult for needle tips to remain in close proximity), that electrical stimulation thresholds correlate only moderately with needle position or block success, and that seeing LA spread around a nerve is the best indicator of a successful block.

There are 4 possible locations of a needle tip prior to injection of LA (Table 5.1) leading to a range of outcomes. Location 2 is ideal, location 3 probably happens more often than we previously thought (ultrasound evidence) but appears to cause surprisingly little damage. Location 4 is the most likely to cause serious neural damage.

Table 5.1 Four possible locations of a needle tip prior to injection of local anaesthetic and their characteristics

Location	Twitch	Resistance	Blockade	Damage
1. Outside epineurium and fascial layer	Unstable 0.5mA or higher	Low, <4psi	Failed	No
2. Outside epineurium within fascial layer	Stable 0.5mA or less	Low, <4psi	Successful	No
3. Inside epineurium	Excellent may be <0.2mA	Moderate, <10–12psi	Very successful, may be prolonged	Possible, may well be no damage
4. Inside perineurium	Ballistic!	High, >25psi	Probably successful	Very likely

Further reading

Chan VWS, Brull R, McCartney CJ, et al. (2007). An ultrasonographic and histological study of intra-neural injection and electrical stimulation in pigs. Anesth Analg, 104(5), 1281–4.

De Andres J, Sala-Blanch X (2001). Peripheral nerve stimulation in the practice of brachial plexus anesthesia: a review. Reg Anesth Pain Med, 26(5), 478–83.

Ercole A (2008). The effect of injectate conductivity on the electric field with the nerve stimulator: a computer simulation. Anesth Analg, 107(4), 1427–32.

Hadzic A, Dilberovic F, Shah S, et al. (2004). Combination of intraneural injection and high injection pressure leads to fascicular injury and neurologic deficits in dogs. Reg Anesth Pain Med, 29(5), 417–23.

Perlas A (2006). The sensitivity of motor response to nerve stimulation and paraesthesia for nerve localization as evaluated by ultrasound. Reg Anesth Pain Med, 31(5), 445–50.

Rigaud M, Filip P, Lirk P, et al. (2008). Guidance of block needle insertion by electrical nerve stimulation. Anesthesiology, 109(3), 473–8.

Tsui BCH, Wagner A, Finucane B (2004). Electrophysiological effects of injectates on peripheral nerve stimulation. Reg Anesth Pain Med, 29(3), 189–93.

Basic physics of ultrasound

Ultrasound waves

Basic principles

Ultrasound (US) waves are sound waves, but are at a much higher frequency (2–15MHz) compared to human audible sound waves (20Hz–20kHz). They can be used to generate an image of body structures.

A sound wave is a pressure disturbance that travels through a medium as vibrations of the molecules along the line of propagation in a series of compressions (high pressure) and rarefactions (low pressure). The distance between 2 consecutive peaks (or troughs) is the wavelength (λ) measured in metres (or mm for US waves). The number of peaks passing a point in 1 second is the frequency (f) measured in hertz (Hz).

These are related by the equation:

Speed of sound = frequency x wavelength ($C = f \times \lambda$)

The speed of sound of the US wave in tissues varies according to the density and the compressibility of the tissues (acoustic impedance). See Table 6.1.

The average speed of sound (and US) for human soft tissue is about 1540m/sec. This gives wavelengths of ~0.5–0.1mm (for frequencies of 3–10MHz).

Table 6.1 Acoustic impedance and speed of US waves through different tissues

Tissue	Acoustic impedance ($kg/m^2/sec$)	Speed of sound through tissues (m/sec)
Air	392	330
Water	1.54×10^6	1480
Blood	1.61×10^6	1570
Liver	1.66×10^6	1580
Muscle	1.64×10^6	1575
Fat	1.31×10^6	1430
Cortical bone	7.8×10^6	2800

Generation of US waves

The pressure disturbances of medical US waves are produced by the expansion and contraction of certain crystals subjected to an electrical voltage. This is the Piezoelectric effect (literally 'pressure-electric'). Most transducers use artificial polycrystalline ferroelectric materials (ceramics) e.g. lead zirconate titanate (PZT). When a voltage spike is applied to the crystal it vibrates at its resonant frequency. The frequency of the transmitted sound wave is determined by the thickness and shape of the piezoelectric material and current applied to it.

Crucially the piezoelectric effect also works 'in reverse'; when subjected to a mechanical stress, i.e. an US wave, the piezoelectric material will produce a small voltage.

Interactions of US waves with tissues

US waves, like all wave motions (including light), will undergo reflection, refraction, and absorption. Reflections of US waves are crucial to the generation of the images as only those waves that are reflected back to the transducer will be able to form the picture.

Interface reflection (specular reflections)

When an US wave meets the interface between two tissues, some of the energy will be reflected back. The greater the difference in acoustic impedance between the two tissues, the more of the US beam is reflected. When a high proportion of US waves are reflected back, this prevents imaging of structures deep to the interface. Conversely with little reflection, the US beam penetrates deep to the interface. Large flat interfaces, perpendicular to the US wave, produce better reflections and are termed 'specular (mirror) reflection' (see Fig. 6.1).

Reflectivity is greatest when the object being visualized is perpendicular to the angle of the US beam. As the angle of incidence (angle of insonation) decreases from 90°, some of the US beam is reflected away from the transducer, and will not form part of the image (see Fig. 6.2). The visibility of certain structures/tissues (including nerves and tendons) can be highly dependent on the angle of insonation; this is called 'anisotropy'.

Refraction

Refraction (bending/distorting) may occur at any interface, but is more common in fatty tissue and when the probe is angulated. In some patients the combination of globules of dense fat in a matrix of less dense fat causes poor visualization (like looking through wobbly bathroom glass).

Attenuation (absorption) of US waves

As US waves pass through tissue, some of the energy is reflected, some is scattered and some absorbed as heat. Energy lost by scattering and absorption is known as 'attenuation'. Eventually the energy of the beam is reduced to the extent that no useful reflections will be detected (depth of view).

The higher the US frequency, the greater the scattering and the greater absorption as heat. Attenuation is directly proportional to the frequency of the US beam; low frequencies are attenuated less and will penetrate tissues better the than high frequencies. This is an important concept in probe selection and machine settings.

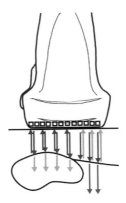

Fig. 6.1 Specular reflection; strong reflection of US waves from tissues when perpendicular to the US beam.

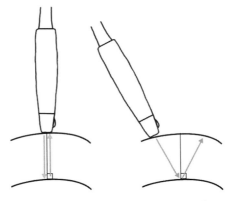

Fig. 6.2 As the angle of incidence decreases from 90°, then the US waves are reflected away from the transducer and do not form part of the image.

Scattering (Rayleigh)

When structures are smaller than the wavelength of the US beam (<0.1mm), for example, cells in tissue parenchyma, the US wave is scattered in all direction and is termed 'Rayleigh scattering'. This gives a speckled appearance of the tissue, but is not a true image of the cellular anatomy as that is too small to be resolved. See Fig. 6.3.

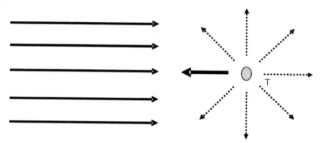

Fig. 6.3 Rayleigh scattering of a US beam by small object.

Generation of ultrasound image

Transducer/receiver

Pulse generation and pulse echo principle

Only very short bursts, just 2–3 cycles, of sound waves are produced by the transducer. This is done by damping the piezoelectric crystal shortly after applying the voltage to it. The probe then switches to 'receive' mode to pick up the sound waves that are reflected back from the tissue (the 'echo').

Only US waves reflected back to the probe can form part of the image.

The cycle of transmission and reception (pulse echo principle) can be repeated up to 7000 times a second.

Scanning (linear array/ curvilinear)

US probes have many piezoelectric crystals which are stimulated in small groups to produce a narrow beam. The US beam is electronically scanned along the length of the transducer, by exciting only small subsets of crystals in order. Scanning across the field of view takes ~0.1sec giving a high 'frame rate' and allowing visualization of moving objects. See Fig. 6.4.

A *linear array* probe has all the elements (crystals), up to 200 of them, along the flat face of the transducer, producing a rectangular field of view. Whereas a *curvilinear-array* transducer has the elements in a convex arc and produces a sector-shaped image.

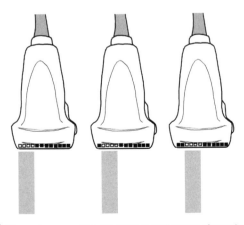

Fig. 6.4 Diagram to represent the stimulation of small sections of piezoelectric crystals in sequence to 'scan' along the transducer to produce sequential lines of the image.

Greyscale
Each returning echo from the tissues is represented by a spot on the image, whose brightness corresponds to the strength of the returning signal. See Fig. 6.5.

The time from pulse to echo is related to the depth of the structure that produced the echo. This is calculated from the equation:

Time = 2 × depth/speed of sound

As already mentioned, the speed of sound is slightly different in all tissues (due to differences in acoustic impedance) but for the purposes of this calculation, the speed of sound *is assumed to be constant at 1540m/sec*.

By representing the strength of the returning echoes from each depth as a spot whose brightness depends on the echo strength and depth position calculated from the time delay, each vertical line of an US image is produced. By placing such lines next to each other as the US beam is scanned along the transducer a complete image of a slice through the tissue is produced. See Fig. 6.6. This is the basis of how US images are generated in 'B mode' (brightness).

Structures that strongly reflect US generate large signal intensities and appear whiter or *hyperechoic*, In contrast, *hypoechoic* structures weakly reflect US and appear darker.

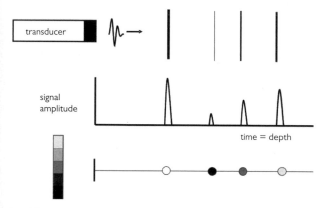

Fig. 6.5 Diagram showing how one line of an image is produced by a grey scale corresponding to the strength of the reflected signal from different depths. Stronger reflections produce signals of greater amplitude which produce a brighter/whiter image.

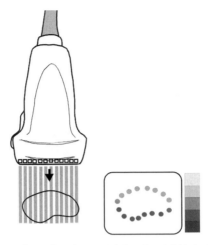

Fig. 6.6 Diagram showing how the image is built up from individual points corresponding to depth and strength of reflections from ultrasound beams scanned along the transducer.

Time gain compensation

One of the principal problems of the greyscale image production is that echoes reflected from deeper structures are weaker than those from closer structures as the US waves have had to travel through more tissue and thus have been subject to more attenuation. This would cause the image to get dimmer at greater depths. To compensate for this during processing of the signal the US machine software applies increasing amplification to the returning echo signals over time. This is known as 'time gain compensation' (TGC). This should in theory provide an image of uniform brightness when scanning a homogeneous organ. A penetration limit still occurs for a given probe when so much gain is being applied that only noise is being amplified, i.e. there are no further echoes to detect.

Resolution

Resolution refers to the US machine's ability to distinguish one object from another. This is in the order of 0.5–1.5mm.

Axial resolution

Axial resolution refers to the ability to discriminate 2 objects within the line of the US beam. This depends on the length of the US pulse and is roughly equal to 1.5x the pulse length. Two objects within the same pulse at the same time will reflect echoes back together and so cannot be resolved. See Fig. 6.7. Good axial resolution therefore requires a short pulse with short wavelengths, i.e. high frequency.

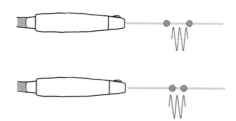

Fig. 6.7 Axial resolution determined by pulse length. In the upper image the two objects are further apart than the US pulse and so will be seen as two separate structures on the image. In the lower image the two objects will only be seen as one as they are closer together than the US pulse width.

Lateral resolution

Lateral resolution refers to the ability to discriminate 2 objects lying across the US beam. This depends on having narrow and well-defined US beams as 2 objects within the same beam will reflect echoes at the same time and not be resolved. See Fig. 6.8. Lateral resolution is always worse than axial resolution, but is also better with higher frequency wavelengths and focusing (see Focusing, p. 69).

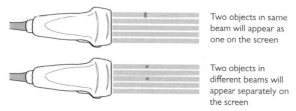

Two objects in same beam will appear as one on the screen

Two objects in different beams will appear separately on the screen

Fig. 6.8 Diagram showing objects need to be in different US 'beams' to be discriminated laterally.

Temporal resolution

Temporal resolution refers to the ability to discriminate 2 different images in time and is directly related to the 'frame rate'. This is a function of the scanning (or sweep speed) along the US transducer. Poor temporal resolution results in movements appearing blurred. Temporal resolution is rarely of concern in regional anaesthesia so long as needle movements and injection of local anaesthesia is slow.

Focusing

Lateral resolution at a particular depth can be further improved by focusing the US beam, similar to focusing a light beam with a lens. Focusing can be achieved electronically in the transducer array. See Fig. 6.9.

On the higher-end US scanners the focal depth can be altered by the user; more basic portable scanners tend to have a fixed focus generally to the centre of the field of view.

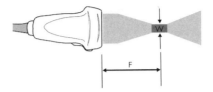

Fig. 6.9 Diagram showing the focusing of an US beam. W = focal width; F = focal distance.

It is important to set that focal depth to the depth of the target of interest since outside that focal zone the width of the beam will be wider and the resolution will be poorer than it would have been if no focusing was applied.

Colour Doppler US

The Doppler effect is the phenomena that produces a change in pitch of a sound as it comes towards you or away from you. It produces a higher note as the sound comes towards you, as the sound waves are effectively 'squashed up' to give a higher frequency with a shorter wavelength. As it moves away from you the sound waves are effectively 'stretched out' to give a lower pitch. See Fig. 6.10.

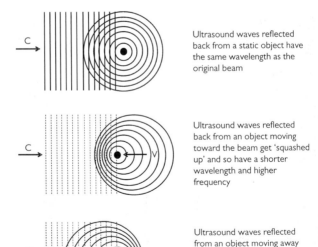

Ultrasound waves reflected back from a static object have the same wavelength as the original beam

Ultrasound waves reflected back from an object moving toward the beam get 'squashed up' and so have a shorter wavelength and higher frequency

Ultrasound waves reflected from an object moving away from the beam get 'stretched out' and have a longer wavelength and lower frequency

Fig. 6.10 Diagram to represent the change in wavelength when an object is moving towards and away from a source of sound waves.

When US reflects from a moving target such as blood or the heart, the frequency of the returning echo is slightly different from the transmitted frequency due to the Doppler shift. This difference in frequency can be detected electronically to enables the velocity of these movements be appreciated and measured.

For target velocities found in the body, the Doppler frequency is in the 0–5kHz range, i.e. within the audible range. The easiest way to detect the Doppler shift is therefore to put the output to a normal loudspeaker or headphones.

However, the velocity information may be shown graphically as a Doppler waveform display, or it may be used to colour an overlay map that is superimposed on the greyscale image. This latter technique is known as colour Doppler ultrasound (CDU) or colour flow mapping (CFM). Flow towards the probe may be shown as red through to yellow for increasing velocities, and flow away from the probe shown as blue through to green for increasing velocities. Only parts of the image where there is movement will show colour. See Fig. 6.11.

If the movement of blood within a blood vessel is at 90° to the direction of the US beam, no colour filling will be seen.

'Power Doppler' or other similar names are used for functions that have a higher sensitivity for flow, but do not give directional information.

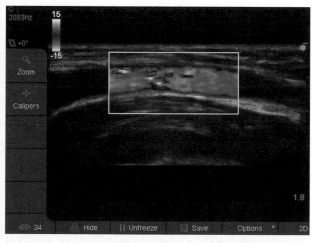

Fig. 6.11 Flow of blood in a blood vessel, shown by colour Doppler.

Artefacts

An artefact is any feature in an image that is not a true or accurate one-to-one depiction of the target being imaged. Because US imaging is formed by interrogating tissue with pulses of sound and detecting echoes that may travel on a long complex path through the intervening tissue, US images are subject to a number of artefacts. The user must understand how these are formed and learn to recognize them in order not to misinterpret the images. Correct diagnosis comes through understanding the physical processes involved, correctly driving the scanner, and a good knowledge of the anatomy being examined.

Contact artefacts

Where shadowing or lack of image appears from the top of the image, it indicates a contact problem between the probe and the skin, e.g. a hollow curved surface of the skin, lack of gel on skin, or at worst a faulty transducer (Fig. 6.12).

Acoustic shadowing

When an acoustically opaque target appears in the line of the US beam, e.g. bone, calcification, or a vessel wall viewed edgeways on (see Fig. 6.13), no US will reach any distal targets and a dark shadow will appear deep to the obscuring target on the image (Fig. 6.14). In the case of calcification, this, together with a bright reflection from the proximal surface, can be diagnostic.

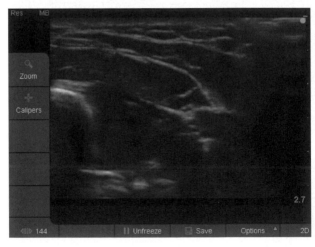

Fig. 6.12 US showing contact artefact. There is a loss of contact in the right hand side of the image with a drop out zone beneath it.

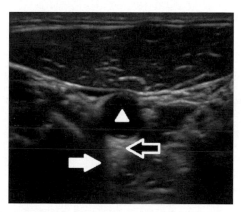

Fig. 6.13 US showing postcystic enhancement and lateral wall shadowing. White triangle, carotid artery; Black arrow, post cystic enhancement; White arrow, lateral wall shadowing.

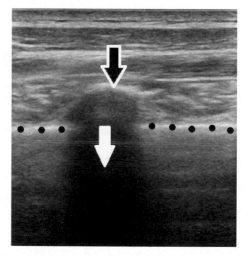

Fig. 6.14 US showing acoustic shadowing. Black arrow, surface of rib; White shadow, acoustic shadow deep to rib; Black dots, pleura.

Post cystic enhancement

This artefact appears as an inappropriately bright area on the image behind a fluid filled structure such as a cyst or blood vessel (Fig. 6.13).

It results from the application of TGC across a region of low echogenicity as is found in a fluid. The TGC continues to increase the gain with depth even though the US pulse is only weakly attenuated. The echoes distal to the cyst then have too much gain applied relative to the adjacent solid tissue and so appear brighter. Although it is an artefact, it is useful in that it is usually diagnostic of a fluid-filled, as opposed to a solid structure and the TGC should not be adjusted.

Note that incorrect adjustment of the TGC and gain controls may itself produce artefact in an image as information is lost or mis-read due to poor technique by the operator.

Reflection artefacts

Some anatomical structures have a large smooth surface and can act as 'mirror' reflectors of US (e.g. diaphragm, bone, pleural). A 2nd or reflected image then appears in a place on the image where anatomically it is unlikely to be. For example, on colour Doppler over the clavicular region, a 2nd image of the subclavian artery is seen in the lungs (Fig. 6.15).

Reverberation

Reverberations occur as the result of US waves bouncing back and forth between 2 strongly specular reflectors. The result is usually multiple linear and hyperechoic areas distal to the reflecting structures.

In regional anaesthesia this predominantly occurs between the needle and probe surface, especially when the needle is perpendicular to the US beam (Fig. 6.16).

Slice thickness artefacts

Slice thickness artefact is the presence of echoes within the image that arise from structures outside the image plane. Although an US image is of a plane cut through the tissue, in reality, the slice through the tissue is not infinitely thin but has a thickness determined by the out-of-plane shape of the US beam.

It is most noticeable when viewing targets such as blood vessels in longitudinal section, when echoes arising from the steeply curved vessel surface outside the image plane show up as echoes within the vessel lumen itself (Fig. 6.17).

This artefact is a limitation of US itself and cannot be avoided, but should be recognized.

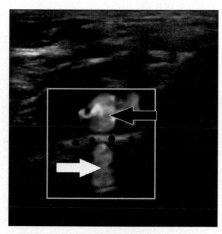

Fig. 6.15 US showing reflection artefact. Black arrow, subclavian artery; White arrow, reflection of subclavian artery below pleura; Black dots, pleura.

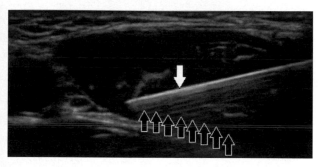

Fig. 6.16 US showing reverberation artefact from a needle, seen as a series of white parallel lines deep to the needle reflection. White arrow, needle; Black arrows, reverberations/multiple reflection artefact of the needle.

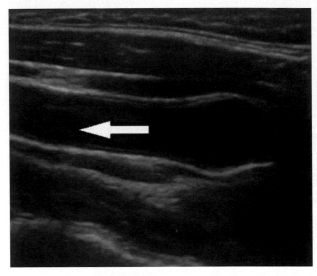

Fig. 6.17 Slice thickness artefact seen as faint shadowing within the vessel lumen. White arrow, slice thickness artefact.

Refraction artefacts

An US image is built up on the assumption that the speed of sound in soft tissue is 1540m/sec. In reality there will be variations of up to 5% around this value. These differences in speed of sound may cause the beam to be bent by refraction at large interfaces with different speeds of sound on either side.

In regional anaesthesia this is commonly seen as a 'bent 'needle as it passes through 2 tissues of different acoustic impedance (e.g. fat and muscle). This has been termed the 'Bayonet artefact' (Fig. 6.18). This does not present difficultly with needling technique as the tip of the needle is accurately represented relative to the surrounding structures, even if the needle has a 'step' in the shaft.

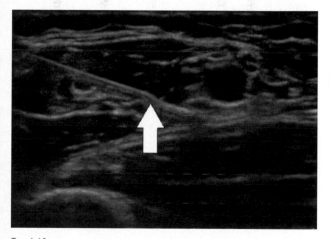

Fig. 6.18 Refraction artefact, seen as a bent needle as it passes through 2 areas with slightly different acoustic impedance; 'bayonet artefact'. White arrow, apparent step in needle contour due to 'Bayonet artefact'.

Further reading

Hangiandreou NJ (2003). AAPM/RSNA physics tutorial for residents. Topics in US: B-mode US: basic concepts and new technology. *Radiographics*, **23**(4), 1019–33.

Sites BD, Brull R, Chan VWS, *et al.* (2007). Artifacts and pitfall errors associated with ultrasound-guided regional anesthesia. Part I: Understanding the basic principles of ultrasound physics and machine operations. *Reg Anesth Pain Med*, **32**(5), 412–18.

Sites BD, Brull R, Chan VWS, *et al.* (2007). Artifacts and pitfall errors associated with ultrasound-guided regional anesthesia. Part II: A pictorial approach to understanding and avoidance. *Reg Anesth Pain Med*, **32**(5), 419–33.

Chapter 7

79

Principles and practice of ultrasound-guided regional anaesthesia

Introduction

The introduction of US to regional anaesthesia has meant the operator is now able to:

- view an image of the target nerve directly
- guide the needle under real-time visualization
- navigate away from sensitive anatomy
- monitor the spread of LA
- block nerves at any point along their course, without relying on previously used landmarks
- make real-time procedural adjustments.

The technology is applicable to most patients requiring regional anaesthesia. It may be particularly useful for patients with obscured anatomical landmarks, coagulopathy, neural pathology or trauma.

US is a highly operator-dependent imaging modality. If ultrasound-guided regional anaesthesia (UGRA) is to become the new gold standard with respect to safety and efficacy, the operator must acquire the appropriate knowledge and skills to be a safe practitioner.

It is important to understand how to obtain and capture an image, differentiate true image from artefact, introduce a needle, place it close to the nerve, and deliver LA to surround the nerve.

The components required to achieve this are:

- Image capture
- Image optimization
- Image interpretation
- Needling techniques.

Image capture

Important factors include:

Machine

Consumer demand and improving computer processing has led to rapid development of good quality portable 'lap top' machines, and progress continues to advance. Many companies now produce machines that offer quality and resolution capabilities adequate for use in regional anaesthesia e.g. Sonosite, Esaote, BK and GE. Machines should include basic image optimization features, technique specific settings (nerve or vascular imaging), Doppler function, image storage features, and a number of enhanced imaging techniques such as tissue harmonics and multibeam technology as standard.

Probe choice

From a clinical perspective there are 2 key concepts: *resolution* and *penetration*. Image resolution increases with US frequency; hence high-frequency probes will give improved image detail. However, higher frequencies are attenuated more rapidly as they pass through tissue. As a consequence they can only be used to image superficial structures (generally under 4–6cm in depth, e.g. brachial plexus, peripheral nerves). To image deeper, a lower-frequency probe is used, sacrificing image resolution for ↑ depth/penetration (e.g. lumber plexus, proximal sciatic nerve). As a general rule, always use the highest frequency probe available for the depth of target structure to be imaged.

The probe's 'footprint' (size of probe face) may limit access (e.g. in the supraclavicular fossa or paediatrics) and in these cases smaller probes may be needed. See Table 7.1 and Fig. 7.1.

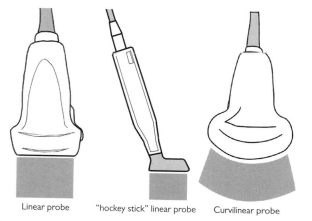

Linear probe   "hockey stick" linear probe   Curvilinear probe

Fig. 7.1 Diagrams of the different probe types.

Table 7.1 Probe characteristics

Probe	Array	Frequency	Field depth	Resolution	Blocks
Linear	Linear	6–13 MHz ('high frequency')	1.5–6cm	0.5 mm axial 1 mm lateral	Brachial plexus Abdominal wall Femoral and distal sciatic Vascular access
Curvilinear	Curved face	2–5MHz ('low frequency')	5–16cm	2mm axial 3mm lateral	Neuraxial Lumbar plexus Proximal sciatic
Phased array		1–5MHz	6–16cm		Abdominal, pleura, cardiac

Acoustic coupling

US waves are rapidly attenuated by air so it is critical that no air exists between the probe and the skin. To achieve this, an acoustic couplant is needed. This has the added advantage of acting as a lubricant for the probe to slide over the skin. Any water-based gel or alcohol skin disinfectant can be used. Manufactures generally advise against the use of oil based couplants as they may cause damage to the transducer. Probe covers are recommended in all cases to protect both probe and patient. These can range from a glove or clear plastic dressing, to a purpose designed cover.

Scanning technique

Three basic hand/transducer movements; *slide*, *tilt*, and *rotation*, are employed to improve view and locate the target structure. See Fig. 7.2.

Slide

Refers to the movement of the probe across the skin to trace the course of a structure. Aids identification and location of optimal entry points for injection.

Tilt

A rocking hand movement that changes the angle the probe makes with the skin. It is useful for obtaining the best view of a structure by altering the angle at which the ultrasound beam hits the target structure thus maximizing the beam signal strength returning to the transducer.

Rotation

Describes a twisting movement, used to obtain a *short-axis* or *long-axis* view of the target structure. Very small rotational movements may be needed to maintain full alignment of the US beam and the needle.

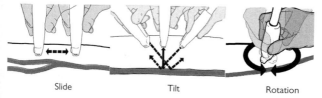

Slide   Tilt   Rotation

Fig. 7.2 Diagram showing slide, tilt, and rotation movements.

Short-axis and long-axis views

These terms relate to how the image of the target structure is visualized
(Fig. 7.3). With the short-axis view, the US beam is perpendicular to the
nerve. Hence the nerve is seen in cross section and will appear round, oval,
or triangular. Rotate the probe through 90°, and the long-axis view is generated where the length of the nerve is visualized. In general, the short-axis
view of a nerve is preferred because of the following:

• Nerve identification is easier.
• Improved view of surrounding structures and planes.
• Facilitates needle access to the nerve, e.g. lateral, medial, deep, and
  superficial aspects can all be targeted.
• Improved assessment and verification of circumferential distribution of
  LA.
• Slight probe movement will still maintain a workable image.

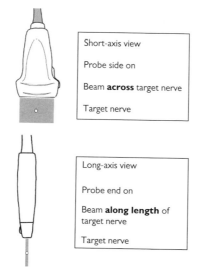

Short-axis view

Probe side on

Beam **across** target nerve

Target nerve

Long-axis view

Probe end on

Beam **along length** of
target nerve

Target nerve

Fig. 7.3 Short-axis and long-axis views.

Image optimization

Once the target structure has been identified it is important to optimize the image by making adjustments to:

Pre-sets

Most machines will come with a range of manufacturer settings, designed to optimize image quality for individual probes and different tissue types. Standard pre-sets are: nerve, vascular, musculoskeletal, breast, and small parts.

Depth

Depth should be adjusted to keep the target structure in the middle of the screen. This allows visualization of all the structures around the target and is also frequently the best focused area of the image.

Gain

Gain, or contrast, should be set so that it is consistent throughout the screen. This is important as echoes from similar structures should give rise to similar screen brightness, regardless of their depth.

Focus

On some machines (e.g. Sonosite) the focus is fixed to the middle of the screen. If not, then it is important to adjust the focus to the depth of the target structure in order to maximize resolution.

Image interpretation

Image interpretation is a critical part of successful UGRA. It requires a good knowledge of anatomy, an understanding of the appearance of different tissues, consideration of how artefact can affect images, and familiarity with the methods available for interrogating a structure to aid its identification. Important factors include:

Echogenicity

The degree to which the US beam reflects from a structure and returns to the probe determines the returning signal intensity. This creates images that are black, white, or varying degrees of grey (Table 7.2 and Fig. 7.4):

- Structures that strongly reflect the US beam generate large returning signal intensities at the transducer and appear white or *hyperechoic*.
- Structures that only weakly reflect US generate lower signal intensities and appear darker or *hypoechoic*.
- Structures that reflect none of the US beam appear black or *anechoic*.

Table 7.2 Echogenicity of different tissues

Hyperechoic (bright structures)	Hypoechoic (dark echoes)
Connective tissues	Fatty tissue
Fascial layers/pleura	Fluid (blood, LAs)
Vessel walls	Muscle
Bony surfaces	
Nerves	Nerves
Tendons	Tendons

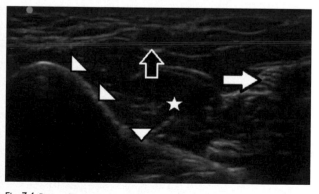

Fig. 7.4 Picture showing varying echogenicities of nerve, muscle, bone, fascial layers—forearm. Black arrow, blood vessel (radial artery); White arrow, nerve (median); White star, muscle; White triangle, bone cortex (radius).

Sonographic appearances

Pattern recognition of the different tissues is critical to identification. This is aided by observing their real-time interaction with the US probe and beam (compression, pulsation, anisotropy, and Doppler shift). See Table 7.3.

Anisotropy

The term is derived from the Greek *anisos* meaning 'unequal' and *tropos* 'turn'. It is used to describe the property of 'now-you-see-me-now-you-don't' which can occur with US imaging. The angle the US beam hits (or insonates) a structure will determine how many of the reflected echoes are detected by the transducer and how many fall out of the sight of the receiving transducer. As the probe angle alters, the appearance of the structure being visualized may change and on occasions the structure may seem to disappear altogether. This alteration in echogenicity of a structure with probe angulation is termed anisotropy. Nerves and tendons classically illustrate this property.

Table 7.3 Sonographic appearance of peripheral nerves and surrounding tissues

Tissue	US appearance
Artery	Anechoic (black circles or tubes)—pulsatile
Vein	Anechoic (black circles or tubes)—compressible, dilate with Valsalva (jugular, subclavian, femoral)
Tendon Fibrillar appearance	Long axis—tubular structure
	Internal architecture, loosely packed continuous blurred bright lines (hyperechoic), pale surface
	Short axis—circular structure with pale halo (tendon sheath)
	Internal architecture hyperechoic (semi-bright) dots (tendon fibrils) loosely packed, within hypoechoic (darkened) surroundings—'granular appearance'
	Anisotropic ++
Nerve Fascicular appearance	Long axis—tubular structures: bright surface. Internal architecture multiple broken bright (hyperechoic) lines
	Short axis—circular structure with bright surface (epineurium). Internal architecture multiple hypoechoic black dots (nerve fascicles) with bright outlines within bright surroundings (connective tissue, perineurium). 'Speckled appearance'. Appearance varies between proximal and distal peripheral nerves (see text)
	Anisotropic +
Pleura	Hyperechoic lines—'sliding lung sign' with respiration
Lung	Normal lung is air filled and therefore not seen, generally characterized by its lack of distinct detail. Reverberation artefacts from pleura (A lines) can be seen
Bones Periosteum Cortex and medulla	Hyperechoic line ++
	Anechoic—black (due to reflection of the majority of the US beam from the periosteum, 'drop out' artefact below)

Peripheral nerves

Identification of peripheral nerves is not always easy. Knowledge of their distinguishing features is important. Nerves can be round, oval, triangular, or even flattened in shape. Along the course of a single nerve all shapes can be seen as the nerve passes between adjacent structures. The larger peripheral nerves demonstrate a 'fascicular' or 'honeycomb' pattern.

In general the more proximal the peripheral nerve the more hypoechoic its appearance, becoming more hyperechoic as it moves distally. This is due, in part, to alterations in the ratio of connective tissue (highly compressed collagen which reflects US beam = hyperechoic) and neural tissue (high lipid content which absorbs US beam = hypoechoic) within each nerve (Fig. 7.5). The ratio tends towards more connective tissue and less neural tissue the more distal the nerve. However, a number of other anatomical and technical factors are important in determining the overall appearance of the target nerve. For example, its size, depth, and surrounding structures (large muscles attenuate the US beam leading to reduced visibility, e.g. sciatic nerve); technical factors such as the frequencies used, probe design, and the angle of the incidental beam (some nerves are highly anisotropic, e.g. sciatic nerve).

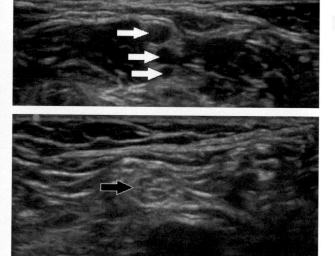

Fig. 7.5 Hypoechoic nerve roots in the interscalene groove and more hyperechoic, speckled appearance of tibial nerve in the popliteal fossa. White arrow, hypoechoic (black) nerve roots in the interscalene groove; Black arrow, hyperechoic (white) speckled tibial nerve in the popliteal fossa.

Artefact
Important to be able to recognize. See Chapter 6.

Interrogation
Along with tissue pattern recognition there are various methods of interrogating a structure to aid its identification:
- Compressibility with the US probe.
- Pulsation.
- Valsalva: aids identification of the large veins in the neck and femoral vessels.
- Artefact effect: anisotropy with nerves and tendons. Post-cystic enhancement with a fluid-filled space.
- Doppler: nerves are often accompanied by vessels. With larger nerves this relationship is usually consistent; however, considerable anatomical variation may be present with smaller nerves. Colour flow will identify flow away from the probe as blue, and towards as red. **Blue away, red towards: 'BART'.**
- Tracing structures: tendons may resemble peripheral nerves, similar in size, shape and their anisotropic nature. Follow their course, tendons change their cross-sectional area and end in muscle or bone. Nerves are relatively uniform along their length.

Needling techniques

Good technique is based on a background of a good understanding of the relevant anatomy and repetitive hands-on practice.

Never advance a needle unless you can identify its tip at all times. If the needle tip cannot be seen with certainty, then withdraw the needle and start again.

Needle visibility

Primarily determined by:

Insertion angle

The more superficial and parallel the needle to the probe face, the better the reflected image (parallelism). A 'steep' needle will reflect much of the US beam away from the transducer. A curvilinear probe may improve this due to the diverging nature of its US beam, improving the angle the beam makes with the needle. Entering the skin close to the transducer, while resulting in a shorter distance to the target structure (less painful), forces a steeper needle angle often with reduced needle visualization. Enhanced needle visualization software now exists that can greatly improve needle visualization at steeper needle angles.

Needle depth

As the needle is inserted deeper it becomes more difficult to see. This is due to signal attenuation with increasing depth.

Needle gauge

Large-bore needles (e.g. 18G or Tuohy) are more readily visible due to their larger cross-sectional area and are preferred for deeper blocks. They also tend to be less flexible and therefore less likely to bend out of the plane of the US beam. Smaller bore needles (e.g. 22G or 24G) are harder to see but adequate for more superficial blocks and insertion is less painful with less tissue damage. Needles tips are better seen when the bevel faces the probe.

Nature of the surrounding tissues

Needle visualization is improved with contrast against surrounding structures. Best visualized on a dark, anechoic background, i.e. in a vessel or after LA deposition.

Needle design

Bevel: standard hypodermic needles are long bevelled and cut to 12° as regulated by British Standards (BS). However the majority of peripheral nerve blocks are performed using short-bevelled or pencil point needles. Short-bevelled needles are not BS regulated and may be cut between 18° and 45°. They are designed to part rather than cut tissues and also offer ↑ resistance to insertion. This allows the operator an improved 'feel' of the needle passing through tissue planes. It is thought that the risk of damaging nerves is reduced with a short-bevelled needle as the nerve fascicles will roll/slide out of the path of the needle tip. However, it is recognized that should the needle enter neural tissue the risk of fascicular injury is probably greater with a short-bevelled rather than long-bevelled needle.

Insulation

Insulated needles are coated and only emit current from the tip. This allows a much lower stimulating current to be used and also more focused stimulation when refining the needle tip position.

Immobility

Once the needle tip is in the desired position it is important that movements such as attaching a syringe, aspirating, and injecting do not displace the needle tip and result in inappropriate LA deposition or neurovascular trauma. For this reason the concept of the 'Immobile Needle' was described by Winnie in 1969. There are various needles which come with pre-attached extension sets that allow syringe manipulation to be done remotely from the needle hub.

Advanced visualization techniques

Various technologies can be used to improve the echogenicity of needles, these include: coating, roughing, scoring, or dimpling the surface. Some manufacturers have done this towards the tip of the needle in order to aid needle tip identification. Others have adapted the whole needle shaft to improve overall visibility on US.

Catheter insertion

For perineural catheter insertion there are various kits available. These are either Seldinger wire, catheter through needle, or cannula over needle in design. It is also possible to obtain stimulating catheters to refine the position of the catheter tip.

In-plane and out-of-plane

These terms describe the relationship between the plane of the US beam and the needle;

• *In-plane (IP) approach*: needle and beam axis parallel.
• *Out-of-plane (OOP) approach*: needle and beam axis at right angles (see Fig. 7.6).

The choice of approach will depend on the site of injection, probe and personal preferences. The IP approach (with a short axis view of the target structure) may be safer for clinicians starting in US as the needle tip is more easily visualized. See Table 7.4.

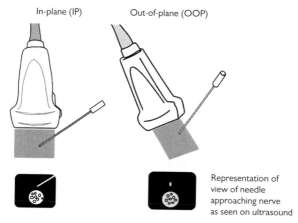

In-plane (IP)   Out-of-plane (OOP)

Representation of
view of needle
approaching nerve
as seen on ultrasound

Fig. 7.6 Images of IP and OOP needle approaches to nerves.

Table 7.4 Advantages and disadvantages of needling techniques.

Needle insertion (with short-axis view of target structure)	Advantages	Disadvantages
In-plane (IP)	Full visualization of needle shaft and tip Good visibility needle–nerve interface	Difficult to perform. Requires precise alignment of the US beam (width 1mm), needle and nerve Longer skin–nerve distance (more tissue trauma) Intramuscular needle passage—painful Unfamiliar needle insertion point (compared to the standard landmark approaches)
Out-of-plane (OOP)	Familiar needle insertion point Short skin—nerve distance Minimal intramuscular needle passage	Difficult to visualize tip clearly Needle only seen as a white 'dot' as it passes through the US beam (beware tip & shaft look similar) Poor visibility needle–nerve interface

Needle location tips

To aid needle tip identification:

Local tissue movement

Small volume (0.1–0.5mL) test injections looking for tissue expansion—hydrolocation (avoid air bubble injection as this will cause acoustic shadowing and reduce visibility at the needle tip).

Dorsal US shadow produced by the needle tip

Even if the needle is not well seen, it will often produce a 'drop out' shadow beneath it, which can aid needle (tip) location.

Triangulation

With OOP techniques, concentrate on the depth of the target structure and the distance that the needle starts from the probe to construct a 'triangulation' type image. Use this to help insert the needle at the correct angle towards the nerve, e.g. a target nerve 2cm deep with the needle entering the skin 2cm from the probe will mean an angle of 45° is needed to ensure the needle tip passes under the US beam at the point where it is just above the nerve.

Alternatively, as the needle is advanced, the probe can be tilted with the tip to follow it as it heads towards the nerve.

If the needle image is lost, always move the transducer to find the needle, not the needle to find the transducer. Beware with the IP approach of a partial needle image. The probe and needle are in line, but for only a certain distance along the needle's length. This results in a false interpretation of the needle tip position as only the proximal part of the needle is visualized.

Needle–nerve position

Never deliberately contact the nerve. Position the needle close to it but not deliberately touching it. This reduces the likelihood of damage and patient discomfort.

Peripheral nerve stimulators (PNSs) can be used in conjunction with US. Place at a low setting, i.e. 0.6mA, and consider only turning the stimulator on when needle is nearing the nerve. Higher more standard settings result in vigorous twitches that lead to moving, poor quality images. The combined use of US and PNS may have some advantages where:

• due to the depth of the intended target nerve there is suboptimal image quality, e.g. lateral infraclavicular, lumbar plexus and proximal sciatic nerve approaches.
• some practitioners feel it may help exclude the possibility of intra-neural needle placement (absent twitches below 0.2mA).
• to aid the identification of specific nerves where they lie in close proximity, e.g. to selectively target specific nerves during an axillary block.
• when learning US-guided techniques. Confirmation/reassurance of nerve identification.

Nerve–local anaesthetic spread

On reaching the target nerve inject 0.5–1mL of LA and observe spread, this should be around the nerve. An improved block with the use of less LA occurs with deposition that surrounds the nerve to create a 'halo' or 'doughnut' sign (Fig. 7.7).

This is most easily achieved using the so-called 'V' technique. This describes the movements of the needle; advancement to one side of the nerve, injection, partial withdrawal, and then redirection to the other side of the nerve.

After injection the probe can be slid along the path of the nerve to check adequate LA distribution.

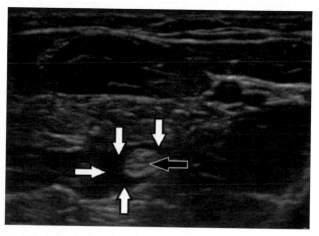

Fig. 7.7 US showing near complete circumferential spread of LA around a nerve; 'halo' or 'doughnut' sign. Median nerve (black arrow) surrounded by local anaesthetic (white arrows).

Local anaesthetic injection

Inject slowly watching the screen at all times. The injection should be painless and resistance free.

LA should be clearly seen, if not consider:
- Intravascular injection. Stop injection and reposition.
- Needle tip not within US beam. Move probe to visualize needle tip and re-inject.

The nerve often appears brighter, and easier to identify after injection (improved contrast).

If the nerve swells, stop injection and consider intraneural placement. Reposition needle.

'Extrafascicular' injection
Needle position beneath epineurium but not inside the fascicles. Superficial swelling of the nerve but no internal disruption. Unlikely to result in permanent nerve damage.

'Intrafascicular' injection
Needle position within the nerve fascicles. Whole nerve swells with internal disruption. ↑ likelihood of permanent nerve damage.

Aseptic precautions

AAGBI guidelines state that peripheral regional blocks demand an appropriate aseptic technique comprising of skin preparation, wearing of sterile gloves, and use of drapes. It is important that the US probe does not become a vector for infection and therefore it should be covered as an absolute minimum with a clear occlusive dressing and the machine wiped clean after each use. Maximal aseptic precautions including the use of a full sterile probe sheath, gown, gloves, mask, and cap are recommended for neuraxial techniques and peripheral nerve catheter (PNC) insertions. Several studies also support the administration of antibiotics for PNC insertion in surgical patients.

Effective topical antiseptic solution is an important component of an aseptic technique. Several studies have compared chlorhexidine gluconate (CHG) with povidone iodine and have led to the American Society of Regional Anaesthesia & Pain Medicine Practice Advisory Panel suggesting 0.5% CHG in 80% ethanol as the most effective solution for aseptic techniques in regional anaesthesia. The alcohol base aids penetration into the stratum corneum and more effectively eradicates microorganisms. Care must be taken to ensure the solution dries and that there is no contamination with needles or catheter equipment due to potential neurotoxicity concerns. 2% chlorhexidine is an alternative for peripheral nerve blocks but should *not* be used for neuraxial techniques.

Performing a block

Preparation

- Explain procedure. Consent patient. Agreement from surgeon
- Consider light sedation
- Position patient and machine ergonomically
- Select probe. Apply sterile cover
- Disinfect skin. Drape area
- Ensure good acoustic coupling with gel or alcohol spray
- Place probe on skin.

Preliminary scan

- Optimize machine settings; pre-sets, gain, and depth (target structure in middle of screen).
- Orientate image on the screen, so probe movement reflects hand movement.
- Find target structure. Interrogate to aid identification.
- Investigate area to identify important related structures (arteries, veins, pleura).
- Slide/tilt/rotate the probe to obtain the best image.
- Make sure the image can be held stable.
- Identify the optimal needle insertion point:
  - avoiding important structures
  - target structure closest to skin.
- Infiltrate entry point with LA.

Needling

- Introduce the needle using either the IP or OOP approach.
- After passing through the skin, identify the needle within the US beam; always find the needle with the probe, and *never* the probe with the needle.
- Advance the needle towards the target structure. Viewing the tip *at all times*. If using PNS in combination with US then turn this on as nearing the target structure (0.6mA).
- Position the needle besides the nerve, *never* deliberately contact the nerve.

Injection

- Inject LA in small aliquots (e.g. 2mL). Observe spread. Inject sufficient to encircle the nerve, repositioning the needle as required.
- Scan along the nerve to ensure LA surrounds it. Doughnut sign.

Golden rules of US-guided regional anaesthesia

- Never advance the needle unless you can identify the needle tip at **all** times.
- Never deliberately contact the nerve. Place the needle next to the nerve.
- Observe injection. If unable to see spread of LA consider intravascular injection or needle tip not in scan plane.
- Injection should be resistance free and painless. If not, **stop**, reposition needle.
- If the nerve swells on injection, **stop**, consider intraneural injection.

Further reading

AAGBI (2008). *Infection Control in Anaesthesia* (2nd edn). London: AAGBI. Available at: ℘ http://www.aagbi.org/sites/default/files/infection_control_08.pdf.

American Society of Anesthesiologists Task Force on infectious complications associated with neuraxial techniques (2010). Practice advisory for the prevention, diagnosis and management of infectious complications associated with neuraxial techniques. *Anesthesiology*, **112**(3),530–45.

Hebl JR (2006). The importance and implications of aseptic techniques during regional anaesthesia. *RAPM*, **31**(4), 311–23.

Hopkins PM (2007). Ultrasound guidance as a gold standard in regional anaesthesia. *Br J Anaesth*, **98**(3), 299–301.

Jeng CL, Torillo TM, Rosenblatt MA (2010). Complications of peripheral nerve blocks. *Br J Anaesth*, **105**(1), i97–i107.

Risks, benefits, and controversies of regional anaesthesia

Risks

- *Risk:* the probability that a specific adverse event will occur in a specific time period, or as a result of a specific situation.
- *Benefit:* a favourable outcome as a result of the intervention.
- *Hazard:* a situation with the potential to cause harm.
- *Side effect:* a predictable and anticipated response to an intervention different from the intended effect. Side effects are usually mild in effect, with a short duration, i.e. Horner's syndrome with an interscalene block, hypotension with an epidural.
- *Complication:* an unanticipated harmful consequence of an intervention. Complications are rare, and may result in long-term harm to the patient; i.e. cardiac arrest resulting from early tourniquet release during bupivacaine Bier's block, VCH with cord compression from epidural catheter insertion.

There are clearly some risks and benefits associated with all regional anaesthetic techniques, and these will be discussed in this chapter (see Table 8.1). Other potential benefits or risks in regional anaesthesia are not clearly identified, either in terms of their rarity or novelty (making statistical proof difficult to ascertain), or of the difference in professional opinion and variation in worldwide practice. Procedure-specific risks, such as postdural puncture headache, or phrenic nerve block, will be discussed within the relevant section for the procedure.

Table 8.1 Incidence of various complications

Complication	Risk
Death	1:50,000 (all techniques) 1:125,000 (neuraxial)
Permanent disability (>6 months)	1:24,000 (neuraxial)
Permanent nerve damage (>6 months)	1:7,000 (peripheral) 1:25,000–100,000 (neuraxial)
Temporary nerve damage (<6 months)	1:1,000–10,000 (peripheral) 1:8700 (neuraxial)
Systemic local anaesthetic toxicity	1:9500 (peripheral) 1:35,000 (epidural)
Failure	1:20 (epidural) 1:50 (spinal) <1:20 (peripheral, nerve stimulator) <1:50 (peripheral, ultrasound)
Haematoma	1:20,000 (periop epidural) 1:60,000 (epidural)
Abscess	1:24,000 (periop neuraxial) 1:20,000 (epidural) 1:10,000 (periop epidural)

Using the evidence

Controversy is generated by lack of evidence and diversity of opinion in how best to interpret that which is available. Evidence is produced by experts within a field, therefore producing bias from the outset, and practitioners established in using different individual techniques in different populations will often disagree on the appropriate technique for any given patient. In addition, evidence produced in any one hospital setting may not be applicable to other environments, as the development of local practice and protocol may enhance the perceived benefit of that technique, and other institutions may not have the benefit of that experience. Furthermore, complications from regional anaesthesia are rare, whereas regional anaesthesia use is common, making it difficult to discern risks and benefits. One size does not fit all, and a careful analysis of risk vs benefit for any given patient in any given environment is paramount prior to administering their anaesthetic. Given these limitations, it becomes difficult to see how even well-conducted systematic reviews and meta-analyses can give an accurate picture of the risks or benefits for any individual patient receiving a regional anaesthesia technique from any individual practitioner.

Generic strategies to reduce risk associated with regional anaesthesia

- Aseptic technique
- Full monitoring and IV access
- Appropriate equipment, to include where relevant:
  - short-bevel needle
  - safe needle length for the intended block
  - use of nerve stimulation and/or US.
- Slow advancement of needle towards the target nerve
- Ensuring negative aspiration prior to injection
- Slow incremental injection avoiding high pressures
- Trained assistant to recognize high injection pressure
- Use of an injection pressure monitor
- *Stop* injection if patient reports pain
- Use appropriate LA considering all factors
- Do not repeat a failed block in the same location
- If it feels wrong, or all is not going as it should, *stop*!

Nerve damage

Definition
Any unresolved neurological symptom or sign within a predetermined time-frame caused directly by a regional anaesthesia technique.

Outcomes
Neurological symptoms as a consequence of either the surgery or the regional anaesthesia technique occur commonly; this manifests itself as discrete areas of altered sensation or reduced strength which return to normal within days.

Temporary nerve damage has no clear definition, although may be considered to be neurological symptoms as a consequence of the regional anaesthesia technique which return to normal within a 6-month period. The incidence of this varies according to the timescale described, and can be loosely quantified as around 1 in 1000 to 1 in 10,000 blocks.

Permanent nerve damage can be considered to be persisting neurological symptoms as a consequence of the regional anaesthesia technique beyond 6 months. The incidence of this is ~ 1 in 7000 peripheral blocks, or 1 in 25,000 neuraxial blocks.

Possible mechanisms
Large-vessel ischaemia, small-vessel ischaemia, physical disruption, LA neurotoxicity (lidocaine spinal anaesthetic compared to bupivacaine causes more neurological complications), pressure neurapraxia, axonotmesis, neurotmesis.

Strategy of investigation/management
Conduct patient interview. Confirm patient symptoms, and clarify the timing. Note the block performed and the operation performed, including awake vs sedation vs GA, patient positioning, and surgical adjuncts (such as tourniquet time or postoperative abduction pillow following rotator cuff surgery.) Specifically ask about paraesthesia (pins and needles), hyperalgesia, allodynia, hypoalgesia. Enquire about pre-existing conditions and confirm the past medical history, with a focus on any chronic neurological symptoms (think multiple sclerosis, mononeuritis multiplex, polyneuropathy states, complex regional pain syndrome, etc.).

Conduct full neurological examination and ensure findings are documented thoroughly in the patient's medical notes. Ensure the surgeon has also seen and examined the patient. Consider neurology referral, a magnetic resonance image (MRI) scan of the block area and affected limb, an MRI of the neuraxis, nerve conduction studies, and electromyography. This should locate the approximate area of nerve injury, and suggest any necessity for further management.

Generally speaking, the patient can be reassured following explanation. The consequences of the nerve injury will determine the extent of appropriate investigation and follow-up. Those leading to loss of function or pain may require referral to specialists in neurology or pain medicine.

Systemic local anaesthetic toxicity

Definition
The development of symptoms and signs of high systemic levels of LA following a regional anaesthetic technique.

Outcomes
Many patients with high circulating levels of LA will have no symptoms. For some patients, as LA levels rise, they will experience initially excitatory, followed by inhibitory symptoms and signs.

Early identification, prevention of acidosis and hypoxia, and intralipid have resulted in full resolution of symptoms and signs with no long-term sequelae. Despite being a myocardial depressant, bupivacaine has cardioprotective effects, so resolution of cardiac function may occur after prolonged resuscitation attempts. Numbers of cases are still small, making statistical analysis inappropriate.

Pathogenesis
IV injection; systemic absorption.

Identification
The development of symptoms or signs of LA toxicity constitutes a life-threatening emergency. If these occur immediately post-injection, neurological and cardiovascular collapse are imminent. Following a large-volume regional anaesthesia technique, peak systemic levels of LA occur at between 5 and 60 minutes depending on the anatomical location (see Table 8.2). For further information see Chapter 4.

Management
See Chapter 4.

Table 8.2 Time to peak serum concentration and the approximate concentration reached for different blocks. This table is comparing approximate 2mg/kg bupivacaine doses

Site of block	Time to peak serum concentration (min)	Peak serum concentration (micrograms/mL)
Cervical plexus	2–5	3
Intercostal	5–15	1.75
Scalp	8–16	1.36
Interscalene	10–20	2
Epidural	15–25	1.35
Paravertebral	15–25	1.45
Combined leg block	25–45	1.66
Axillary	50–60	1.52

Infection

Definition
A localized or systemic infection resulting from a regional anaesthesia technique.

Outcomes
Variable. Colonization of an indwelling catheter technique may not lead to any symptoms or signs. Cellulitis may cause pain and discomfort, and may spread or cause lymphangitis. Abscess formation may lead to permanent neurological dysfunction. In the epidural space, abscess formation may raise the pressure in the spinal canal resulting in paraplegia if not rapidly identified and decompressed. Prompt recognition, diagnosis, and treatment will improve outcomes in patients with epidural abscesses.

Pathogenesis
Colonization, cellulitis, abscess; poor aseptic technique, delayed removal of catheter, systemic or local infective process at time of insertion.

Identification/management
Any patient who develops symptoms or signs of infection (pyrexia, pain, and redness at regional anaesthesia site, pus exudate, leucocytosis, raised C-reactive protein) following a regional anaesthetic technique should have assessment and documentation of any neurological abnormality. Any perineural or neuraxial catheter should be removed at the earliest safe opportunity. The catheter tip, any exudate, and venous blood samples (if pyrexial) should all be sent for microbiological analysis, culture, and sensitivity.

Investigate any alternative infection sites—midstream/catheter specimen of urine culture, chest X-ray, etc. Broad-spectrum antibiotics to cover skin flora (i.e. *Staphylococcus/Streptococcus*) should be commenced pending confirmatory culture and sensitivity; it is also often helpful to discuss the choice of antibiotics with a microbiologist.

Contact the anaesthetist who performed the procedure, or the on-call anaesthetist if unavailable.

Consider MRI of infected site, MRI neuraxial, surgical decompression.

Clinical notes
Following neuraxial blockade, prolonged or progressive abnormal neurology in conjunction with signs of infection may suggest epidural abscess. This is a neurosurgical emergency and warrants immediate imaging and neurosurgical consultation.

Haematoma

Definition

A localized collection of clotted blood following performance of a regional anaesthesia technique.

Outcomes

Variable. An enlarging haematoma within an enclosed space such as the spinal canal may rapidly lead to neurological injury if not decompressed urgently. Prompt recognition, diagnosis, and treatment of patients with a VCH will improve outcome. Haematomas from PNBs are less likely to cause neurological problems, but can be significant leading to hypovolaemia, transfusion, and surgical intervention.

Risk factors

Anticoagulant drugs, antiplatelet drugs (not aspirin or NSAIDs), coagulopathy (see Chapter 9), identified vessel puncture, female gender, increasing age, history of bruising, wider needle gauge and difficult needle placement, hip surgery, catheter technique, multiple attempts; may occur spontaneously.

Identification/management

Any patient with persistent or progressive neurological symptoms/signs following regional anaesthesia should have urgent assessment and documentation of their neurological abnormality. Check coagulation status and date/time of last anticoagulant; consider reversal. Up to 50% of haematomas from epidurals may be related to the removal of the catheter. Inform the anaesthetist who performed the procedure. Further management differs according to technique:

- Neuraxial block: urgent MRI neuraxial; neurosurgical referral and surgical decompression.
- Peripheral block: consider US; consider MRI of affected region; consider appropriate surgical referral for decompression. PNB haematoma is unlikely to cause neuropraxia due to pressure.

Clinical notes

Following neuraxial blockade, prolonged or progressive abnormal neurology may suggest epidural haematoma. This is a *neurosurgical emergency* and warrants immediate imaging and neurosurgical consultation.

Failure

Definition
Following performance of a regional anaesthesia technique, an absence of analgesia/anaesthesia in the intended distribution.

Outcomes
If identified, results in an alternate anaesthetic approach. If unidentified, results in unsatisfactory analgesia, pain, or potentially awareness during anaesthesia, and patient dissatisfaction. Incidence is difficult to accurately assess, as a functional analgesic block may not function as an anaesthetic block, and neuraxial/plexus blocks may result in near total anaesthesia/analgesia and function with adequacy but not totality. Spinal anaesthesia may fail in <1%, even with appropriate care and attention to procedural detail. Epidural catheters may give an inadequate block in ~1 in 10 insertions, and fail completely in up to 1 in 20. For trainees in regional anaesthesia, ~1 in 20 blocks fail, whereas for the experienced regional anaesthetist, perhaps 1 in 50 to 1 in 100 will fail.

Pathogenesis
Needle mislocation, anatomical variation, poor anatomical knowledge, poor technique, wrong drug, wrong volume or concentration; epidural or plexus septae or scar tissue.

Identification/management
Good practice mandates the testing of a block to ensure it has worked prior to surgery. In the awake patient this is mandatory, but this is often overlooked in a patient who already has had, or subsequently will get, a general anaesthetic. Some blocks are amenable to troubleshooting (both neuraxial and peripheral).

The key to troubleshooting any problematic block is to be absolutely sure how to test it! The presence of a definite block in well-defined areas allows the regional anaesthetist to mentally map which areas are missed, and thus how best to top-up. Neuraxial blocks may mandate further boluses or doses, a change of position, or withdrawal of epidural catheter. Peripheral nerve blocks may require additional 'top-up' blocks distal to the initial location of block.

Wrong-site surgery

Definition
The performance of a procedure at a site different to that intended. This is most often opposite side, same location surgery.

Outcomes
Although surgery at the wrong site may be disastrous, wrong-sided regional anaesthesia results in purposeless anaesthesia/analgesia at the cost of risks of a complication occurring. Further, the subsequent performance of the correct-side block may itself cause harm; ↑ local anaesthetic dose, risk of bilateral epidural spread from proximal blocks, risk of bilateral phrenic nerve palsy causing respiratory insufficiency with interscalene blocks, risk of bilateral pneumothoraces with supraclavicular blocks, etc. This may also result in immobility requiring admission—a poor outcome if ambulatory surgery was anticipated.

Prevention
Every individual performing a procedure on a patient has the responsibility that they are performing the correct procedure at the correct site and side on the correct patient. This has recently been the target of patient safety initiatives in the UK and across the world, with the Correct Side Surgery, WHO Surgical Safety Checklist and 'stop before you block'.

A simple series of checks and marking, and a chain of repetition from ward to theatre, can easily prevent this.

Extra caution should be taken with:
- Patients who are unable to consent.
- Patients who are sedated or under general anaesthesia.
- Moving patients once checked in, but before administration of the block.
- Patients seen by or marked by other anaesthetists.
- Patients with bilateral surgical disease.
- List errors/documentation errors.
- Emergency patients.

Miscellaneous other risks

Drug allergy

LAs very rarely cause allergic reactions. However, most solutions contain additives or preservatives of some kind, and allergy to these may induce life-threatening anaphylaxis. The ester-based LAs have a higher incidence of allergic reaction, usually in the form of urticaria or other skin reactions; this is partially why there are very few available in the UK. Any patient claiming an allergy to LA must be taken seriously, but in the majority of cases the history will indicate a 'reaction to local' during a dental procedure. Dental syringes do not allow dentists to aspirate and thus intravascular injection of epinephrine is usually the cause of the reaction. Preservative-free solution could be used in cases where the history is not conclusive.

The insensate limb

Patients receiving regional anaesthesia for ambulatory surgery take responsibility for their insensate limb until the block has resolved. It is paramount to ensure that the blocked limb is protected for the duration of the block.

Inform the patient of the anticipated effects of the block and the duration. Give specific instructions, e.g. you are not allowed near the hob or fire, do not use the iron, keep your arm in the sling until it feels like your normal arm again, do not smoke whilst your arm is in a nylon sling, etc. Back this up with written information where possible.

Equipment problems

Occasionally, as with any field of medicine, the equipment malfunctions. The results of this vary. A malfunctioned nerve stimulator should be apparent, as most have failsafe mechanisms in place, but may result in 'pepper-potting' of the nerve. Needles are generally sound, but may break, and are particularly likely to at the junction of hub and needle. Indwelling catheters, such as epidural or perineural catheters, may shear, knot, or coil. Simply pulling hard is likely to cause damage and worsen the situation; suitable imaging, interventional radiology ± surgery may be required. US machines are often blamed for giving a poor image. Usually the US machine is only doing what you have told it to do, and the error is one of 'user error'. First look for the problem at the proximal end of the needle...

Drug errors

Administering the wrong drug in the direct vicinity of nervous tissue is likely to result in permanent neurological damage. Absolute vigilance is necessary; check all drugs yourself and insist on seeing all ampoules, and if in doubt, draw it up again yourself. Adjuncts are another source of error, particularly epinephrine as it comes in several different concentrations.

Non-anaesthesia neurological damage

Most commonly neurological damage is a consequence of other factors rather than the anaesthesia, including patient positioning, surgical retractors, the surgery itself, tourniquet with prolonged or high pressures, prolonged labour or compartment syndrome, or unmasked neurological disease.

Benefits

Pain relief

The most consistent and apparent benefit from regional anaesthesia techniques is pain relief. Many studies, looking at central and peripheral techniques across almost all surgical specialties, have shown this benefit, either in terms of pain scores, immediate opiate consumption, total opiate consumption, or other surrogate markers of pain.

Pre-emptive analgesia

Thoracotomy, breast surgery, and hernia surgery studies have shown a reduction in analgesia requirements in the postoperative period when regional anaesthesia was established before the incision was made. The evidence for other types of surgery is less convincing. Animal studies have shown that regional anaesthesia can reduce spinal cord excitation and thus reduce analgesia requirements.

Intraoperative

Regional anaesthesia compared to general anaesthesia has unfortunately produced very few benefits in the intraoperative period, excluding analgesia requirements. In high-risk vascular patients undergoing carotid surgery evidence has failed to show superiority of one technique over the other.

Surgical stress response

Neuraxial anaesthesia established prior to surgery has been shown to minimize the extent and duration of the surgical stress response during major abdominal surgery, including the reduction in serum cortisol and catecholamine levels. There is also less disturbance in blood glucose levels in diabetic patients.

Blood loss

Use of regional anaesthesia has been associated with reduced blood loss in a variety of lower limb surgical techniques.

Post-operative

Superior analgesia

Single injections or continuous infusions are superior to traditional analgesia techniques for outpatient shoulder and knee surgery. Continuous femoral nerve catheters provide clinical advantages for hip and knee replacement regarding analgesia and earlier mobilization for knee replacements.

Nausea and vomiting

Regional anaesthesia allows a reduction in both volatile anaesthetic usage, and opiate usage, both significant contributors to PONV rates. Minimizing opiate consumption may also reduce other related opiate side effects, such as pruritis, reduced gut motility, respiratory depression, confusion/drowsiness, urinary retention.

Respiratory function

Neuraxial regional anaesthesia techniques have been shown to better preserve pulmonary function, functional residual capacity, oxygenation and reduce infective respiratory complications for a variety of procedures (mostly in thoracotomy and major upper gastrointestinal surgery). This has reduced postoperative morbidity and perhaps mortality.

Cardiac mortality/morbidity
Thoracic epidural analgesia for open abdominal aortic aneurysm repair reduces postoperative mortality and myocardial infarction. Large-scale studies of a link between epidural analgesia and reduced mortality in other major surgery have not conclusively demonstrated a mortality benefit.

Early mobilization/physiotherapy
Good quality postoperative analgesia allows early mobilization and physiotherapy. This can lead to early improved function following certain procedures; particularly upper and lower limb orthopaedic procedures.

Bowel function
Postoperative ileus is reduced with epidural analgesia, which increases gut motility.

Cognitive function
This may return to normal faster with the use of regional techniques. The reduction in opiate consumption is a significant factor in the elderly. Regional anaesthesia may remove the need for general anaesthesia completely.

Long-term function
Use of postoperative perineural interscalene catheters for shoulder surgery in combination with physiotherapy regimens have resulted in improved long-term functional outcome following certain types of shoulder surgery.

Time to discharge
Benefits such as those described in this topic have been demonstrated to allow early discharge from hospital. This benefit can best be realized in hospitals set up to optimize care using these techniques; this requires a consistent approach to the use of regional anaesthesia and training of surgical and nursing staff. Shorter intensive care stays for the high-risk group have been reported.

Deep venous thrombosis
A hypercoaguable state is part of the normal stress response to surgery. Use of regional anaesthesia has been associated with a reduction in deep venous thrombosis following lower limb orthopaedic surgery and prostatectomy. The thrombosis of vascular grafts in the immediate postoperative period may be reduced with the use of regional anaesthesia. This effect may already be less significant, because of greater emphasis on postoperative thromboprophylaxis.

Procedure specific
Peripheral blocks complement ambulatory surgery, providing better analgesia, reduced postoperative nausea, and earlier discharge.

Neuraxial blocks in obstetric patients have shown superior analgesia in labour and reduced maternal mortality compared to general anaesthesia.

Contraindications

Whether or not to use regional anaesthesia for an individual patient requires a balanced consideration of the risks and the benefits, the clinical scenario, and the operator's experience.

Absolute contraindications

Patient refusal

As the clinician performing the procedure, it is your responsibility to obtain fully informed consent from an autonomous patient. Regional anaesthesia may offer significant risk reduction in a specific situation and this should be discussed with the patient and surgeon. Therefore, it is also your responsibility to be informed, and to be able to give accurate information (to the best of your knowledge) to allow the patient to make the correct decision for themselves regarding their management. However, if the patient declines the offered regional technique after a discussion of the risks and benefits, then the technique is clearly contraindicated.

Coagulopathy

See Chapter 9 for more details.

Full anticoagulation

This is a contraindication for neuraxial techniques. The development of spinal/epidural bleeding and haematoma formation is a major concern. The risk of haematoma formation is higher if an anticoagulant is present, if multiple and traumatic punctures were attempted, with a larger needle size and with administration of thromboprophylaxis within 1 hour.

The risks for haematoma formation are similar for neuraxial catheter removal as during insertion.

Intraoperative anticoagulation

Typically heparin and common during vascular surgery; the insertion of pre-operative epidural and spinal catheters does not seem to result in neurological problems. This appears to be an acceptable risk provided catheter insertion is >1 hour before heparin administration and not in the presence of other causes of coagulopathy.

Partial anticoagulation

In the form of antiplatelet drugs commonly prescribed to patients. Aspirin and NSAIDs do not appear to increase the risk of haematoma formation. More potent antiplatelet drugs, such as clopidogrel (thienopyridines) should be stopped electively 7 days preoperatively. For emergency surgery an analysis of the risks and benefits would be required, but most clinicians would avoid a neuraxial block and may consider peripheral techniques a safer option. Low-molecular-weight heparins (LMWHs) do pose a significant bleeding risk in particular for the insertion and removal of epidural catheters. LMWH should only be administered 4 hours after neuraxial catheter insertion or removal and the insertion or removal of neuraxial catheters should occur at least 12 hours after a dose of LMWH.

Blood results and markers of potential coagulopathy are frequently presented to clinicians for consideration. These markers are difficult to interpret because they do not represent the whole coagulation cascade.

Thrombocytopenia of <100 and an INR of >1.5 may indicate ↑ risk, but platelet function and coagulation may be well preserved. The use of peripheral techniques or a single injection spinal anaesthetic may be preferred in these circumstances. Deep and paravertebral blocks, e.g. lumbar plexus blocks, require the same caution with coagulopathy criteria as central neuraxial techniques.

Infection

Local infection at the site of needle insertion poses the risk of spreading the infection. Systemic sepsis is only a contraindication if antibiotic therapy has not been instituted.

Relative contraindications

Patient comorbidities

- Respiratory failure requires caution with the use of interscalene (and supraclavicular) blocks, as they frequently block the phrenic nerve and critically impair hemidiaphragmatic function. Lower volume injection with US can reduce the incidence but not eliminate it. A high spinal/ epidural or bilateral paravertebral blocks may also be contraindicated in these patients.
- The reduction in systemic vascular resistance caused by the sympathetic blockade of a neuraxial block may not be tolerated by patients with severe cardiac stenotic valvular disease such as aortic stenosis (or other causes of a fixed cardiac output) or with significant hypovolaemia.
- Patients with raised intracranial pressure may not tolerate the increase in CSF pressure with epidural injections or CSF leakage after a spinal block.
- Patients with neurological deficits such as multiple sclerosis and diabetic neuropathy require careful examination and documentation. In unstable progressive disease processes it may be best to avoid a regional block, but a risk/benefit analysis should be undertaken for each individual; regional anaesthesia should be considered in stable conditions.
- Patients with learning difficulties and those in an agitated and uncooperative state may prove difficult to manage perioperatively, even with an excellent block. Language barriers may make it difficult to explain the rationale and risks to a patient; it is important to use an interpreter in these circumstances so informed consent can be obtained.

Controversies

Awake versus general anaesthesia blocks

The decision to perform a neuraxial or regional anaesthesia block in an awake or anaesthetized patient has been one of the most controversial subjects in this field of anaesthesia. Anaesthetists are acutely aware of the medicolegal implications involved in postoperative nerve injury. Blame is unjustly and automatically attributed to the regional technique, despite numerous other factors resulting in neurological sequelae unrelated to anaesthesia, e.g. surgical retraction, patient position, and tourniquet pressures. There are no randomized controlled studies that can give us definite answers concerning this dilemma. Our own clinical practice and beliefs are also diverse. We accept the practice of regional blocks in anaesthetized children; commonly perform lower limb blocks on anaesthetized patients under general or spinal anaesthesia; perform rescue blocks on partially insensate limbs and all these issues have not resulted in a higher incidence of neurological problems. In the last 15 years, the attitudes, beliefs, and practice of anaesthetists have changed. Recent surveys have demonstrated that more neuraxial blocks are performed on awake patients and more peripheral blocks are performed on anaesthetized patients compared to practice 10–15 years ago.

Pain on injection

Current recommendations are based on the premise that intraneural injections are extremely painful and that an awake patient would therefore be the best monitor to avoid neurological injury. This belief is unfortunately unreliable. The majority of both neuraxial and peripheral nerve blocks resulting in nerve injury have been reported in awake patients and most have not been associated with pain on injection. Conversely a large proportion of patients (21%) reporting discomfort on injection have not resulted in neurological problems. The intensity of the pain on injection and the interpretation of that pain by each individual patient and anaesthetist are also very subjective. Normal pressure paraesthesia described by Winnie, has resulted in permanent nerve injury in some cases. Another complicating factor is that in some case reports, nerve injuries occurred despite the operator repositioning the needle when pain was reported on the initial injection. This suggests that nerve disruption occurs with the initial small volume (<1mL) injection and the nerve was damaged at the point of the patient reporting discomfort. Obviously our reporting systems will lead to bias, because we are unaware of how many nerve injuries have been prevented by patients reporting pain during the procedure and warning the clinician.

Local anaesthetic toxicity

Some experts argue that in an awake patient early recognition and treatment of systemic toxicity results in a better outcome. There are no reports of LA toxicity in adult patient under GA, in fact the anticonvulsant effects of sedation and GA may offer protection. Cardiovascular collapse can occur without CNS symptoms and the time to peak plasma levels may be variable depending on anatomical site (see Table 8.2). We often induce GA within a few minutes of administering the LA. The traditional treatment of LA toxicity would include securing the airway with a high fraction of inspiratory oxygen and haemodynamic support. One could argue that an anaesthetized patient is potentially better placed when it comes to treatment of toxicity. The one group of patients where LA toxicity is potentially of greatest concern is the paediatric group because of mg/kg dose requirements; in this group, regional anaesthesia in anaesthetized children is universally accepted practice.

Conscious sedation
Regional anaesthesia techniques may involve passage of the needle through significant amounts of tissue, especially for deeper blocks, that may cause a patient discomfort which can lead to limited acceptance and dissatisfaction in regional techniques. Sedation can in the majority of cases provide excellent conditions for an anxious patient that reduces the discomfort and stress and increases the acceptance of regional blocks. The emphasis should be on conscious sedation, where the patient can maintain an airway, respond to verbal commands, and react appropriately to physical stimuli. The North Americans often refer to this as monitored anaesthesia care (MAC). A wide range of conscious sedation techniques are available, including single dose, target controlled infusions, and even patient controlled sedation. Most anaesthetists would use benzodiazepines (midazolam) and propofol sedation, but ketamine, clonidine, fentanyl, and remifentanil techniques are well described.

Recommendations
This lack of conclusive evidence has left us with recommendations by experts that are based on case reports and anecdotal experience. Blanket statements like 'all thoracic epidurals have to be done awake' as for some European countries are based on 2 case reports and personally I do not find them useful. The medicolegal repercussions may be severe for clinicians. The tragic case reports by Benumof, where 4 patients suffered cervical paraplegia after interscalene blocks were performed during GA, should obviously be noted, but further reading reveals that outdated techniques were used and probably inappropriate needle lengths. However, this still led ASRA to recommended that interscalene blocks only be performed on awake or lightly sedated patients. When things go wrong, a clinician will be measured against their peers and what general consensus considers good practice, despite the lack of evidence. In my opinion the majority of anaesthetists would *endeavour to perform regional blocks on awake or conscious sedated patients and blocks on anaesthetized patients should be the exception*. There seems to be a trend to suggest that procedures closer to the CNS demands an awake/sedated approach, e.g. epidurals, spinals, interscalene; and more peripheral, painful, or deeper blocks are performed on asleep patients. Every patient, clinician's experience, and environment is different and all these factors should be considered every time a regional technique is employed.

Nerve localization technique

Historically, clinicians performing PNBs relied upon surface anatomy to identify the injection point, and manipulation of the inserted needle to elicit paraesthesia in an appropriate sensory distribution to ensure correct needle position. The use of electric current to stimulate nerves was introduced in the 1960s. Needle quality improved and the technology in nerve stimulators became more sophisticated, such that by the 1980s this had become routine practice, allowing the tip of a regional anaesthesia needle to very closely approximate the intended nerve; sequential reduction in the threshold stimulating current implying reducing distance to the nerve.

The last 10 years have seen a rapid improvement in microprocessors and radiological imaging equipment. This has spurred interest in the use of portable US to image the anatomy, and visualize both the needle approaching the nerve and the subsequent spread of local anaesthetic. All 3 of these techniques are capable of providing a nerve block that works, but there is currently controversy regarding which of the latter 2 is 'better'.

An ideal regional anaesthesia technique produces a rapid blockade of the intended axonal traffic (pain, sensation, and/or motor) every time without discomfort, side effects, or complications.

Nerve stimulation

Nerve stimulation to approximate the needle tip to the nerve has been associated with very high success rates (>97%) and a rapid onset of block, and modern, insulated regional anaesthesia needles are between 20G and 23G in size, minimizing discomfort. There is extensive (>40 years') experience with this technique of nerve localization and considerable, well-conducted, research to support its use.

The required equipment is small, portable, and reasonably priced. However, the techniques described for nerve stimulator-guided nerve block have tended to use large volumes of LA to improve success but increasing the possibility of side effects and complication. The techniques are 'blind', relying upon a surrogate endpoint of threshold current, so there may be situations in which the needle tip is 'tenting' a fascial plane to generate a low-threshold current, yet LA injects away from the nerve. There is also no way of identifying variants from normal anatomy, which may explain why this technique does not reach a 100% success rate. Finally, nerve stimulation usually relies upon the stimulation of motor nerve fibres, which are only a proportion of nerves (sensory fibres, connective tissue, blood vessels etc.). It is easy to appreciate either that the needle may be in an ideal position and not elicit an appropriate response, or that a needle may be in a nerve before a motor response is achieved. This can lead to failure, or worse, nerve damage.

Ultrasound-guided regional anaesthesia

Ultrasound is used to identify the anatomy (including variants from normal), visualize the needle throughout the technique, and visualize the spread of LA. There is evidence to suggest a reduction in procedure time, and a more rapid onset of block using much lower volumes of LA (i.e. 5mL LA vs 40mL LA for interscalene block; 10mL LA vs 40mL LA for axillary block.) Side effects can be reduced (phrenic nerve block with interscalene block = 50%) and the ability to visualize the needle and its tip theoretically prevents direct axonal trauma or unintended intraneural injection. Meta-analysis also confirms a reduced failure rate or need for conversion to GA. An additional benefit is the ability to teach trainees the anatomy relevant to the intended block and show why the surface anatomy is there, and how it correlates with the 'real' anatomy underneath. However, UGRA requires the purchase of a US machine with appropriate capability, an initial outlay of ~ £20,000. Users need education in how US works, and the limitations of the technology. Each block needs to be 're-learnt' to accommodate this new tool, and there is a definite learning curve with each block, as well as with the in-plane and out-of-plane needling techniques. There is no evidence to demonstrate a reduction in (what are already low) complication rates and the abolishment of complications is unlikely.

Current amplitude

When using a nerve stimulator as a nerve location tool, the aim is to locate the needle tip at a distance close enough to the nerve for injected LA to distribute around the intended nerve, whilst not being within the nerve itself. The threshold current at which this occurs varies between patient, anatomical location, with comorbidity such as diabetes mellitus or neuropathies, and opinion differs between experts in the field.

General opinion suggests that a threshold of <0.2mA is highly likely to result in intraneural injection, which may result in nerve damage. Some experts mandate a threshold of 0.3–0.5mA for brachial plexus blocks, particularly interscalene and supraclavicular blocks. Lower threshold currents also result in a greater success rate for some blocks, although this is not the case for nerves within their own type of 'sheath': femoral, sciatic, axillary. Higher thresholds have been correlated with equal success rates for some blocks (sciatic, femoral, axillary); thresholds of <0.5mA have also been linked to intraneural injection, particularly in hyperglycaemia. The combination of US guidance and nerve stimulation regularly demonstrates a needle tip location very close to the nerve, or within an appropriate sheath, with no motor stimulation at all.

Outcome and epidurals

Epidural analgesia has some clear theoretical and practical benefits:
- Excellent analgesia.
- Reduction in stress response.
- Prevention of surges in heart rate, blood pressure, and myocardial oxygen demand.
- Improvement of postoperative respiratory function.

Unfortunately several large-scale trials have not shown these benefits to translate into mortality reduction for high-risk patients undergoing major surgery. Many practitioners have interpreted and used this data as a reason to avoid the use of epidural analgesia, claiming no benefit at the risk of causing harm. The counter argument is that these data have clearly shown epidural analgesia to provide the best analgesia and patient satisfaction, with comparable mortality and a side effect/complication profile similar to or better than patient-controlled analgesia (PCA).

Qualification/accreditation

Regional anaesthesia has developed significantly over the last 40 years, with the advent of new techniques, new equipment and a deeper knowledge base around all aspects of patient safety. Many practising anaesthetists will have spent years administering blocks on orthopaedic lists without any notion of having to be 'qualified' or 'accredited' to a regional anaesthetic body. There is a fundamental medical professional obligation to ensure that the management we deliver is safe for the patient. In the current climate of reduced trainee hours, reduced training case load, and a changed educational environment, trainees and consultants will be increasingly expected to be able to demonstrate their competence at particular techniques. ESRA have an increasingly popular diploma qualification and the University of East Anglia has launched an MSc in RA; RAUK and AAGBI have developed guidelines on the quality, content, and accreditation of UGRA courses; and increasingly regional anaesthesia fellowships are becoming available in England, comparable to their North American counterparts. Trainee logbooks displaying numbers are no longer considered valid within regional anaesthesia; the important differentiation is one of, for example, 50 safe successful blocks versus 50 unsafe, failed blocks causing permanent harm. Both will display the same using the RCOA logbook; an outcome-based logbook tool will demonstrate the difference. Cumulative sum analysis can provide a simple outcome-based logbook with an easy-to-interpret graph. See Chapter 15.

Further reading

Auroy Y, Benhamou D, Barguee L, *et al.* (2002). Major complications of regional anesthesia in France. *Anesthesiology*, **97**(5),1274–80.

Cook TM, Counsell D, Wildsmith JAW (2009). Major complications of central neuraxial block: report on the Third National Audit Project of the Royal College of Anaesthetists. *Br J Anaesth*, **102**(2), 179–90.

Enneking FK, Chan V, Greger J, *et al.* (2005). Lower-extremity peripheral nerve blockade: essentials of our current understanding. *Reg Anaesth Pain Med*, **30**(1), 4–35.

Neal JM, Gerancher JC, Hebl JR, *et al.* (2009). Upper extremity regional anaesthesia. essentials of our current understanding 2008. *Reg Anaesth Pain Med*, **34**(2), 134–70.

Rigg JA, Jamrozik K, Myles PS, *et al.* (2002). Epidural anaesthesia and analgesia and outcome of major surgery: a randomized trial. *Lancet*, **359**(9314), 1276–82.

Regional anaesthesia in patients taking anticoagulant drugs

Background

Introduction

Increasing numbers of patients are taking drugs that impair normal coagulation and this causes concern about the risk of perioperative bleeding events. The anaesthetist is particularly concerned about compressive vertebral canal haematomas, which may occur after spinal or epidural anaesthetic techniques. Fortunately, the risk of this feared complication is very low but the major risk factors are coagulopathy or technical difficulties with the block. There is also concern about perineural haematomas, which may be associated with peripheral nerve blocks (PNBs) and this chapter attempts to put the risks of these complications into context with reference to different classes of anticoagulant drugs.

Risk of vertebral canal haematoma

The advantages of central neuraxial block (CNB) are well known to all anaesthetists. However, the worry that devastating vertebral canal bleeding may occur if these techniques are used in patients who are receiving anticoagulant drugs, is a common clinical dilemma.

The incidence of vertebral canal haematoma (VCH) associated with CNB is extremely low. Tryba estimated the risk as 1 in 150,000 epidural anaesthetics and 1 in 220,000 spinal anaesthetics after reviewing 1.5 million patients who had undergone one of these techniques. However, the risk is almost certainly higher in patients who have received drugs that impair coagulation.

In 1994, Vandermeulen carried out a comprehensive literature review to identify case reports of VCH associated with CNB and found only 61 cases published between 1906 and 1994. 46 of these cases were associated with epidural techniques and 32 involved a catheter. The remainder, 15, occurred after spinal anaesthesia. 68% of the cases occurred in patients who were taking anticoagulant drugs (most commonly IV unfractionated heparin) or had a coagulopathy. The other common risk factor identified was technical difficulties with block performance. Coagulation abnormalities and/or technical difficulties were associated with over 87% of these cases.

Since Vandermeulen's review was published there have been over 70 case reports of VCH associated with CNB in patients taking LMWH. These cases projected this issue into the limelight and led to understandable caution by anaesthetists wishing to use regional anaesthetic techniques.

The American Society of Anesthesiology Closed Claims Database Project published a review of 1005 complications associated with regional anaesthesia that had completed the medico legal process over the period 1980–1999. 84 cases of injuries to the neuraxis were identified, of which the commonest complication was epidural or spinal haematoma, which accounted for 36 of the 84 cases. Only 3 of these cases occurred in obstetric patients and 32 (89%) patients were left with permanent neurological deficits. 72% of cases occurred in patients with abnormal clotting, most commonly due to perioperative administration of anticoagulant drugs.

The Royal College of Anaesthetists' National Audit Project 3 found 8 VCH in a 12-month period (September 2006–August 2007), on a background of just over 700,000 CNB, about 1 in 90,000, with the risk of permanent harm 1 in 140,000. 7 of the 8 patients had received some form of anticoagulation medication and all were found in perioperative epidurals (giving a 1 in 12,000 risk in this setting). 50% of symptoms were first reported/noted at the time of, or after, catheter removal.

Peripheral nerve block and anticoagulants

Most reports of serious bleeding events associated with PNB have followed psoas compartment (lumbar plexus) blocks or lumbar sympathectomy. Several large retroperitoneal haematomas have occurred following these techniques. One case was associated with perioperative administration of heparin and warfarin, 2 with LMWH, and 2 with thienopyridine antiplatelet drugs (1 clopidogrel which proved fatal, 1 ticlodipine). Major bleeding was of greater significance than neural compression in all these cases.

The guidelines in Table 9.1 could be applied to PNB performance, but some regional anaesthetists would argue that this would be unnecessarily restrictive. Careful consideration of the risks and benefits of a PNB on an individual patient basis is the most logical way to practice.

Table 9.1 Recommendations relating to drugs used to modify coagulation

Drug	Time to peak effect	Elimination Half-life	Acceptable time after drug for block performance	Acceptable time for next drug dose after block	Acceptable time after drug dose for catheter removal	Acceptable time after catheter removal for next drug dose
Heparins						
UFH s.c. prophylactic	<30min	1–2h	4h and normal APTT	1h	4h and normal APTT	1h
UFH i.v. treatment	<5 min	1–2h	4h and normal APTT	4h	4h and normal APTT	4h
LMWH s.c. prophylactic	3–4h	3–7h	12h	4h	12h	4h
LMWH s.c. treatment	3–4h	3–7h	24h	4h	24h	4h
Heparin alternatives						
Lepirudin	0.5–2h	2–3h	10h	4h	10h	4h
Desirudin	0.5–2h	2–3h	10h	4h	10h	4h
Bivalirudin	5 min	25 min	10h	4h	10h	4h
Argatroban	<30 min	30–35 min	4h	2h	4h	2h
Fondaparinux[a]	1–2h	17–20h	>36h	12h	42h	12h
Antiplatelet drugs						
NSAIDs	1–12h	1–12h	No additional precautions			
Aspirin	12–24h	Not relevant	No additional precautions			6h
Clopidogrel	12–24h	Irreversible effect	7 days	After block performance	7 days	6h

Ticlopidine	8–11 days	24–32h but 90h in chronic use	10 days		10 days	6h
Tirofiban	<5 min	4–8h	8h	After block performance	8h	After catheter removal
Eptifibatide	<5 min	4–8h	8h	After block performance	8h	After catheter removal
Abciximab	<5 min	24–48h	48h	After block performance	48h	After catheter removal
Dipyridamole	75 min	10h	No additional precautions			6h
Oral anticoagulants						
Warfarin	3–5 days	4–5 days	INR <1.4	After catheter removal	INR <1.4	1h
Rivaroxaban[a]	3h	7–9h	21h	5h	a	a
Dabigatran[b]	0.5–2.0h	12–17h	36h	6h	b	b
Thrombolytic drugs						
Alteplase, anistreplase	<5 min	4–24 min	Contraindicated	Contraindicated	Not applicable	10 days

Notes: the data used to populate this table are derived from the German guidelines adopted by ESRA, the ASRA guidelines and data presented by drug manufacturers. Ticlopidine no longer has a UK licence. These recommendations relate primarily to neuraxial blocks.

APTT, activated partial thromboplastin time; INR, international normalized ratio; IV, intravenous; LMWH, low-molecular-weight heparin; NSAIDs, non-steroidal anti-inflammatory drugs; SC, subcutaneous; UFH, unfractionated heparin.

[a] Manufacturer recommends caution with use of neuraxial catheters.

[b] Manufacturer recommends that neuraxial catheters are not used.

Anticoagulant drugs

Aspirin and NSAIDs

These drugs impair platelet function by inhibiting platelet cyclo-oxygenase (COX). Aspirin inhibits COX irreversibly while NSAIDs do so reversibly. This means that the antiplatelet effect of aspirin will persist until a new platelet population is manufactured which will take at least 7 days whereas platelet function will return to normal within 3 days after stopping a NSAID. Despite the widespread use of these drugs for many years, there have only been 5 case reports of VCH in patients receiving aspirin or NSAIDs alone. It is therefore safe to proceed with CNB in patients taking these drugs, a view that has been endorsed by ASRA, ESRA, and AAGBI.

COX-2 inhibitors

This class of anti-inflammatory drugs selectively inhibit COX-2 which is not expressed in platelets and therefore do not affect platelet function. While being safe when used alone, they can potentiate the effect of warfarin by increasing the prothrombin time. There is not an ↑ risk of VCH in patients on COX-2 inhibitors.

Clopidogrel

This thienopyridine derivative is a potent antiplatelet agent. ADP-induced platelet aggregation is inhibited as is platelet–fibrinogen binding. These effects are irreversible and platelet function will not return to normal until at least 7 days after stopping the drug. Clopidogrel is recommended in combination with aspirin in patients with acute coronary syndrome. Clopidogrel should be continued for 4 weeks after insertion of bare metal coronary stents and for a minimum of 12 months after drug-eluting coronary stent to reduce the risk of stent thrombosis.

There have been many case reports of ↑ and even fatal surgical bleeding complications associated with clopidogrel. In one observational study in patients undergoing CABG, the re-exploration rate for bleeding in patients taking clopidogrel and aspirin was 10.4% vs 2.2% in those on aspirin alone. Non-urgent surgery should be postponed if possible in patients who are taking clopidogrel. If an antiplatelet effect must be maintained (e.g.in patients with coronary stents) aspirin can be continued.

To date, there have been 3 case reports of VCH associated with CNB in patients taking clopidogrel and also 2 cases of major bleeding following lumbar sympathetic block (1 fatal). This is concerning, and the clopidogrel datasheet states that it should be discontinued 7 days before surgery. This interval should also be observed before carrying out any central neuraxial or peripheral block. It is recommended that individual hospitals adopt policies to ensure that clopidogrel is discontinued before surgery.

Platelet GP IIb/IIIa antagonists

Abciximab, eptifibatide, and tirofiban are recommended by the UK National Institute for Health and Care Excellence (NICE) to prevent coronary ischaemic events in high-risk patients. CNB should be avoided until platelet aggregation has returned to normal, which will be a minimum of 8 hours after tirofiban and eptifibatide and 24–48 hours after abciximab dosing. The data sheets for these drugs states that they are contraindicated within 4–6 weeks of trauma or major surgery.

Unfractionated heparin

Unfractionated heparin (UH) has been used for many years both for thromboprophylaxis and therapeutic anticoagulation. SC thromboprophylactic doses have rarely been associated with bleeding complications and are not considered to significantly increase the risk of vertebral canal haematoma. Expert opinion recommends performing CNB 4 hours after UH administration and delaying administration for 4 hours after a block. However, it is likely to be safe to give a low-dose bolus (up to 5000 IU) of UH 1 hour after CNB. Doubt exists about the timing of higher doses, e.g. for cardiopulmonary bypass. Patients who have been receiving UH for >4 days should have a platelet count, as the incidence of heparin-induced thrombocytopenia is about 3%.

Therapeutic anticoagulation with heparin is a contraindication to regional block and an IV heparin infusion should be discontinued for 4 hours and the APTT should be normal before attempting a block or removing a catheter.

Low-molecular-weight heparin

LMWHs have longer half-lives than UH which makes once-daily administration possible. They have fibrinolytic properties as well as anti-Xa activity. Measurement of anti-Xa plasma levels is not useful in clinical practice. Over 40 cases of vertebral canal haematoma following CNB in patients receiving LMWH occurred in North America in the late 1990s. This may have been because North American dose guidelines were for twice-daily LMWH administration, meaning there was no 'safe' time to perform a block or remove an epidural catheter. A similar cluster of cases had not been reported in Europe despite the fact that LMWH had been available for 4 years longer, suggesting that the once-daily administration regimen used there was safer.

Current guidelines recommend waiting at least 12 hours after LMWH administration before CNB or catheter removal. Postoperative LMWH dosing has been shown to provide acceptable thromboprophylaxis, which makes this option attractive for both anaesthetist and surgeon. It is recommended that the first dose is given within 6 hours of surgery.

If high-dose LMWH is used for therapeutic anticoagulation it will take about 24 hours for coagulation to return to normal. Therefore, in this situation, an interval of 24 hours should elapse before attempting CNB or PNB.

Fondaparinux

This thromboprophylactic drug is a synthetic pentasaccharide, which has potent anti-Xa activity. It has a much longer elimination half-life than LMWH of 17 hours in young patients and 21 hours in healthy elderly patients. It is administered 6 hours after surgery, which makes decisions with respect to regional anaesthesia easier. However, its long half-life means that it should be used with caution in patients with neuraxial or peripheral nerve catheters *in situ*. An interval of at least 36 hours should elapse before removal of neuraxial or peripheral nerve catheters.

Warfarin

Warfarin is indicated for thromboembolic prophylaxis in an increasing range of cardiovascular conditions. A significant proportion of older patients presenting for surgery are on long-term warfarin therapy. This presents a challenge to both the surgeon and anaesthetist. In the vast majority of patients, the risk of perioperative bleeding greatly exceeds the risk of thrombotic events. Warfarin should therefore be stopped and the INR allowed to fall to <1.5. This normally takes about 4 days. If more rapid INR correction is necessary, small doses of vitamin K should be used. An INR of <1.5 is associated with normal haemostasis and it is therefore safe to proceed with CNB or PNB. There are a small number of patients who are at high risk of perioperative thrombotic events and they should be bridged with LMWH therapy. This 'high-risk' group are those who have a history of arterial thrombotic events, venous thrombotic events within 3 months or those with non bioprosthetic or multiple replacement heart valves. If a LMWH has been administered in place of warfarin, the recommended intervals discussed previously should be observed before performing any block.

Oral thrombin blockers

Rivaroxaban and dabigatran have recently been introduced into clinical practice and are currently licensed for thromboprophylaxis after hip and knee arthroplasty. It is likely that this class of drugs will replace warfarin in the future. Their major advantages are that they have predictable pharmacokinetics and dynamics and have no significant drug interactions. This means that clinical monitoring of their efficacy is unnecessary and will be associated with significantly less morbidity than warfarin. They are commenced after surgery and continued for 2–5 weeks. The rivaroxaban datasheet recommends an interval of 18 hours after dosing before removing an epidural catheter and delaying the next dose for 6 hours to reduce the risk of VCH, but it is best avoided altogether in patients with epidural catheters. The dabigatran datasheet does not recommend its use in patients with indwelling epidural catheters. There are currently no recommendations for patients with perineural catheters but adopting the same practice as for epidural catheters seems reasonable.

Further reading

Horlocker TT, Wedel DJ, Benzon H, et al. (2003). Regional anesthesia in the anticoagulated patient: defining the risks (the second ASRA Consensus Conference on Neuraxial Anesthesia and Anticoagulation) Consensus Development Conference. *Reg Anesth Pain Med*, **28**(3), 172–97.

Lee LA, Posner KL, Domino KB, et al. (2004). Injuries associated with regional anesthesia in the 1980s and 1990s. *Anesthesiology*, **101**(1), 143–52.

Regional Anaesthesia in Patients with Abnormalities in Coagulation. A guidance document produced by a Joint Working Party of the Association of Anaesthetists of Great Britain & Ireland (AAGBI), Obstetric Anaesthetists' Association (OAA), Regional Anaesthesia UK (RA-UK). 2011. Available at: ℘ http://www.aagbi.org/sites/default/files/RAPAC%20for%20consultation.pdf.

Tryba M (1993). Regional anaesthesia and low molecular weight heparin: pro (German). *Anaesth Intensivmed Notfallmed Schmerzther*, **28**(3), 179–81.

Vandermeulen EP, Van Aken H, Vermylen J (1994). Anticoagulants and spinal-epidural anesthesia. *Anesth Analg*, **79**(6), 1165–77.

Preparation and care of the awake patient during surgery

Background

Introduction

Regional anaesthesia offers a number of advantages over general anaesthesia especially in day stay surgery. However, adequate planning, patient education, a skilled anaesthetist, and skilled assistant are required. An enlightened surgeon and surgical team are helpful.

General considerations

- Early knowledge of the planned surgery, duration of surgery, and possible problems allows careful planning of the correct technique.
- Assess the patient's ability to lie still for the duration of the operation.
- Always have an alternative plan if the block is inadequate.
- Regional anaesthesia should always be for the patient's benefit and not for the anaesthetist's.

Influences on selected technique

Characteristics of the patient

- Supra or infraclavicular approach rarely suitable if the patient has significant respiratory compromise.
- Morbid obesity can make neuraxial techniques difficult.
- Risk of compartment syndrome would make limb blocks other than very short acting unsuitable.
- Pre-existing neuropathy is a relative contraindication.
- Uncooperative patients, e.g. dementia, may need significant sedation.

Characteristics of the surgery

- Duration of block must be adequate, operating conditions must be met, e.g. a still and cooperative patient, surgical field and limb tourniquet area must be adequately analgised.
- Day surgery requires short-acting agents and no ongoing lower limb motor block.

Anaesthetist expertise

- Only techniques which are familiar to the anaesthetist present for the procedure are appropriate.

Surgeon support

- Surgeon's support for regional techniques is more likely to be forthcoming when effective/efficient blocks are delivered.

Other issues

- Techniques may need to be modified to fit with local protocols e.g. postoperative ward protocols for specific LAs at specific concentrations. Ward staff may not have the expertise to provide adequate care for every regional technique.
- Equipment: US, nerve stimulator, stimulating needles and catheters may not always be available at the required time.

Preoperative

Anaesthetic assessment

- As for all anaesthetic reviews: medical history, physical examination, medications, medical and anaesthetic records. Then as required: electrocardiogram (ECG), pathology results, imaging studies, respiratory and cardiac function tests.
- BMI is an important factor in providing regional anaesthesia. Although it is less important if US guidance is used rather than landmark and nerve stimulation.
- Ordering pathology tests is only necessary for high-risk patients or high-risk procedures (e.g. patient recently taking anticoagulants). See Chapter 9.
- Assess patient's ability to lie in the position required for performance of the block and that required for surgery.
- Provide written information in addition to verbal education about what the patient will experience in theatre, and expected postoperative care:
  - how the block will be performed—nerve stimulator or US
  - what are the benefits and the potential risks. See Chapter 8
  - how much of the body will be numb
  - what they will be able to see and hear
  - what drapes will be used, i.e. clear or opaque
  - what they should do if they are uncomfortable or sore
  - how long the block will last and how to look after the anaesthetized limb
  - what analgesia to take and when.
- There should be a discussion about what level of sedation the patient would like, for both the performance of the block and during surgery.
- Consent should be obtained. If there is no specific consent form for regional anaesthesia, a note of the topics discussed and the risks described should be made, including failure.

Indications

- Avoidance of GA desirable—poor health, severe PONV, desire for early discharge from hospital.
- Early return to normal diet—diabetic.
- Analgesia for very painful procedure, to allow physiotherapy.
- Improvement of blood supply to surgical area.
- Early immobilization of operative area, such as tendon repair.

Contraindications

- Absolute contraindications include: patient refusal, infection over needle puncture site. LA allergy—very rare.
- Relative contraindications include: coagulopathy, general sepsis (for neuraxial block), uncooperative patients, and peripheral neuropathy.

Theatre visit

Block performance

- The block should be performed in an area with full resuscitation facilities. Ideally this would be an anaesthetic room or dedicated block room, with full monitoring to Harvard/AAGBI standards.
- Personnel: an anaesthetist, anaesthetic assistant (ODP, anaesthetic nurse) and person to provide emotional support for the patient.
- Equipment: this depends upon which block and which technique is used. US with appropriate frequency of probe, resuscitation drugs including Intralipid®, nerve stimulator, insulated short-bevel needle, continuous oxygen.
- The area to be anaesthetized should have been marked by the operating surgeon or deputy, who should be in theatre. The anaesthetist should confirm with the admitting nurse, the consent form and the patient, if possible, which area and which side is being anaesthetized. *Stop before you block!*
- The dose of LA allowable for that patient should be calculated before starting the procedure and a decision made on the addition of epinephrine or other adjuvant.
- Sedation in the form of short-acting opiate such as fentanyl and/or a benzodiazepine such as midazolam should be administered, if needed.

Intraoperative care

- Adequate numbness and, if necessary, paralysis of the limb should be tested prior to inflation of the tourniquet or first surgical incision. Nipping the skin in view of the patient can often give them confidence that there will be no pain with surgery. Avoid long-bevel needles as these are often not painful and can leave the area bleeding.
- A suitable screen should be used to separate the patient from the surgical site. An inquisitive patient moving to see the operation site can make the surgery very challenging.
- Full monitoring should be used as with a GA. Risks of late LA toxicity or intraoperative complications should not be underestimated.
- A nervous patient may need a hand-holder, with or without additional sedation. Sedation is not a treatment for an inadequate block and it should only be used to treat anxiety.
- Even with a dense upper limb block, the patient will rarely tolerate a tourniquet for more than an hour and a half. Regularly check that the patient is comfortable and provide additional analgesia/anaesthesia if problems occur.
- Always be prepared to convert a LA to a GA, unless a definite plan is made that this would be unacceptable. A plan regarding abandoning surgery may need to be made in such circumstances.

Postoperative

Postoperative care

- The operation site should be adequately protected from injury that may occur postoperatively from the loss of sensation. Upper limbs should be protected in a sling till motor and sensory block wears off. Lower limb blocks that limit weight bearing are unsuitable for day surgery, unless special provision is made for home care.
- Patients need to have adequate information regarding return of sensation and appropriate preloading with analgesia.
- Patients should have a contact number to phone in case of concerns regarding the anaesthetic or surgery during the postoperative period. Ideally they should be phoned by a member of the team to ensure complete resolution of the block. This can offer opportunities for audit.

Long-term follow-up

Any patients with complications that may be due to the anaesthetic should be reviewed by appropriate specialists. Surgeons and even neurophysiologists can wrongly blame the anaesthetist for complications of the surgery.

Further Reading

Ironfield CM, Barrington MJ, Kluger R, et al. (2014). Are patients satisfied after peripheral nerve blockade? Results from an International Registry of Regional Anaesthesia. *Reg Anesth Pain Med*, **39**(1), 48–55.

Lee A, Gin T (2005). Educating patients about anaesthesia: effect of various modes on patients' knowledge, anxiety and satisfaction. *Curr Opin Anaesthesiol*, **18**(2), 205–8.

Safe Anaesthesia Working Group (2011). Wrong site blocks during surgery. ℜ http://www.rcoa. ac.uk/standards-of-clinical-practice/wrong-site-block

Wound infiltration and catheter techniques

Introduction

The use of LA for wound infiltration is both an established aspect of clinical practice, and important facet of multimodal analgesia. Direct blockade of nociceptive and sympathetic afferents results in analgesia, a reduction in peripheral and central sensitization, and anti-inflammatory effects. Wound infiltration is achieved by single shots, a wound catheter with intermittent boluses, or a wound catheter with continuous wound infusion (CWI).

Overall CWI is an effective modality for the management of acute and postoperative pain. Compared to placebo it is associated with:
- ↓ pain scores at rest and with activity
- ↓ opioid requirements and risk of PONV
- ↑ patient satisfaction with ↓ length of stay in hospitalized patients.

In addition to these benefits CWI has a number of other advantages:
- Simple
- Safe
- Easy to perform
- Minimally invasive
- Well tolerated with few side effects
- Feasible in the majority of patients.

Clinical application

One of its major applications may be in those patients in whom a peripheral nerve or neuraxial technique is contraindicated.

The requirements for postoperative resources and levels of supervision are less, compared to epidural analgesia or IV PCA.

Although the use of local wound infiltration is commonplace, CWI is not in widespread clinical use, which may be due to:
- Lack of information and a perceived lack of evidence
- Fear of septic complications
- Lack of familiarity with the technique
- Over-reliance on already established practices.

Factors influencing success
- Site and duration of catheter placement
- Correct drug, volume, dosage
- Method of infusion.

Methods of infusion

- *Single-shot* injections are limited by the duration of action of LA whereas intermittent boluses may require greater resources and training, to ensure safety and appropriate delivery.
- *Continuous infusions* may not reach a level of analgesia suitable for activity and mobilization and a *combination* of techniques may be more appropriate. Electronic and elastometric pumps are available. The former are accurate and expensive, and the latter less accurate and cheaper. Disposable devices may be best for day case procedures.

Adjuvant analgesia

- Adjuvant drugs (e.g. NSAIDs, steroids, clonidine, and epinephrine) are used to augment analgesia via additional mechanisms of action.
- It is important to consider the potential side effects of these agents both locally, and systemically. Epinephrine has been used as an adjuvant relatively safely in a number of disciplines. This may not necessarily be extrapolated to all situations or patients (e.g. ↑ risk of chondrolysis if given intra-articularly with bupivacaine).
- Intra-articular morphine confers no benefit compared to placebo after knee arthroscopy. The use of adjuvants via local or systemic administration varies widely, and no firm recommendations are made.

Type of catheter

The use of multi-holed catheters facilitates the diffuse spread of LA which is important for efficacy. The optimum design may be specific to the type and extent of surgery, as well as the method of infusion (bolus vs continuous). In a comparison of a bolus via a triple-orifice epidural catheter versus a multi-hole catheter (40 holes, 3.5mm apart, over 15cm) placed subfascially after hip arthroplasty, there was no significant difference in spread observed. There are a number of commercially designed catheters available.

Location of catheter

Innervation of the abdominal wall, peritoneum, and viscera is highly complex, and CWI is unlikely to provide complete analgesia. As such, the location of the catheter may influence the degree of efficacy. Superficial wound infusion of LA after midline colorectal surgery confers no difference in outcome compared to an infusion of saline. Placebo-controlled randomized controlled trials (RCTs) of a continuous infusion of LA into the preperitoneal space, after open colorectal surgery may offer advantages such as improved pain relief, reduced opioid consumption, faster recovery of bowel function, and a reduction in hospital length of stay.

In addition, after elective Caesarean section a catheter placed below the transversalis fascia results in reduced pain at rest, and total opioid consumption (15.7mg, 95% confidence interval (CI) 9.7–20.7mg) compared to a catheter above the fascia (26.4mg, 95% CI 18.1–34.7mg), and provides analgesia and levels of satisfaction comparable to the use of a postoperative epidural. The use of single-shot infiltration is also effective in the short term. After abdominal hysterectomy intraperitoneal levobupivacaine has been shown to have opioid-sparing effects, and the use of a patient-controlled wound catheter showed greater efficacy above the superficial abdominal fascia. The optimum site of placement may therefore vary for different procedures through the same skin incision.

Safety

Safety concerns of CWI include:
- LA toxicity
- Wound sepsis
- Myotoxicity
- Chondrolysis.

Some LAs have been shown to have bacteriostatic and bactericidal properties and in a meta-analysis of >2000 patients, there were no reports of LA toxicity, and a lower rate of wound infection (0.7%), compared to controls (1.2%). Although intra-articular infusions of bupivacaine have been associated with chondrolysis, this appears both time and dose dependent, and a single dose has been considered safe.

Catheter or pump failure occurs relatively infrequently (1.1%). The catheter may become blocked or dislodged, and the pump may be inaccurate in the rate of delivery. Meticulous attention to technique, process, and technological design is therefore paramount for analgesic success and safety.

Cost-effectiveness

A recent study has demonstrated that CWI is cost effective (€6460) after open-abdominal surgery when compared to epidural (€7500) or patient-controlled opioid analgesia (€7273), with analgesic success (77.4%) at least equivalent to the epidural group, (72.9%) and more favourable than the PCA group (53.9%). Therefore CWI may be a viable economic and clinical alternative to traditional methods of postoperative pain control.

Type of surgery

Studies of CWI are heterogeneous, and may be viewed in isolation for specific circumstances. Nevertheless, the meta-analysis of studies involving cardiothoracic, general, urology, gynaecological, and orthopaedic surgery showed an overall combined clinical benefit, when compared to placebo, in terms of a reduction in pain at rest and activity, opioid consumption, PONV, length of hospital stay, and patient satisfaction.

Cardiothoracic surgery

There is an overall statistically significant ($p < 0.05$) reduction in pain scores and opioid use for CWI after cardiothoracic surgery, although studies are diverse with regards to the type of procedure and catheter location. Epidural or paravertebral analgesia is very effective, and associated with a reduction in both pulmonary and cardiac morbidity. CWI may therefore have a place in patients in whom such techniques are inappropriate, or for minimally invasive procedures. Sternal catheters are an effective and well-tolerated method of analgesia after traumatic fracture.

General/gynaecological surgery

Wound infiltration has been applied in a variety of situations. Day case inguinal hernia repair is a simple example in which LA is infiltrated with excellent results with reduced morbidity compared to the use of neuraxial techniques. CWI has been shown to be superior to placebo after appendicectomy, improves analgesia after iliac crest bone graft harvest, and may be as effective as a single-shot paravertebral block after radical mastectomy. There is evidence to suggest that pre-emptive instillation of intraperitoneal LA improves early postoperative pain after laparoscopic cholecystectomy, and preoperative infiltration reduces the stress response to surgery in children prior to inguinal herniorrhaphy.

Orthopaedic surgery

Minor diagnostic and minimally invasive arthroscopic procedures can usually be performed with a single bolus of intra-articular LA; however, analgesia is limited by the duration of action of the drug.

Major joint replacement surgery

In major joint replacement surgery the use of LA infiltration and postoperative intra-articular wound catheters has many potential advantages, including the ability to engage with physiotherapy and fully mobilize within a few hours postoperatively. Infiltration obviates the need for a femoral nerve block which may delay mobilization. In addition there may be a reduction in overall analgesic consumption with improved pain scores for up to 2 weeks, reduced joint stiffness, and an improvement in patient satisfaction and length of hospital stay, with many services being offered as day case procedures.

Shoulder surgery

Subacromial infusion of LA is as effective as a continuous interscalene catheter technique after rotator cuff repair, is simpler to perform, and reduces the risks of brachial plexus injury.

Summary

Future trends and novel therapies

The development of further sophisticated therapies may add a new dimension to postoperative and acute pain management. These include the use of liposomes or microcapsules to deliver sustained-release LAs, and permanently charged LAs, with a long duration of action due to trapping within neurons. However, none are as yet, in clinical use.

Conclusion

LA wound infiltration appears to be a safe, simple, and cost-effective analgesic strategy, with accumulating evidence of efficacy. Future studies to refine techniques will be useful to reinforce its use in clinical practice. CWI may be especially indicated in some procedures where other forms of regional anaesthesia are contra-indicated or unavailable, or to facilitate early mobilization after major joint replacement surgery.

Further reading

Andersen LØ, Kristensen BB, Madsen JL, et al. (2010). Wound spread of radiolabeled saline with multi- versus few-hole catheters. Reg Anesth Pain Med, 35(2), 200–2.

Beaussier M, El'Ayoubi H, Schiffer E, et al. (2007). Continuous preperitoneal infusion of ropivacaine provides effective analgesia and accelerates recovery after colorectal surgery: a randomized, double-blind, placebo-controlled study. Anesthesiology, 107(3), 461–8.

Gupta A (2010). Wound infiltration with local anaesthetics in ambulatory surgery. Curr Opin Anesthesiol, 23(6), 708–13.

Liu SS, Richman JM, Thirlby RC, et al. (2006). Efficacy of continuous wound catheters delivering local anesthetic for postoperative analgesia: a quantitative and qualitative systematic review of randomized controlled trials. J Am Coll Surg, 203(6), 914–32.

Macintyre PE, Scott DA, Schug SA, et al. (2010). PCA, regional and other local analgesia techniques. In Macintyre PE, Scott DA, Shug SA, et al. (eds), Acute pain management: Scientific evidence (3rd edn), pp. 175–224. Australian and New Zealand College of Anaesthetists and Faculty of Pain Medicine, 2010. Available at: ℘ http://www.anzca.edu.au/resources/books-and-publications/acutepain.pdf

O'Neill P, Duarte F, Ribeiro I, et al. (2012). Ropivacaine continuous wound infusion versus epidural morphine for postoperative analgesia after cesarean delivery: a randomized controlled trial. Anesth Analg, 114(1), 179–85.

Rackelboom T, Le Strat S, Silvera S, et al. (2010). Improving continuous wound infusion effectiveness for postoperative analgesia after cesarean delivery: a randomized controlled trial. Obstet Gynecol, 116(4), 893–900.

Scott NB (2010). Wound infiltration for surgery. Anaesthesia, 65(1), 67–75.

Tilleul P, Aissou M, Bocquet F, et al. (2012). Cost effectiveness analysis comparing epidural, patient-controlled intravenous morphine, and continuous wound infiltration for postoperative pain management after open abdominal surgery. Br J Anaesth, 108(6), 998–1005.

Whiteman A, Bajaj S, Hasan M (2011). Novel techniques of local anaesthetic infiltration. Contin Educ Anaesth Crit Care Pain, 11(5), 167–71.

Dermatomes and myotomes

Dermatomes and myotomes

Fig. 12.1 shows a dermatome and nerve map of the anterior body.

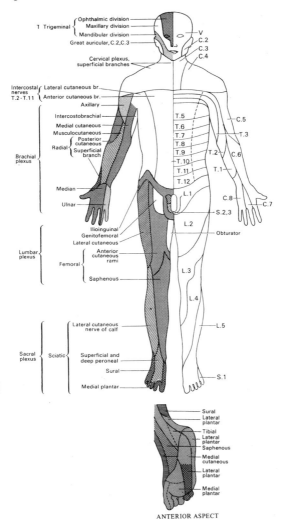

ANTERIOR ASPECT

Fig. 12.1 Dermatome and nerve map of the anterior body.

Fig. 12.2 shows a dermatome and nerve map of the posterior body.

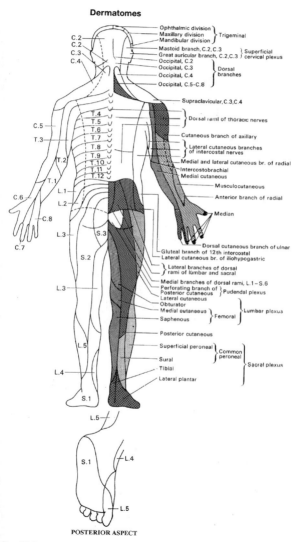

Fig. **12.2** Dermatome and nerve map of the posterior body.

Muscles and their innervations

Table 12.1 and Table 12.2 show the actions and innervations of the major muscles of the upper and lower limbs.

Table 12.1 Major muscles of the upper limb: their actions and innervations

Muscles	Movement	Nerve roots	Cord	Nerve
Deltoid	Shoulder abduction	C5, C6	Upper trunk Posterior cord	Axillary
Biceps	Elbow flexion	C5, C6	Upper trunk Lateral cord	Musculocutaneous
Triceps	Elbow extension	C7, C8	Posterior	Radial
Pronator teres	Forearm pronation	C6, C7	Lateral	Median
Extensor carpi radialis (longus and brevis)	Wrist extension	C6, C7	Posterior	Radial
Extensor carpi ulnaris		C7, C8		
Extensor digitorum	Finger extension	C7, C8	Posterior	Radial
Extensor pollicis longus	Thumb extension	C7, C8	Posterior	Radial
Extensor pollicic brevis				
Abductor pollicis longus	Thumb abduction	C7, C8	Posterior	Radial
Flexor carpi radialis	Wrist flexion	C6, C7	Lateral	Median
Palmaris longus		C8	Medial	Median

Muscle	Action	Root	Cord	Nerve
Flexor digitorum profundus	Finger flexion	C8, T1	Medial	Median/ulnar
Flexor digitorum superficialis		C7, C8, T1	Medial/lateral	Median
Flexor pollicis longus	Thumb flexion	C8, T1	Medial	Median
Oppones pollicis	Thumb opposition	C8, T1	Medial	Median
Flexor pollicis brevis	Thumb flexion			
Abductor pollicis brevis	Thumb abduction			
Lumbricals	MCPJ flexion	C8, T1	Medial	Ulnar/median
	PIPJ and DIPJ extension			
Flexor carpi ulnaris	Ulnar flexion of wrist	C8	Medial	Ulnar
Dorsal interossei	Abduct fingers	C8, T1	Medial	Ulnar
Palmer interossei	Adduct fingers			
Adductor pollicis	Thumb adduction	C8, T1	Medial	Ulnar
Abductor digiti minimi	Little finger flexior and abduction	C8, T1	Medial	Ulnar
Flexor digiti minimi				
Opponens digiti minimi				

DIPJ, distal interphalangeal joint; MCPJ, metacarpophalangeal joint; PIPJ, proximal interphalangeal joint.

Table 12.2 Major muscles of the lower limb: their actions and innervations

Muscles	Movement	Nerve roots	Plexus	Nerve
Psoas major	Hip flexion	L2, L3	Lumbar	
Iliacus	Hip flexion	L2, L3	Lumbar	Femoral
Pectineus	Hip flexion and adduction	L2, L3, L4	Lumbar	Femoral
Piriformis	Lateral rotation and abducts hip	S1, S2	Sacral	
Obturator internus	Lateral hip rotation	L5, S1, S2	Sacral	
Gemelli		L4, L5, S1		
Quadratus femoris				
Gluteus maximus	Hip extension and adduction	L5, S1, S2	Sacral	Gluteal
Gluteus medius		L4, L5		
Gluteus minimus				
Tensor fascia latae	Hip flexion and medial rotation	L4, L5, S1	Sacral	Gluteal
Obturator externus	Lateral hip rotation	L3, L4	Lumbar	Obturator
Adductor magnus	Hip adduction (medial rotation)	L3, L4	Lumbar	Obturator
Adductor brevis		L2, L3		
Adductor longus		L2, L3		
Gracilis	Hip adduction, flexion of knee	L3, L4	Lumbar	Obturator

Muscle	Action	Roots	Plexus	Nerve
Semimembranosus	Hip extension, knee flexion	L5, S1, S2	Sacral	Sciatic
Semitendinosus		S1, S2		
Biceps femoris				
Sartorius	Hip flexion, adduction and lateral rotation. Knee flexion (medial rotation)	L2, L3	Lumbar	Femoral
Quadriceps femoris	Knee extension	L3, L4	Lumbar	Femoral
Peroneus longus	Ankle plantar flexion and eversion	L5, S1	Sciatic	Superficial peroneal
Peroneus brevis				
Tibialis anterior	Ankle dorsi-flexion	L4, L5	Sciatic	Deep peroneal
Extensor digitorum longus	Toes extension and ankle dorsi-flexion	L5, S1	Sciatic	Deep peroneal
Extensor digitorum brevis				
Extensor hallucis				
Gastrocnemius	Ankle plantar flexion and knee flexion	S1, S2	Sciatic	Tibial
Soleus		L5, S1, S2		
Tibialis posterior	Ankle plantar flexion	L5, S1	Sciatic	Tibial
Flexor digitorum longus	Toe flexion and ankle plantar flexion	S1, S2	Sciatic	Tibial
Flexor hall. longus				
Small muscle of foot (except extensor digitorum brevis)	Toes movements	L5, S1, S2	Sciatic	Tibial (plantar)

The brachial plexus

Fig. 12.3 shows a diagram of the brachial plexus.

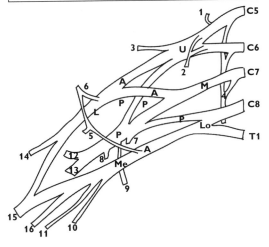

Fig. 12.3 The brachial plexus. **1** dorsal scapular nerve; **2** nerve to subclavius; **3** suprascapular nerve; **4** long thoracic nerve; **5** medial pectoral nerve; **6** lateral pectoral nerve; **7** upper subscapular nerve; **8** lower subscapular nerve; **9** thoracodorsal nerve; **10** medial cutaneous nerve of arm; **11** medial cutaneous nerve of forearm; **12** axillary nerve; **13** radial nerve; **14** musculocutaneous nerve; **15** median nerve; **16** ulnar nerve.

The lumbar plexus

Fig. 12.4 shows a diagram of the lumbar plexus.

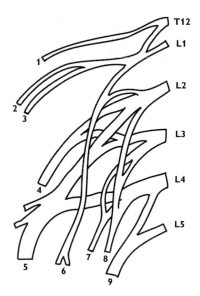

Fig. 12.4 The lumbar plexus. **1** T12 segmental nerve; **2** iliohypogastric nerve;
3 ilioinguinal nerve; **4** lateral cutaneous nerve of the thigh; **5** femoral nerve;
6 genitofemoral nerve; **7** accessory obturator nerve; **8** obturator; **9** lumbar nerve
root contribution to sciatic nerve.

Paediatric regional anaesthetic techniques

General considerations

Overview and safety

- The benefits of regional anaesthesia are well documented and include outstanding intra- and postoperative analgesia, attenuation of the stress response, opioid-sparing effects, and earlier extubation. Therefore, a LA technique should be used for all operations unless contraindicated.
- Although all blocks used in adult practice are feasible in children, many blocks are underused or avoided. This is largely from fear of complications and failure, and limited experience with complicated techniques. Despite this, regional anaesthesia is becoming increasingly popular.
- In the UK, almost all blocks in children are performed under GA with no evidence of a higher complication rate. The principal concern with this practice is the masking of signs and symptoms of intravascular and intraneural injection. However, children <8 years of age will not reliably report symptoms of toxicity even if awake. Therefore, the anaesthetist is more reliant on monitoring which must be commenced prior to the procedure.
- In the uncommon scenario of an awake technique, prior to theatre, a sedative and LA gel applied to the proposed needle puncture site may be useful. The presence of a parent and/or play therapist, distraction techniques, and Entonox® can be helpful during block insertion.
- Compared to central blocks, peripheral blocks can provide more intense and targeted analgesia, greater suppression of the stress response, a safer profile, and are generally more acceptable to patients and parents.
- The main complication is a failed block. Therefore, it is prudent to have a 'Plan B'. A failed block should be recognized intraoperatively, and supplemented with LA infiltration and/or IV analgesia.
- Preoperatively, a history should be taken to elicit any contraindications to LA techniques. If possible, the area where the block is to be sited should be examined and the patient's weight noted to calculate the maximum safe dose of LA.
- An attempt should be made to describe the postoperative sensation to the child, e.g. 'pins and needles' as they can find paraesthesiae distressing.
- Consent should be obtained for all nerve blocks. It may be verbal but should be recorded in the case notes and include a discussion of frequent and serious risks versus the benefits.
- Short-bevelled needles are used for PNBs. It is helpful to first nick the skin to avoid missing the feel of the underlying fascia during the puncture.
- A LA with a prolonged duration of action is preferred, e.g. levo-bupivacaine (Chirocaine®). Adequate postoperative analgesia is usually achieved with a concentration of 0.25%.
- The safe practice of slow incremental injection with repeated aspiration is compulsory for all blocks.
- Never exceed the calculated maximum LA dose.
- Landmark techniques for mixed nerve location can be aided by PNS as in adults.

- More recently US has been used as an imaging modality; allowing real-time needle guidance and monitoring of LA distribution; leading to improved success rates with reduced doses of LA. US imaging in children is generally of high quality as nerves are more superficial compared to adults, thereby enabling the use of higher-frequency probes.
- Continuous catheter techniques are particularly useful for prolonged blockade. The problem of dislodgement can largely be overcome by subcutaneous tunnelling and application of a tissue glue, e.g. Dermabond®.
- In recovery, it can be difficult to distinguish between pain and agitation. If in doubt, pain should be assumed and dealt with swiftly (use fentanyl or ketamine for rapid control of the situation).

Contraindications

Depend on the block to be performed but fall into broad categories:

Absolute
- Patient or parent refusal
- Local/systemic infection
- Allergy to LA
- Coagulopathy (central block).

Relative
- Coagulopathy (peripheral block)
- Neuromuscular disease
- Risk of masking compartment syndrome (discuss with surgeon).

Pharmacology
- Age-related differences in pharmacology and physiology must be considered for safe and effective practice (Table 13.1).
- In children, fibrous sheaths around the nerves are not well developed and myelination is incomplete until around 12 years of age. Thus, immature nerves are more sensitive to LA and less concentrated solutions can be used.
- The elimination half-life of amide LA is at least twice the adult value, reflecting an ↑ volume of distribution and possibly a reduced clearance.
- LAs are bound to plasma proteins, although alpha1-acid glycoprotein has a higher affinity for LA, a larger mass of drug is bound (albeit weakly) to albumin.
- Acidosis decreases protein binding and, therefore, increases the proportion of free drug, hence increasing the risk of toxicity.
- Less than 6 months of age, immature hepatic metabolism of amide drugs and reduced alpha1-acid glycoprotein lead to higher free plasma levels of drug. *The recommended dose in neonates is half the adult maximum, for both bolus doses and infusions.* Children >6 months of age receive the same dose in mg/kg as adults.
- The choice of LA for nerve blockade is a matter of personal preference depending on the desired duration of action. However, confounding factors such as hepatic metabolism, potential for IV injection or rapid absorption, or prolonged infusion requirements, dictate the use of conservative doses of one of the less toxic racemates.

Table 13.1 Pharmacology of local anaesthetics given in regional anaesthetic blocks

	T½ (min)		Onset (min)	T max (min)	Duration of action (min)
	Infant <6 months	Child >6 months			
Lidocaine	?	120	5–10	25–45	90–200
Bupivacaine	120–420	120–300	10–15	15–30	180–600
Ropivavaine	300	120–300	10–15	30–115	180–600

Drugs (Table 13.2)

Bupivacaine
- Potent amide LA
- Hepatic metabolism produces slightly active metabolites, which are significantly less toxic than the parent drug
- Longer half-life than in adults and may accumulate with infusions
- Preferred concentration for children is 0.25–0.5% for peripheral nerve blocks and 0.1% for infusions.

Levobupivacaine
- Single stereoisomer S(−) bupivacaine
- Equipotent to but less toxic than racemic bupivacaine
- Pharmacologically assumed to behave like bupivacaine
- Not licensed for children in UK, except for ilioinguinal or iliohypogastric blocks.

Ropivacaine
- Amide LA, single isomer
- Maximum concentration seen 30–115 minutes after injection perhaps due to local vasoconstriction
- Potential for vasoconstriction makes ropivacaine unsuitable for blocks involving end-arterial blood supply
- Not licensed for children <12 in the UK.

Lidocaine
- Amide LA, achiral
- Addition of 1:200,000 epinephrine slows vascular absorption and prolongs its effects.

Prilocaine
- Should be avoided <3 months of age due to risk of methaemoglobinaemia
- Maximum dose 5mg/kg.

Table 13.2 Suggested doses of local anaesthetics given in regional anaesthesia blocks

Drug	Bolus (mg/kg)		Infusion (mg/kg/h)	
	Infants <6 months	Child	Infants <6 months	Child
Lidocaine	3	5	0.8	3
Lidocaine (with epinephrine)	5	7	1	N/A
Bupivacaine	1.5–2	2.5	0.2	0.4
Levobupivacaine	1.5	2.5	0.2	0.5a
Ropivacaine	1.5–2	3	0.2–0.5	0.5

a Up to a maximum of 25mg/h.

Local anaesthetic additives

Additives are not appropriate for neonatal LA infusions.

Epinephrine
- Reduces vascular absorption, increasing duration of action
- Reduces peak plasma levels (lidocaine)
- Reduced benefit in long-acting LA, e.g. bupivacaine
- Less effective in epidurals
- Effective concentration 5 micrograms/mL (1:200,000), max. dose 200 micrograms
- Avoid in the vicinity of end arteries.

Clonidine
- Alpha-2 agonist.
- Acts on the brain to cause sedation and has analgesic effects on the central and possibly the peripheral nervous systems.
- There are minimal haemodynamic changes or sedation unless administered spinally.
- Dosage 2 micrograms/kg in epidurals, followed by an infusion of 0.1–0.3 micrograms/kg/h.

Opiates
- Acts on spinal/ peripheral opiate receptors.
- Proven synergism with LA in epidurals/spinals.
- All opioids have been used, suggested doses are for boluses; morphine 50 micrograms/kg, diamorphine 30 micrograms/kg, and infusion fentanyl 0.2–0.6 micrograms/kg/h.
- Debatable effect in peripheral blocks.

Ketamine
- NMDA receptor antagonist with weak LA properties.
- Now less commonly used due to the potential risk of neurotoxicity. When used it is usually in caudal epidurals in children over 1 year of age (dose 0.5mg/kg).
- Preservative-free drug essential.

Toxicity

- Often presents with cardiovascular collapse.
- There is some evidence that young infants have a higher threshold for neurotoxicity of LA but may have a lower threshold for cardiotoxicity.
- ECG may show T wave or ST segment changes.
- Management of LA toxicity includes:
  - stop LA injection, call for help, maintain & secure the airway, 100% O_2, start CPR
  - control seizures with a benzodiazepine, thiopentone, or propofol in small incremental doses
  - manage arrhythmias:
    —magnesium (50mg/kg over 15min, followed by an infusion of 25mg/kg/h)
    —phenytoin (5–10mg/kg)
    —amiodarone (5mg/kg IV over 3min, followed by infusion of 5–15mg/kg/min)
    —Intralipid® 20% (1.5mL/kg over 1min, repeated twice at 5min intervals, whilst continuing infusion of 0.25mL/kg/min). See AAGBI guidelines (see Fig. 4.1).

Using a peripheral nerve stimulator

- Set up and use as in adults.

Ultrasonography in paediatric regional anaesthesia

- General principles are the same as in adults.
- Due to their size, most structures are very superficial allowing the use of high-frequency probes and setting (>10MHz).
- For visualization of deeper structures, e.g. lower limb blocks in older, obese children, it may be necessary to use a lower-frequency transducer.
- With smaller children, the 'footprint' of the probe can be problematic and often a 25mm 'hockey stick' probe is used.
- Whilst the paediatric population is generally easy to scan there are exceptions. One particularly difficult patient group is those with neuromuscular conditions, e.g. cerebral palsy. Image interpretation can be difficult due to the absence of some muscles, fixed flexion deformities, or fibrosis. The latter causing a whiteout obscuring the nerve.
- A unique feature of US in paediatrics compared to adults is the lower level of ossification; this is particularly relevant for spinal imaging in infants. By the age of 21 years the spine is fully ossified and the echo windows into the spine decrease by 30–60%.

Regional anaesthetic techniques: peripheral blocks

Infiltration and field block

Indications
- Surgery where a specific nerve or plexus block is impossible.

Anatomy
- LA is injected subcutaneously or intradermally.

Technique
- Infiltration involves the injection of a LA subcutaneously into the wound edges.
- A field block involves the injection of LA into the skin around the operative site.
- After initial aspiration of the syringe, the needle is kept moving as LA is injected thus reducing the risk of intravascular injection.
- It can be performed preoperatively so allowing a lighter GA. Though this may distort the wound, e.g. the vermillion border of the lip.
- Alternatively, LA is injected or instilled into the incision prior to closure. A gradual emergence from GA is preferred as it allows the LA to take effect.
- In the awake child injection can be painful. This is minimized by distraction techniques, application of a topical LA, e.g. EMLA® or LET (lidocaine, epinephrine, tetracaine mix), warmed LA, use of a 27G needle and slow injection.

Complications
- Intravascular injection
- LA toxicity
- Haematoma.

Ilioinguinal/iliohypogastric block

This block provides analgesia to the skin only; simple analgesics should also be given.

Indications
- Herniotomy
- Orchidopexy (if a low scrotal incision is made, supplement with infiltration or pudendal nerve block)
- Varicocoele ligation
- Hydrocele.

Anatomy
- Both nerves originate from the primary ventral ramus of L1 in combination with a branch of T12.
- The nerves lie between the internal oblique and transversus abdominis muscles at the level of the anterior superior iliac spine (ASIS).
- At the level of the ASIS or more ventral the iliohypogastric nerve pierces the internal oblique muscle to lie beneath the external oblique muscle.
- The distance between the ASIS and the nerves is not related to age or weight. Both cadaver and US studies have shown the nerves to be closer to the ASIS than most traditional techniques presume.

Contraindications
- General
- Relative—obstructed hernia.

Landmark technique
- The various methods described and the 30% failure rate suggest that this is not a simple block to perform effectively. This is due to anatomical variation between patients.
- Patient supine.
- Prepare the skin with 0.5% chlorhexidine in 70% alcohol. Wait until the skin is dry.
- A 22G short-bevelled needle is inserted at a point 2.5mm medial along a line between the ASIS and the umbilicus.
- When performed blind a single fascial click technique is advised (50% of patients have only 2 muscles at the level of the ASIS). This decreases the risk of intraperitoneal injection (the average nerve–peritoneum distance is 3.3mm).
- 0.25% levobupivacaine 0.3–0.5mL/kg is injected slowly.
- A deep plane of GA is maintained until peritoneal, spermatic cord, or testicular manipulation is complete.

US-guided technique
- US machine is placed on the opposite side of the operator.
- Patient supine.
- A linear probe is held in a transverse plane with one end of the probe resting on the ASIS and orientated tangentially 45–60° to the sagittal plane towards the umbilicus.
- Muscle layers and peritoneum are identified.
- Moving the probe medially towards the umbilicus, the nerves are seen as hypoechoic ellipses sandwiched between the internal oblique and transversus abdominis muscles.
- Prepare the skin with 0.5% chlorhexidine in 70% alcohol. Wait until the skin is dry.
- Both the out-of-plane and in-plane (medial to lateral direction) approach have been described. The advantage of the latter is greater needle visibility, therefore diminishing the risk of intraperitoneal injection. (Coming lateral to medial in an IP technique can result in a steep needle angle and difficultly coming over the ASIS.)
- Usually in blocking the ilioinguinal nerve the LA also spreads to block the iliohypogastric nerve.
- Using US, blocks can be performed with as little as 0.075mL/kg of LA whilst maintaining a superior success rate.
- An improvement on this technique is to scan posteriorly around the flank just above the ASIS. The nerves are more consistently in the same plane and less likely to have divided. Thus making identification easier.

Complications
- Femoral nerve block is described in up to 11% of patients. In ambulant patients this should be tested for prior to discharge
- Intraperitoneal injection

- Bowel perforation
- Failed block
- Pelvic haematoma.

Rectus sheath block

Indications

- Umbilical and periumbilical surgery
- Pyloromyotomy (need visceral analgesia)
- Duodenal atresia repair (need visceral analgesia).

Anatomy

- The rectus muscles extend from the xiphisternum to the pubis.
- The lateral border of the rectus muscle is called the semilunaris. In small infants it may be difficult to define.
- The rectus muscles meet in the midline—linea alba.
- A fascial sheath encloses each rectus muscle. The sheath is formed by the aponeuroses of the lateral abdominal wall muscles (external oblique, internal oblique, and transverses abdominis). Below the umbilicus the lateral aponeuroses all pass anterior to the rectus muscle. This is known as the arcuate line, and it is at this point the inferior epigastric artery enters the rectus muscle.
- The posterior wall of the sheath is loosely connected to the rectus muscle.
- There are 3 tendinous intersections within the rectus muscle, which are attached to the anterior fascia: 1 at the level of the xiphisternum, 1 at the umbilicus and 1 between the 2.
- The 9th–11th intercostals nerves run between the posterior rectus sheath and the posterior wall of the rectus muscle. Ultimately, they penetrate the sheath to supply the periumbilical skin.

Landmark technique

- Patient supine.
- Prepare the skin with 0.5% chlorhexidine in 70% alcohol. Wait until the skin is dry.
- The needle is inserted just medial to the semilunaris at the umbilical level. The needle is inserted at an angle of 60° aiming towards the umbilicus.
- If the semilunaris is not identifiable, then introduce the needle 2–3cm lateral to the umbilicus.
- The needle is felt to 'pop' as it passes through the anterior sheath into the rectus muscle. The needle tip needs to reach the space between the muscle and the posterior sheath as this allows optimal spread of LA. This is felt as a 'scratch' by gently moving the needle from side to side.
- The procedure is then repeated for the opposite side.
- The depth of insertion is not related to age or weight. In children <10 years of age the needle should not be inserted >1cm.
- 0.2–0.4mL/kg per side 0.25% levobupivacaine is injected.

US-guided technique
- Patient supine.
- Operator stands on the opposite side to the US machine.
- A linear probe is positioned in a transverse plane just above the umbilicus. In a neonate the probe will straddle the linea alba and both rectus sheaths can be imaged and blocked without moving the probe. In larger patients, the probe is positioned over each side separately.
- Initially identify the transversus abdominis, internal and external oblique muscles and the formation of the rectus sheath by their aponeurosis.
- Use the colour Doppler to identify the inferior epigastric artery within the rectus muscle. The artery is most easily found in the hypogastric region and can then be tracked cephalad.
- Prepare the skin with 0.5% chlorhexidine in 70% alcohol. Wait until the skin is dry.
- The needle is inserted (bevel up) at the semilunaris; using an IP approach (lateral to medial) until the tip reaches the posterior sheath.
- To confirm needle position a small volume of saline or LA is injected and the sheath is seen to peel away from the muscle. As little as 0.1mL/kg per side 0.25% levobupivacaine is effective.
- If the tip is not quite in position the test dose will cause the muscle to 'fluff up ', carefully advance the needle a fraction further, a 'pop' is often felt.
- If the probe is turned 90° to a sagittal plane the spread of LA caudad and cephalad beneath the tendinous intersections can be monitored.

Complications
- Haematoma
- Intraperitoneal injection
- Visceral perforation.

Penile block

Indications
- Circumcision
- Distal hypospadias repair (discuss with surgeon).

Anatomy
- The ilioinguinal and genitofemoral nerves supply the penile base.
- The dorsal penile nerves (S2–4) supply the rest of the penis.
- The dorsal nerves pass under the pubis ramus within the subpubic space.
- The subpubic space is separated into left and right compartments by the suspensory ligament.
- The anterior border of the subpubic space is formed by Buck's fascia.
- The dorsal penile arteries, superficial and deep veins are in the midline. The dorsal nerves run lateral to these vessels.
- The ventral branches of the dorsal penile nerves originate in the subpubic space.

Contraindications
- LA containing epinephrine.

Technique 1—subpubic block

- Advantage of this method is ↓ risk of neurovascular or corpus cavernosum damage.
- Patient supine.
- Locate the symphysis pubis in the midline.
- The penis is pulled down ensuring the subpubic skin is taut.
- A 22–25G short-bevelled needle is inserted just through the skin in the midline (remember the vessels are in the midline), aiming posteriorly, 10° caudal and 20° lateral.
- A slight 'pop' is felt as the needle first breeches the superficial fascia, then a more definite 'pop' is felt on traversing the deep (Buck's) fascia (depth between 8–30mm, independent of patient weight or age).
- After injection, withdraw the needle to just under the skin and redirect it to the contralateral side.
- 0.25% levobupivacaine 0.1mL/kg/side, maximum 5mL each side. The volume injected is limited to diminish the possibility of vascular compromise. Ropivicaine should be avoided due to its vasoconstricting properties.
- Success rate may be improved by infiltrating subcutaneously around the root of the penis onto the lateral side of the scrotum, blocking branches from the ilioinguinal and genitofemoral nerves (1–5mL 0.25% levobupivacaine, depending on the size of the child).

Technique 2—ring block

- A simpler method
- LA is injected subcutaneously around the base of the penis.

Complications

- Intravascular injection
- Superficial haematoma
- Deep haematoma potentially causing vascular compromise.

Regional anaesthesia techniques: central blocks

Anatomy

- In the neonate the conus medullaris terminates at the L2 vertebral level (range from T10 to L3).
- In the preterm neonate the conus can terminate as caudad as the L4 vertebral level.
- The sacral hiatus occurs where the 5th and occasionally the 4th posterior neural arch fail to fuse.
- The sacral hiatus is roofed by the sacrococcygeal membrane, which is formed anteriorly from the ligamentum flavum and posteriorly from the sacral ligaments.
- The distance to the epidural space is <2cm, in neonates it is often <0.5cm.
- In neonates the dural sac is located at the S3/4 vertebral level, at 3 years of age it is found at the S2 vertebral level.
- The spinal canal in children is relatively wide; the lumbar interpedicular diameter in a neonate is 70% of the adult size. This creates a larger canal volume, hence the 4mL/kg of cerebrospinal fluid (twice that of an adult). This may explain the higher dose of LA per body weight required for infant subarachnoid block compared to adults.

Sonoanatomy of the spine

- The spinal canal can be visualized through an US window that consists of the interspinous and interlaminar spaces. The vertebrae become increasingly ossified (and thus echogenic) with age and these US windows therefore diminish in size. The size of the US windows increase from cranial to caudad.
- The neuraxial structures in the neonate are very superficial, the posterior dura being as little as 1cm from the skin; thus the highest-frequency probes (15MHz) can be used to provide the highest resolution image (Fig. 13.1).
- The spinal cord is hypoechoic with a hyperechoic outline, within the cord can be seen the central canal complex. The central canal complex has a hyperechoic border, during the first 2 days of life its termination may be normally dilated.
- The spinal cord lies a half to a third of the distance from the anterior to the posterior vertebral canal walls, if it lies more dorsally then this suggests tethering of the cord. Other US signs that may indicate spinal cord tethering are:
  - A lack of pulsations within the spinal cord
  - A thickened filum terminale (>2mm thick).
- At conus medullaris the cauda equina is visualized as numerous hyperechoic lines. All these structures are bathed in CSF which is anechoic.
- Surrounding these structures are the dura and ligamentum flavum, both seen as hyperechoic layers, often not differentiable.

Posterior/superficial

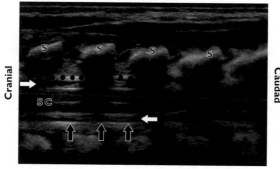

Anterior

Fig. 13.1 Paramedian sagittal oblique view of the paediatric lumbar spine. S, spinous process; SC, spinal cord; Black dots, posterior dura; White arrows, CSF; Black arrows, anterior dura.

Subarachnoid blocks

Indications

• Limited to quick subumbilical surgery in the ex-premature infant.

Introduction

• The application of this technique is nearly solely in the scenario of the preterm neonate undergoing quick subumbilical surgery; where there is a perceived risk of post general anaesthesia apnoea.
• With modern anaesthetic agents e.g. Desflurane the risk of apnoea may be overstated. Administration of any sedative drugs to facilitate placement of the block negates the proposed advantages of the subarachnoid block.
• The technique is the province of experts only as it a difficult technique to perform.
• The anaesthetist must be ready to convert to general anaesthesia as block duration is short and highly variable. The short duration of block may be due to the higher cardiac index, and the higher regional blood flow in the spinal cord and epidural space.
• (Levo)bupivacaine can be expected to last 60–90 minutes.
• Ensure the theatre team are scrubbed and ready to start promptly.

Anatomy

• See ➜ Anatomy, p. 160.

Contraindications

• General
• Note: a ventricular shunt is not a contraindication.

Landmark technique
- Palpate spine to assess L4/5 or L5 /S1 intervertebral space.
- Apply Ametop® or EMLA® to proposed puncture site.
- Position neonate sitting up, ensure airway is not obstructed.
- Full aseptic precautions should be used, including gown, gloves, hat, mask, and 0.5% chlorhexidine in 70% alcohol and drapes on the patient.
- A 25mm length 27G atraumatic tip needle should be used.
- When CSF begins to flow insert the needle 1mm deeper.
- Establish that the CSF flows readily.
- Slowly inject 0.3–1mL/kg (levo)bupivacaine (baricity is unimportant). At the end of the injection ensure CSF still flows as it is easy for the needle to become misplaced during the injection.
- Reinsert the stylet and wait for a couple of seconds before withdrawing the needle as this may help stop the LA tracking out along the puncture route.
- The spinal column is flat so the LA tends to spread quite evenly often reaching the mid thoracic level.
- Do not raise the lower limbs, e.g. to apply a diathermy plate, as this can cause more cephalad LA spread and consequently respiratory compromise.

Ultrasound technique
- US may be used prior to performing the landmark technique to assess the level of the conus medullaris, depth, and angle of insertion to reach the dura.
- Real time US guidance is possible with a small linear probe held in the sagittal paramedian position; with the needle inserted out-of-plane in the midline.

Complications
- Failure rates as high as 28% have been published.

Lumbar and thoracic epidural

Indications
- Major abdominal surgery
- Open thoracic surgery
- Bilateral lower limb surgery
- Spinal surgery (inserted by surgeon at operation).

Anatomy
- See ➲ Anatomy, p. 160.

Sonoanatomy
- See ➲ Anatomy, p. 160.

Contraindications
- General.
- Note: a ventricular shunt or Baclofen pump is not a contraindication.
- Beware cutaneous stigmata of spinal dysraphism and presence of anorectal malformation. Prior to insertion this should be assessed by US, and MRI if necessary.

Landmark technique
- Generally the technique is the same as in adults; but there are a few key differences.
- Epidurals in children should only be performed by trained paediatric anaesthetists.
- All epidurals are placed with the patient under GA as it is difficult for a child to cooperate with the procedure.
- Patient positioned in left lateral position with hips flexed.
- When assessing neonatal intervertebral space level the intercristal line is more caudad at the L5 level.
- Full aseptic precautions should be used, including gown, gloves, hat, mask, and 0.5% chlorhexidine in 70% alcohol and drapes on the patient.
- For neonates a 19G Tuohy needle should be selected, and for infants and older children an 18G is appropriate. Usually a 5cm length needle is used; the needle should have 5mm depth markers.

Formulae for estimation of depth to epidural space include:
- Lumbar epidural space:
  - depth (mm) = (weight in kg + 10) × 0.8
  - depth (mm) = (age in years × 2) + 10.
- Thoracic epidural space:
  - depth (cm) = 2.15 + (0.01 × months of age)
  - depth (cm) = 1.95 + (0.045 × weight in kg).
- 1mm/kg body weight for children between 6 months and 10 years of age. These formulae are only a guide.
- Loss of resistance to saline is the preferred method of locating the epidural space; intravascular injection of air being more likely to cause a significant air embolism in this population.
- A bolus of 0.5mL/kg of 0.25% (levo)bupivacaine is used to start the epidural. In neonates 0.125 % (levo)bupivacaine is preferred as it provides effective and safe analgesia: this is possible because the spinal cord is yet to be myelinated.
- Tunnelling the catheter may improve fixation.
- Remember, in neonates the epidural infusion should be limited to 48 hours due to the risk of LA toxicity.
- Where there is an inability to place a thoracic/lumbar epidural catheter then consideration should be given to placing the catheter caudally (see Caudal epidural catheter insertion, p. 164).

Ultrasound technique
- US-guided real-time epidurals remain the province of a few institutions. And as such cannot be recommended at this point.
- However, US can be useful in providing the following prepuncture information: depth and angle of needle insertion, level of the conus medullaris, and post-catheter insertion assessment of LA spread.
- Both the transverse and longitudinal (paramedian usually better than median) planes are used for imaging.

Caudal epidural catheter insertion

Indications
- Best limited to children <1 year of age
- Major abdominal surgery
- Open thoracic surgery.

Introduction
- Successful analgesia depends on the epidural catheter tip infusing LA at the level of the operation; thus minimizing both the amount of LA required and the necessity for epidural opioids. This can be achieved by threading the epidural catheter from the caudal space.
- This is considered a safer technique, however, there is probably a greater risk of catheter misplacement.

Anatomy
- See ➔ Anatomy, p. 160.

Sonoanatomy
- See ➔ Anatomy, p. 160.

Contraindications
- General.
- Note: a ventricular shunt or baclofen pump is not a contraindication.
- Beware cutaneous stigmata of spinal dysraphism and presence of anorectal malformation. Prior to insertion this should be assessed by US, and MRI if necessary.

Landmark technique
- Patient is positioned in the left lateral position with hips flexed.
- Full aseptic precautions should be used, including gown, gloves, hat, mask, and 0.5% chlorhexidine in 70% alcohol and drapes on the patient.
- Specific kits are available, or an 18G IV cannula can be used to access the caudal space through which a 20G epidural catheter can be threaded. Some kits have styletted catheters; these are more easily imaged with X-ray and US.
- Prior to threading the catheter, the expected length of catheter required is estimated by holding the catheter up against the child's spine. This is usually an underestimate of the length that is actually required.
- The caudal space is accessed as for a single-shot caudal block (see ➔ Single-shot caudal, p. 165).
- Generally, threading the epidural catheter is easy, if there is resistance then gently flex or extend the patient's spine.
- The epidural catheter tip position should be assessed; ease of insertion does not equate to correct positioning.
- If the epidural catheter tip is too high then respiratory compromise may result, and too low a position may not provide adequate analgesia.
- Numerous methods have been described to assess catheter tip position: X-ray with and without radio opaque contrast, a modified ECG technique, nerve stimulation, and US.
- Tunnelling the catheter cephalad decreases colonization.

Ultrasound technique

- As described for the landmark technique but with the advantage of observing the progress of the catheter as it is threaded.
- The US machine is placed on the opposite side of the patient to the operator.
- A linear probe with a large footprint is selected as this gives a wider field of view when trying to identify and follow the catheter. Select a frequency of 10 MHz or greater.
- This is easier to perform with an assistant, as the assistant threads the catheter; the primary operator monitors the course of the catheter.
- The catheter tends to move in and out of alignment with the US probe; as such it is necessary for the US operator to scan between the median and both paramedian longitudinal positions to track the catheters' course.
- This is a straightforward process in neonates, but with increasing patient age (and hence ossification) the catheter becomes obscured by the spinous processes.
- Note the epidural catheter may travel in either the anterior or posterior epidural space; the former tends to occur when the introducing cannula has been inserted too far into the caudal epidural space, so causing the catheter to follow the concave curve of the sacrum.
- If the catheter tip is proving difficult to identify then its position may be inferred by the injection of a small volume of saline (<0.1mL/kg).
- Tunnelling the catheter cephalad away from the perineum may decrease catheter colonization.
- Once the correct level has been attained a small volume of saline (<0.1mL/kg) is injected to discount intravascular placement.

Single-shot caudal

Indications

- Mainly indicated in infants for subumbilical surgery.

Anatomy

- See ◆ Anatomy, p. 160.

Sonoanatomy

- See ◆ Anatomy, p. 160, Fig. 13.2, and Fig. 13.3.

Contraindications

- General.
- Note: a ventricular shunt or baclofen pump is not a contraindication.
- Beware cutaneous stigmata of spinal dysraphism and presence of anorectal malformation. Prior to insertion this should be assessed by US, and MRI if necessary.

Landmark technique

- Patient in left lateral position with hips flexed.
- Prepare the skin with 0.5% chlorhexidine in 70% alcohol. Wait until the skin is dry.

- Specific needles are available, or an IV cannula can be used to access the caudal epidural space (24G for neonates, 22G thereafter).
- Palpate the sacral hiatus in the midline. It is identified as the apex of an equilateral triangle made up of it and the 2 superior posterior iliac spines.
- Introduce the needle perpendicular to the skin at the most cranial aspect of the sacral hiatus.
- Once resistance is felt, flatten out the angle of entry to ~ 45°. A 'give' may be felt as the needle punctures the sacrococcygeal membrane. In neonates needle entry should be flatter.
- The needle should not be advanced more than a few millimetres; where an IV cannula is used, this should easily slide over the needle into the caudal epidural space.
- To assess for intravascular or intrathecal placement gently aspirate using a 2mL syringe, then leave the cannula open to air for 10 seconds (the latter is necessary as even gentle aspiration will cause vein collapse).
- Other tests to assess correct needle placement include the addition of epinephrine to the LA, PNS, and auscultation. None of these tests have gained universal acceptance. US is showing promise as a reliable test of needle placement.
- US is used to identify the injection of <0.1mL/kg of saline expanding the epidural space causing the posterior dura to displace anteriorly.
- The following volumes of LA have been suggested: 0.5mL/kg for sacral root coverage, 1.0mL/kg for lumbar, and 1.25mL/kg for low thoracic coverage (lower concentration to stay within dose limit).
- 0.25% (levo)bupivacaine is used (use 0.125% for neonates).
- During injection watch for superficial swelling indicating misplaced needle position.
- Injection should be easy; resistance may indicate a subperiosteal needle placement.
- In children >1 year of age an additive should be considered (2 micrograms/kg clonidine or 0.5mg/kg of preservative-free ketamine).

Ultrasound technique
- US is rarely required to guide the needle as the landmark technique is simple and reliable.
- A preblock scan is performed using a large linear probe in both the transverse and midline longitudinal planes (see Fig. 13.2 and Fig. 13.3).
- The larger probe allows the operator to monitor a greater number of vertebral levels.
- The following should be elucidated:
  • angle of needle insertion
  • depth of caudal epidural space from skin
  • level of termination of the dural sac.
- An in-plane technique is appropriate.
- After confirming correct needle placement the LA is injected and its level of cephalad spread monitored with US.

Complications
- Intravascular injection
- Intraosseous injection
- Total spinal
- Perforation of rectum.

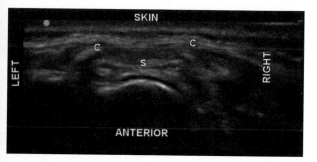

Fig. 13.2 Transverse view of neonatal sacrum. C, sacral cornua; S, sacrococcygeal membrane.

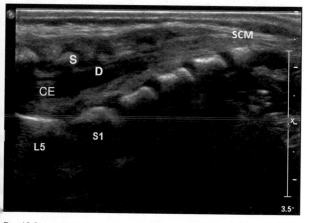

Fig. 13.3 Longitudinal median view of neonatal sacrum. CE, cauda equina; D, dura; S, spinous process; SCM, sacrococcygeal membrane; L5 and S1, vertebral bodies.

Further reading

Chawathe MS, Johnes RM, Gildersleve CD, et al. (2003). Detection of epidural catheters with ultrasound in children. *Paediatr Anaesth*, **13**(8),681–4.

Dadure C, Capdevila X (2012). Peripheral catheter techniques. *Paediatr Anaesth*, **22**(1), 93–101.

Dadure C, Bringuier S, Raux O, et al. (2009). Continuous peripheral nerve blocks for postoperative analgesia in children: feasibility and side effects in a cohort study of 339 catheters. *Can J Anaesth*, **56**(11), 843–50.

Ecoffey C, Lacroix F, Giaufre E, et al. (2010). Epidemiology and morbidity of regional anaesthesia in children: a follow up one year prospective survey of the French-Language Society of Paediatric Anaesthesiologists (ADARPEF). *Paediatr Anaesth*, **20**(12), 1061–9.

Guruswamy V, Roberts S, Galvez I (2005). Caudal injectate can be reliably imaged using portable ultrasound – a preliminary study. *Paediatr Anaesth*, **15**(11), 948–52.

Kim JE, Hong JY, Han SW (2009). Occult spinal dysraphism: detection during ultrasound for epidural blockade in children. *Anaesthesia*, **64**(9), 1026–8.

Lonnqvist PA (2012). Toxicity of local anaesthetic drugs: a paediatric perspective. *Paediatr Anaesth*, **22**(1), 39–43.

Sandeman D, Dilley A (2007). Ultrasound guided dorsal penile nerve block in children. *Anaesth Intensive Care*, **35**(2), 266–9.

Tsui B, Suresh S (2010). Ultrasound imaging for regional anaesthesia in infants, children and adolescents. *Anaesthesiology*, **112**(2), 473–92.

Tsui BCH, Gupta S, Finucane B (1998). Confirmation of epidural catheter placement using nerve stimulation. *Can J Anaesth*, **45**(7), 640–4.

Tsui BCH, Seal R, Koller J (2002). Thoracic epidural catheter placement via the caudal approach in infants using electrocardiographic guidance. *Anesth Analg*, **95**(2), 326–30.

Willschke H, Bösenberg A, Marhofer P, et al. (2006). Ultrasonographic-guided ilioinguinal/iliohypogastric nerve block in pediatric anesthesia: what is the optimal volume? *Anesth Analg*, **102**(6), 1680–4.

Willschke H, Marhofer P, Bosenberg A (2006). Epidural catheter placement in children: Comparing a novel approach using ultrasound guidance and a standard loss of resistance technique. *Br J Anaesth*, **97**(2), 200–7.

Peripheral nerve catheters

Background

In 1946, Ansbro described a technique for continuous block of the brachial plexus but it was not until the 1970s that fine plastic catheters became available that allowed regional anaesthetists to start using these techniques. The technique became more popular in the mid to late 1990s when the equipment became more user-friendly. Before this, the equipment that was commercially available was awkward to use and the technique was only practised by a few enthusiasts.

Anaesthetists saw the potential benefit of continuous peripheral nerve blockade which peripheral nerve catheters could facilitate. The maximum duration of single-shot PNB is about 24 hours and more usually 8–16 hours, using long-acting LA drugs such as bupivacaine or ropivacaine. The blocks were usually used for postoperative analgesia rather than surgical anaesthesia after procedures associated with high levels of pain such as shoulder or knee arthroplasty. When the block regressed, the patient rapidly experienced severe pain requiring administration of systemic opioids, with all their well-known undesirable side effects. There was a need to extend the duration of block in some patients.

In the mid 1990s, a number of regional anaesthetic needle manufacturers developed high-quality catheter-through-needle systems. This made placing micro-catheters close to nerves easier and the catheter-through-needle technique was familiar to most anaesthetists trained in epidural anaesthesia. At this time, the target nerves or plexi were normally **located** using nerve stimulation. Once the needle tip was in an acceptable position, the micro-catheter was passed through the needle and advanced a few centimetres beyond.

Equipment

Needle design

Contemporary kits for placing peripheral nerve catheters use the catheter-through-needle technique. Most anaesthetists favour a needle with a blunt, curved Huber tip like those found on an epidural needle. This curved top allows the catheter to be placed alongside the target nerve or nerve plexus. Some systems such as the Pajunk Stimulong® have a fine catheter with a wire stiffener to make placing the catheter in tissue planes easier. The wire is removed once the catheter is in the desired position.

Catheter design

Catheters can have a single end hole or multiple holes. The former is ideal for perineural placement to optimize LA distribution. Multi-hole catheters increase the chance of LA emerging in tissue planes remote from the perineural area.

Stimulating catheters

Kits incorporating catheters that can be connected to nerve stimulators are also available. These systems either have a metallic spiral or fine wire within the catheter wall to allow optimization of catheter placement. In practice, they have not been shown to be superior to conventional systems, are more time consuming to use and are significantly more expensive. US guidance has superseded stimulating peripheral nerve catheters.

Catheter fixation

Peripheral nerve catheters easily become dislodged in clinical practice so the fixation technique used is important. Catheters in the neck or groin are particularly susceptible to this problem and a wide range of fixation techniques are used. Subcutaneous catheter tunnelling, use of steri-strips, tissue glue, and bespoke dressings such as the Epi-Fix® device increase catheter survival.

Clinical application

PNBs have many advantages compared with opioid-based analgesia techniques. The well-known adverse effects of opioids such as sedation, nausea and vomiting, pruritus, hallucinations, and constipation can be avoided. The quality of analgesia with PNB is undoubtedly superior. Studies suggest that patients can mobilize more rapidly and length of hospital stay may be reduced.

Single-shot PNBs will typically regress after 8–16 hours and rarely last >24 hours. Continuous block is possible if a perineural catheter is correctly placed. This is useful for extending postoperative analgesia after painful surgery such as total shoulder or knee arthroplasty. It is also useful after upper or lower limb amputation. Furthermore, placing a perineural catheter allows more options with regard to using dilute LA concentrations.

LA infusions for continuous PNB

Motor block is an undesirable consequence that occurs when blocking major nerve plexi such as the brachial or lumbar plexus or the sciatic nerve. Patients find muscle weakness or paralysis unpleasant and if it involves lower limb muscle groups may inhibit mobilization. This may defeat the objective of the exercise and methods of minimizing motor block while maximizing analgesia should be explored. Loss of proprioception in the lower leg and foot also makes walking difficult. This is a particular problem in patients who have continuous sciatic nerve block, as the sciatic nerve is particularly sensitive to motor and proprioceptive block.

Most studies of continuous peripheral nerve blockade used LA concentrations extrapolated from epidural analgesia work. For example, infusion of ropivacaine 2mg/mL at 10mL/h or levobupivacaine 1.25mg/mL via a femoral nerve catheter will result in significant motor weakness of the quadriceps muscles, inevitably hindering walking. A recent study found that lumbar plexus infusion of 12mg/h of ropivacaine administered either as 0.1% at 12mL/h or 0.4% at 3mL/h reduced quadriceps strength by 64–68% and concluded that the main determinant of effect of continuous PNB is the mass of LA delivered rather than its concentration or volume.

Another study calculated the minimum effective local anaesthetic concentration (MLAC or ED50) of levobupivacaine (using an up down sequential dose concentration design) for continuous femoral (0.024%) and sciatic (0.019%) blocks in total knee arthroplasty. At these ultra-low concentrations it is possible to achieve differential sensory and motor block as Aδ sensory nerves (1–5nm) are more susceptible to block than the larger Aα motor nerves (13–20nm). These concentrations are nearly a factor of 10 less than were used in earlier studies and can facilitate patient rehabilitation with minimal postoperative pain.

Infusion devices

Any commercially available medical infusion pump can be used to infuse LA solution perineurally via a peripheral nerve catheter, but compact and portable devices are best as they allow patients to move about without restriction. There are a range of such devices currently available and fall into 2 main categories:

Elastomeric pumps

These devices have no moving parts, do not need a power source, are portable and disposable which makes them attractive for use in this setting. The driving force for the pump is the elastic recoil in the wall of the distended pump reservoir. A pinhole flow restrictor, which may be fixed, or variable determines flow rates. There are even versions with a patient controlled bolus facility.

Elastomeric pumps were originally designed for delivering out-of-hospital IV chemotherapy, but are now widely used for a wide range of indications including continuous PNB. Many centres discharge patients home with an elastomeric pump to continue PNB for a few days after major surgery. This can be a useful way of reducing patient length of stay.

Electronic pumps

There are also portable electronic pumps such as the Ambit® device. These pumps are programmable so allow a greater versatility than elastomeric pumps.

Advantages and disadvantages of continuous peripheral nerve block

Advantages
Extending the duration of PNB will extend the duration of analgesia after major surgery and minimize or avoid opioid-induced side effects. Placement of a perineural catheter also allows use of bespoke low LA concentrations, minimizing postoperative motor block. It has also been shown to accelerate rehabilitation and to facilitate earlier patient discharge from hospital.

Disadvantages
Motor block can occur and may inhibit patient rehabilitation and is unpopular with patients, physiotherapists, nurses, and surgeons. Sometimes the infusion has to be stopped to allow motor function to return. Lower limb peripheral block has unfortunately been associated with postoperative patient falls which can be disastrous. Mobilizing patients with knee splints can reduce the risk of falling by compensating for quadriceps weakness associated with continuous femoral or lumbar plexus block.

Loss of lower limb proprioception also makes walking more difficult even if there is little or no motor block. This is why continuous sciatic nerve block is not recommended after total knee arthroplasty.

Problems and complications

Problems

Secondary block failure

This occurs when the initial LA bolus used to establish the block wears off and the continuous infusion fails to maintain the block. The cause is usually that the block needle delivered LA around the target nerves, but the catheter tip is not correctly positioned. The block wears off and bolus top-ups fail to re-establish it. This can occur in up to 20% of cases, and is more likely in unskilled hands. Mechanisms for dealing with 2° block failure have to be established to prevent the health care team losing confidence in the technique. Input from an effective acute pain service is very useful in these situations.

Technical problems

These are common. An audit of 1416 patients with continuous PNBs reported catheter technical difficulties in nearly 18%. Catheter dislodgement, kinking, or blocking was common as was leakage of LA at catheter insertion site. There were also frequent problems with the infusion devices.

Catheter dislodgement is a real problem. Dressings come loose when patients move or sweat and catheters are then dislodged. Catheter dislodgement is more likely with exit sites in the neck above the clavicle, the axillary region, and the femoral or popliteal areas. Infraclavicular or lumbar plexus (psoas compartment) catheters are easier to preserve.

Complications of continuous peripheral nerve block

Infection

This is a concern when catheters are left *in situ* in patients. Between 23% and 57% of peripheral nerve catheters may become colonized with up to 3% causing localized infection. The majority of positive catheter tip cultures are coagulase-negative staphylococci and represent catheter tip contamination by normal skin commensals at time of catheter removal. *Staphylococcus aureus* is associated with infections or abscess formation. Clinically significant infection is uncommon but risk factors include:

- Catheter is left in place for >48 hours
- Femoral or axillary site
- Lack of antibiotic prophylaxis
- Diabetes
- ICU admission.

Scrupulous surgical aseptic precautions must be taken when placing peripheral nerve catheters (hat, mask, gown, gloves, procedure pack, etc.). Serious infective complications such as psoas abscess after continuous lumbar plexus block have been reported but are rare.

Neurological injury

A French audit reported that 3% of patients experienced persistent sensory block, 2% had persistent motor block, and 1.5% had paraesthesia during the continuous PNB period. The overall incidence of postoperative neurological injury was only 0.2%.

The future

Outcomes

The big question is, do continuous PNBs improve short- and long-term outcomes after major surgery? The only evidence to date has failed to demonstrate any difference in quality of life indices up to 12 months after hip arthroplasty. More research in the impact of continuous PNBs on clinical outcomes after major surgery is required.

Drugs, doses, and infusion rates

More research data on the ideal LA drugs to use, optimal concentrations, and infusion rates is also needed. This will help to refine the techniques and make them more clinically useful. MLAC studies will be helpful in finding answers to these questions.

Further reading

Capdevila X, Bringuier S, Borgeat A (2009). Infectious risk of continuous peripheral nerve blocks. *Anesthesiology*, **109**(1), 182–8.

Capdevila X, Dadure C, Bringuier S, *et al.* (2006). Effect of patient controlled perineural analgesia on rehabilitation after ambulatory orthopaedic surgery *Anesthesiology*, **105**(3), 566–73.

Ilfeld B, Ball ST, Gearen PT, *et al.* (2009). Health-related quality of life after hip arthroplasty with and without an extended-duration continuous posterior lumbar plexus nerve block: a prospective, 1-year follow-up of a randomized, triple-masked, placebo-controlled study. *Anesth Analg*, **109**(2), 586–91.

McLeod GA, Dale J, Robinson D, *et al.* (2009). Determination of the EC50 of levobupivacaine for femoral and sciatic perineural infusion after total knee arthroplasty *Br J Anaesth*, **102**(4), 528–33.

Muraskin SI, Conrad B, Zheng N, *et al.* (2007). Falls associated with lower-extremity-nerve blocks: a pilot investigation of mechanisms. *Reg Anesth Pain Med*, **32**(1), 67–72.

Training and assessment in regional anaesthesia

Background

Regional anaesthesia always works, provided you put the right dose of the right drug in the right place. To achieve these goals, a thorough academic understanding of anatomy, pharmacology, physiology, and medical physics needs to be blended with the practical skills of good hand–eye coordination and fine motor control.

The safe and effective use of regional anaesthesia requires commitment to learning the underlying science and dedication to practice the skills in suitable situations. Debate exists as to whether regional anaesthesia, and UGRA, is the remit of all anaesthetists, or should be in the hands of sub-specialist experts. Regardless of this, what is clear is that anyone using regional anaesthesia techniques should be appropriately trained and supervised until competency is attained.

To help clarify these points, recent guidance has been produced to detail what is considered appropriate training, both for anaesthetists in training and those looking to incorporate regional anaesthesia, or especially UGRA into their existing practice. Defining, and assessing, competence or competency has been troubling medical educationalists for some time and is no easier in regional anaesthesia. Neither one-off direct observation of a procedure or assessment of success or failure of a list of procedures constitutes competence, but they, along with other techniques, such as attendance at courses and examinations have their place.

Basic sciences

Anatomy

Anatomy is the cornerstone of successful regional anaesthesia, indeed some have commented that regional anaesthesia is just applied anatomy. However, other knowledge and skills sets are also required. There are no short cuts to learning anatomy, and US in itself does not demonstrate the anatomy, it will only show the anatomy that the user knows. As well as the gross anatomy, initially learnt at medical school from textbooks and cadavers, surface anatomical markers and relationships are important for landmark/nerve stimulator techniques, and cross-sectional sonoanatomy is becoming increasingly important with the growth of UGRA.

Settings and techniques of teaching and learning anatomy are numerous:

- Basic medical training. This has been a fundamental of medical schools for centuries, although modern teaching is often more through models, computer media, and cross-sectional imaging rather than cadaveric prosection and dissection.
- Informal clinical teaching. In theatre practical regional anaesthesia teaching should always start with ensuring adequate anatomical knowledge.
- Exam preparation. Postgraduate anaesthesia examinations are an important method of assessing basic anatomical knowledge and preparation for these should include relevant anatomy teaching.
- Electronic media. This more recent development has huge potential. DVD, Internet-based, or smartphone applications can all show gross anatomy, including the options to look at or subtract specific tissue groups from the image, to rotate the image in 3D and to simultaneously look at various cross-sectional images.
- Courses. Across the world there are countless regional anaesthesia courses, the majority of which will provide anatomy teaching, in the form of lectures, cadaveric prosections or sonoanatomy, live model sonoanatomy and electronic media.
- Sonoanatomy clubs. Numerous clinical centres have introduced a variety of informal educational sessions to teach and learn regional anaesthesia and UGRA, often centring on sonoanatomy.

Pharmacology and physiology

It would be expected that these topics are adequately taught and assessed during undergraduate and postgraduate training. It would suffice to mention here that training in regional anaesthesia is not limited to anatomy and the hands-on practicalities of this specialty and these topics are covered as part of the Royal College of Anaesthetists curriculum for CCT.

Medical physics and ultrasound

A thorough understanding of the principles and function of the equipment used is important to utilize them appropriately and safely. It is important to understand the appropriate settings of a PNS and its limitations (see Chapter 5).

The introduction of small, portable, high-fidelity US machines has radically altered regional anaesthesia in recent years and many argue that UGRA is the 'gold standard' now. All the recent and current guidelines on US training are explicit in stating that an understanding of the physical principles of US machines and sound waves are a prerequisite to using US in medicine (see Chapter 6). These features include:

- US wave generation and interaction with tissues (reflection)
- Selecting appropriate probes
- Controlling depth, focus, gain, and TGC
- Use of colour Doppler
- Recognition and understanding of common artefacts
- Recording and storing images.

Practical skills and patient care

Practical skills

Inserting needles into patients, close to nerves, without causing damage requires good manual dexterity and the haptic feedback of needles passing though subtle tissue planes. In addition, UGRA needs bimanual co-ordination to find, optimize, and hold a steady target image while allowing continual visualization of the needle tip and spread of injected LA. To attain these skills requires training, repetition, and supervision.

The use of commercial and 'home-made' phantoms and simulators do provide valuable training opportunities for those learning regional anaesthesia. In particular the use of phantoms to practise needling techniques and US visualization of the needle in both the in-plane and out-of plane approaches should be encouraged and form part of the ASRA/ESRA guidelines on UGRA training. They are also very useful to demonstrate competence (as for assessments) in correct US and needling technique in a safe environment, prior to performing blocks on patients.

Perioperative care

The Royal College curriculum in particular and the AAGBI US training guide place significant emphasis on training and assessment of 'non-technical' competencies, including important factors such as:

- Risk/benefit
- Contraindications
- Pre-op assessment
- Obtaining consent
- Recognizing and managing complication
- Documentation
- Predicting difficulties
- Care of the patient during a block, during surgery, and postoperatively
- Communication with the patients
- Management of regional anaesthesia list
- Follow-up
- Supervision and teaching of regional anaesthesia techniques to less experienced trainees.

Supervision and experience

In the UK the Royal College of Anaesthetists curriculum does not stipulate a minimum number of blocks to perform and it appears theoretically possible to complete training with minimal practical experience of regional anaesthetic techniques, especially peripheral nerve blocks. Other countries have a more proscriptive approach and have detailed the minimum number of blocks to be performed. In the USA, a minimum of 50 epidurals, 40 spinals, and 40 PNBs during residency are required as stipulated by the Residency Review Committee for Anesthesiology. However, previously up to 40% of residents were failing to achieve this, especially for the PNBs.

Similarly in Germany, the requirements are 100 neuraxial blocks and 50 PNBs.

Fundamentally it remains the responsibility of the clinician not to undertake procedures without proper training and supervision. For trainees/residents this is usually fairly straightforward, with direct supervision from senior colleagues, but for established practitioners it is still unacceptable to just 'have a go'. The ASRA/ESRA guidelines describe two distinct pathways of training in UGRA, one for residents and one called the practice pathway for established practitioners. For the latter it recommends spending time with experienced individuals observing and learning UGRA and that a novice's initial clinical experience be mentored and supported by an individual experienced in UGRA. If there is no one locally, most national societies of regional anaesthesia will be able to help, and RA-UK has agreed to support this arrangement in the UK.

A further recommendation in most of the guidelines for UGRA, is to record video or still clips of blocks performed and most modern machines have such capabilities. Reviewing such footage with experienced colleagues can be very educational and helpful for when no direct supervision is practical. This is an excellent routine for all who practise UGRA, not just novices. In an ideal world all US footage would be recorded, but the practicalities of this often prevent it occurring.

Postgraduate higher qualification

ESRA created a diploma in regional anaesthesia and pain therapy (EDRA) in 2005, with the stated aim of establishing standards in regional anaesthesia in Europe. The number of diplomas awarded has risen from 3 in 2007 to 50 in 2011 and continues to attract significant numbers of candidates. The exam is in 2 parts sat in consecutive years at the ESRA annual congress. Part 1 is a written exam of 100 multiple choice questions and entry requirements are a minimum of 2 years in a recognized training post, attendance at 1 ESRA approved workshop or course, and current ESRA membership. Part 2 of the exam is a 30-minute viva, which may involve demonstrating landmarks and block-related sonoanatomy on models as well as discussions about techniques and other aspects of regional anaesthesia, such as clinical uses, contraindications, and evidence-based practice. To sit part 2, candidates need to have passed part 1 of the exam, performed at least 150 neuraxial, 75 upper limb, 75 lower limb, and 30 trunk blocks, attended 3 appropriate courses and be a current ESRA member. (Please check ESRA website ℘ http://esraeurope.org for latest details on the diploma). Whilst popular, the EDRA has attracted some criticism, as the process perhaps lacked the rigor and standardization expected for a postgraduate qualification. Some of these issues have been addressed but the diploma may still lack some academic credibility. My view is that it does require considerable effort and commitment to complete which does demonstrate that regional anaesthesia is a significant sub-specialist interest. I would also recognize the learning experience gained by attending the required courses and the annual congress.

Until this year, the EDRA was also the only postgraduate qualification specific to regional anaesthesia available. However, the Faculty of Health at the University of East Anglia launched an MSc in Regional Anaesthesia in September 2012. It is a 2-year distance/online course with modules of 16 weeks, covering anatomy, physiology, pharmacology as well as clinical, governance and research topics. A certificate is awarded for 4 modules, a diploma after 6, and an MSc after also successfully completing a research dissertation. These qualifications, being awarded by a reputable university, may overcome some of the shortcomings of the EDRA and become a highly valued postgraduate qualification and a benchmark to define a 'regional anaesthetist'. I would also like to hope that the submission of research dissertations will stimulate an increase in the output of high-quality research in regional anaesthesia from the UK, which perhaps is currently below that of other European and North American countries.

Logbooks and CUSUM

All the training recommendations suggest practitioners keep a logbook or a record of blocks performed, and many of us will already be doing this as part of an overall logbook. However, there are additional benefits to keeping a separate logbook of blocks performed, especially if it includes the outcome of the procedure, i.e. the success or failure of the techniques. It is accepted that all regional anaesthesia techniques do have a failure rate. Collecting such data is a useful tool for reflective practice and can be helpful in the process of demonstrating and assessing competency.

For novices, such data can be arranged to produce learning curves and derivatives of these which fall under the umbrella term of Cumulative Sum, or CUSUM analysis. There are a variety of different graphs used from simple box plots to sequential tests of significance. All of them can be, and are, used for essentially the same purpose, but they do all have subtly different characteristics and interpretations and they are not necessarily interchangeable.

Due to the emerging importance of these logbooks it is worth devoting some time to explaining how they are derived and to clarify the differences between them. To illustrate this let us consider the same sequence of 19 observations (blocks), with failures on the 2nd, 4th, 8th, and 14th tasks.

Learning curve

A basic learning curve plots sequential results, starting at (0, 0) and increasing by 1 on the x-axis for a success and by one on the y-axis for a failure. Percentage failure lines can be added to guide interpretation but are fairly crude. For a novice it would be expected that there would be comparatively more failures early on and then fewer as more experience was gained. Hence the graph will have a steep gradient in the early part and then flattening out. This characteristic shape to the curve gives them their name. See Fig. 15.1.

Alternatively, the number of observations can be plotted on the x-axis and the cumulative number of failures on the y-axis. See Fig. 15.2. This produces a very similar shaped graph to Fig. 15.1, and the information, and interpretation are essentially the same. The only advantage is that this layout forms the basis of the more complex CUSUM analysis that will be shown later.

Mathematically speaking, this is a plot of a function of X, f(X), against the number of observations, n. The function is simply the cumulative number of failures, or mathematically;

$$f(X) = \sum(Xn),$$

where $X = 0$ for a success and $X = 1$ for a failure.

i.e. the plot increases by 1 for a failure and by 0 (stays the same) for a success. Fig. 15.3 is the same as Fig. 15.2 but as a point plot rather than coloured squares.

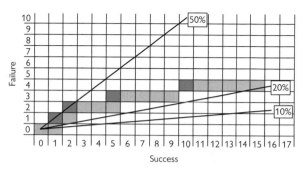

Fig. 15.1 Basic learning curve, showing failures on 2nd, 4th, 8th, and 14th tasks.

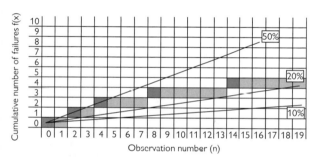

Fig. 15.2 Plot of number of observation against cumulative number of failures. This produces a similar shaped graph, or learning curve to Fig. 15.1.

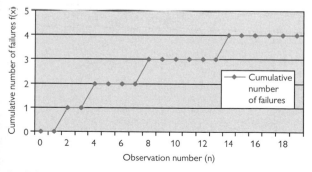

Fig. 15.3 This is the same graph as Fig. 15.2, but using a point plot rather than coloured boxes.

Cumulative score graph

A further layer of information can be added to the graph, by subtracting a value for the acceptable failure rate, 'p0', sequentially from each point. For the purpose of these examples *only*, this will be 20% or 0.2. The actual value used in a clinical setting will need careful consideration.

Then:

$$f(X) = \Sigma(Xn-p0)$$

Where $X = 0$ for a success and $X = 1$ for a failure and p0 = acceptable failure rate.

So the graph will fall by 0.2 ($0 - 0.2 = -0.2$) for a success and increase by 0.8 ($1 - 0.2 = 0.8$) for a failure. If overall direction of the graph is downward this suggest observed failure rate < acceptable failure rate. If there is a general upward trend this suggests observed failure rate > acceptable failure rate. See Fig. 15.4.

This allows continual visual assessment of performance against the set failure rate but provides no statistical interpretation.

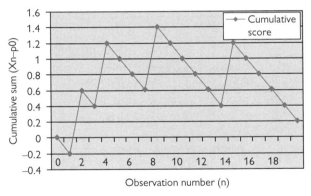

Fig. 15.4 Cumulative score graph.

Sequential test of significance (or sequential probability ratio test)

A sequential test of significance allows analysis to be carried on the data after each observation, rather than at the end of data collection of a predetermined sample size. It can be used for testing for a difference of proportions (i.e. a binomial distribution). In this case it is the proportion of unsuccessful attempts, or the failure rate. Thus sequential tests of significance can be used to assess when an operator's failure rate is statistically the same as, or different to, a standard. After each observation 1 of 3 results is delivered:

• The Null hypothesis is accepted (there is no difference or change).
• More observations are required to make a decision.
• The Null hypothesis is rejected and the alternative hypothesis is accepted (a difference or change has been detected).

These decision limits are calculated statistically and when plotted on the graph produce boundary lines ($X0$ and $X1$) which divide the graph into 3 areas corresponding to the 3 outcomes previously described. See Fig. 15.5. The boundary lines are calculated using 4 variables:

- The α error
- The β error
- $p0$: the acceptable percentage of failures
- $p1$: the unacceptable percentage of failures.

This can be applied to the data used earlier (from Fig. 15.3) on the graph of cumulative number of failures against observation number, producing Fig. 15.6.

As can be seen, the cumulative number of failures crosses the boundary line $X0$ after the 19th observation. At this point, the null hypothesis is accepted; there is statistically no difference between the observed failure rate and the acceptable failure rate (within the power of the test, i.e. the β error).

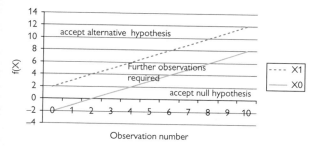

Fig. 15.5 Graph showing boundary lines dividing the graph into 3 'outcome' areas for a sequential test of significance.

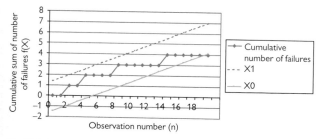

Fig. 15.6 Sequential test of proportions. This shows the lower boundary line being crossed by the plot after the 19th observation.

Crossing the upper boundary line, X1, would lead to the conclusion that the observed failure rate is statistically worse than the unacceptable failure rate (within the power of the test, i.e. the α error). At these points the statistical test is ended. Staying between the lines means more observations are needed to reach a conclusion.

However, a further variation on this graph can allow the user to continue to monitor performance, even when a boundary line has been crossed.

Assuming the α and β errors are the same (they usually are), then the 2 boundary lines are straight lines and parallel to each other. Their gradient is designated as 's'. Therefore if 's' is serially subtracted from the boundary lines then they become horizontal and equidistant from the x-axis (and are now referred to as h0 and h1). Mathematically 's' also needs to be serially subtracted from each of the observations. Hence:

$$f(X) = \Sigma(Xn{-}s)$$

where X = 0 for a success, X = 1 for a failure and s = gradient of boundary lines X1 and X0.

Importantly, the value of 's' is *not the same* as the value of p0 (the acceptable failure rate) and so the 'cumulative score graph' (Fig. 15.4) and the 'continuous CUSUM graph' (Fig. 15.7) are similar but different. This difference is where much variability and potential confusion has occurred in publications about CUSUM analysis.

The benefit of producing horizontal boundary lines is that when a boundary line is crossed, the test does not have to be stopped, as further boundary lines can be added and the test reset/continues. The boundary line crossed becomes the 'new' x-axis, a new boundary line is calculated as 2 × h0 (termed 2h0) or 2h1 as appropriate and the original x-axis becomes the upper or lower boundary line as needed. The tests can continue *ad infinitum*, with further boundary lines added as appropriate (e.g. 3h0, 4h0, …). See Fig. 15.8.

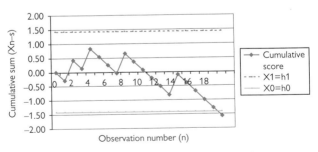

Fig. 15.7 Continuous CUSUM graph showing horizontal boundary lines.

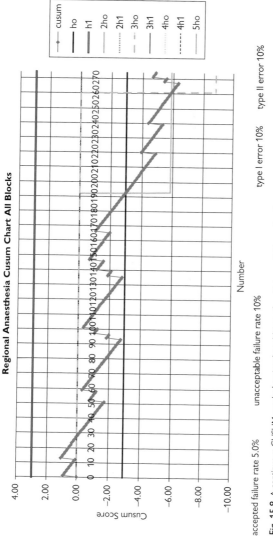

Regional Anaesthesia Cusum Chart All Blocks

Cusum Score

Number

| cusum |
| ho |
| h1 |
| 2ho |
| 2h1 |
| 3ho |
| 3h1 |
| 4ho |
| 4h1 |
| 5ho |

accepted failure rate 5.0%   unacceptable failure rate 10%   type I error 10%   type II error 10%

Fig. 15.8 A continuous CUSUM graph showing the addition of multiple parallel boundary lines.

Constructing a continuous CUSUM graph

Required variables:
- p0 = acceptable failure rate
- p1 = unacceptable failure rate
- α = alpha error
- β = beta error.

Calculations:

$a = \ell n(1 - \beta)/\alpha$

$b = \ell n(1 - \alpha)/\beta$

$P = \ell n(p1/p0)$

$Q = \ell n(1 - p0)/(1 - p1)$

$s = Q(P+Q)$

$h0 = -b/(P+Q)$

$h1 = a/(P+Q)$

CUSUM score $= \Sigma (Xn - s)$ (where $X = 1$ for a failure and $X = 0$ for a success).

Important considerations

There are several important points to take into consideration when using any of these processes:

Defining success and failure

This may not be as easy as it seems. Rarely do we work in an environment that permits us the opportunity to wait for the full onset of a block and to test each dermatome and myotome in all the corresponding nerve territories, unless it is the sole anaesthetic technique. Even then, for example, performing an axillary approach to the brachial plexus for hand surgery, it may not be a failure of the technique if the radial nerve is not adequately blocked if the surgery is in the ulna nerve territory. Would this scenario constitute a success or failure? Or if a block required a top-up but was then adequate for surgery?

The important factor is to be consistent in applying whatever definitions are used. Personally, I use a pragmatic definition of 'does the block do what I intended it to achieve' (e.g. if for awake surgery, was the patient pain free = success, if needed additional analgesia or conversion to GA = failure). I also class any complication as a failure (e.g. intravascular or intraneural injection).

Assesses only one aspect of block performance

There are many different requirements to performing successful, safe and professional regional anaesthesia, including appropriate patient selection, consent, sterility, appropriate drugs and doses, ergonomics, and needling technique, etc. A single dichotomous endpoint of the success or failure of an individual block does not encompass assessment of any of these other aspects.

Setting acceptable and unacceptable failure rates

There is currently no agreed level of acceptable and unacceptable failure rate for regional anaesthesia techniques and I feel that they are probably different for different blocks and for different clinicians at different stages of their careers. A sensible approach is to adopt some less stringent rates initially and when analysis shows adequate performance at this level to then use lower failure rates and confidence limits. As a suggestion for peripheral regional anaesthesia (nerve blocks): a starting point of 10% acceptable and 20% unacceptable failure rates and α and β errors of 10%, moving to a 5% acceptable and 10% unacceptable failure rates, with A and B errors of 5%.

Understanding the nature of learning curves

It is important for novices, and trainers, to understand and accept the natural progression of learning new skills. It is to be expected that there will be failures in the early phase, and thus any sort of learning curve or cumulative sum assessment will reflect this. It is important not to be downhearted about this phase, but to use these tools to make sure that the learning process is not 'out of control'. This is also why it is important to set the parameters appropriately at the outset.

Crossing boundary lines and competence

CUSUM analysis was developed for manufacturing processes, principally for quality assurance and ensuring manufacturing within set tolerances. It was not designed for medical training and assessment. It is important not to get confused between crossing a boundary line and competence at performing a task as they are not the same thing. CUSUM analysis can be useful for identifying when the learning process is out of control and further training and supervision may be beneficial, and when satisfactory results are being achieved. CUSUM analysis may fall down when scrutinized as a formative or summative assessment tool in medical education, but I think it still remains as a useful adjunct to monitoring and assessing performance and competence.

Summary

It has been calculated that it takes 10,000 hours of effective practice to become an expert in a particular field. This is perhaps a fanciful aim for regional anaesthesia, but may highlight the dedication required to ensure safety and effectiveness in using regional anaesthesia for patients' benefits. There are no shortcuts to learning anatomy, physiology, and pharmacology and skilful needle, and US, control only come with practice. However, this needs to be appropriate and supervised, especially in the early stages. Learning and improvements do not stop when 'competency' is attained, and we should all endeavour to continually improve and learn from each other, no matter what stage of our careers. Being prepared to subject yourself to reflective practice, peer review, and to monitor outcome data and are key to this mentality.

Further reading

AAGBI (2011). *Ultrasound in anaesthesia and intensive care; a guide to training*. July 2011. Available at: ℘ http://www.aagbi.org/sites/default/files/Ultrasound%20in%20Anaesthesia%20and%20 Intensive%20Care%20-%20A%20Guide%20to%20Training.pdf

Norris A, McCahon R (2011). Cumulative sum (CUSUM) assessment and medical education: a square peg in a round hole. *Anaesthesia*, **66**(4), 250–4.

Royal College of Anaesthetists. *2010 CCT curriculum*. Available at: ℘ http://www.rcoa.ac.uk/ careers-training/training-anaesthesia/the-training-curriculum/CCT2010

Sites BD, Chan VW, Neal JM, et al. (2010). The American Society of Regional Anesthesia and Pain Medicine and the European Society of Regional Anaesthesia and Pain Therapy Joint Committee Recommendations for Education and Training in Ultrasound-Guided Regional Anesthesia. *Reg Anesth Pain Med*, **35**(2), S74–S80.

Part 2

Head and Neck

Regional anaesthesia for ophthalmic surgery

Background

Landmarks ▬▬▬◄

Indications
- Intraocular procedures
- Extraocular orbital procedures.

Anatomy
- The orbit is a bony pyramid with its base pointing anteriorly. It contains the globe, extra-ocular muscles, lacrimal apparatus, fat, a rich network of blood vessels and nerves.
- The nerves which must be blocked to ensure painless ophthalmic surgery are the ophthalmic and maxillary divisions of the trigeminal nerve (cranial nerve V). These supply the conjunctiva, cornea, sclera, iris, ciliary body and upper and lower eyelids.
- The retina, which is supplied by the optic nerve, does not contain pain fibres.
- Motor nerves to the extra-ocular muscles are from the occulomotor nerve (cranial nerve III), trochlear (cranial nerve IV) and abducens nerve (cranial nerve VI). The facial nerve (cranial nerve VII) supplies motor to the orbicularis-oculi which assists in closing the eye.
- The Tenon's fascia is part of the sling mechanism providing support for the globe in the orbit. It originates at the back of the eye at the annulus of Zinn then sweeps forwards ensheathing the extra-ocular muscles, before attaching to the sclera around the limbus of the eye. Anteriorly, the Tenon's fascia is fused to the conjunctiva. From it's most anterior portion it is reflected back around the globe then runs posteriorly around the optic nerve.
- The length of the globe may affect the anaesthetic technique. The average eye is 23mm in length. Sharp needle blocks where the globe is longer than 26mm are associated with a higher incidence of globe penetration. This may be related to a higher incidence of staphyloma (out-pouchings of sclera) or because longer eyes have thinner sclera so recognition of impending globe perforation is more difficult as the needle passes easily into the eye.

Specific contraindications
Absolute
- Patient refusal
- Inability to communicate
- Young age
- Severely impaired coagulation
- Local infection
- Uncontrolled hypertension
- Severe movement disorders
- Allergy to LAs.

Relative
- Difficulty lying flat
- Previous vitreo-retinal surgery with ocular buckle.

Equipment

- A 25mm 25 gauge needle is adequate for all sharp needle blocks, although some advocate the use of even shorter 11mm needles for peribulbar blocks.
- The classical 38mm Atkinson needle is no longer recommended as it allows the delicate structures at the back of the eye to be penetrated in up to 20% of orbits.
- Sub-Tenon blocks may be performed with a variety of cannulae, varying in length and material of construction. Blunt metal 19–20 gauge Steven's cannulae are commonly used. These have a pre-formed curve which allows easy positioning within the sub-Tenon space.
- The use of short plastic cannulae (e.g. Greenbaum) or metal irrigation cannulae for sub-Tenon's block (STB) has been described. The shorter sub-Tenon cannulae provide adequate anaesthesia, but are associated with an increased incidence of chemosis and sub-conjunctival haemorrhage.
- The elderly frequently become hypoxic when supine. Supplemental oxygen should be administered to all but the fittest patients.
- Monitoring of the patient should be done and documented by an individual with that sole responsibility. It should include continuous assessment of comfort, respiration and circulation. A pulse oximeter is extremely useful in this setting.

Sedation

- Some anxious patients require sedation.
- Sedation should be kept to an absolute minimum as complications are more frequent in sedated patients.
- No sedative agents have been shown to have clear benefits over the others.

Topical local anaesthetics

- Topical LA agents are often used to anaesthetize the conjunctiva prior to performing ophthalmic LA injections.
- Topical agents are ester LAs and have limited penetration.
- Tetracaine stings when dropped onto the conjunctiva so oxybuprocaine 0.4% or proxymetacaine 1% are often administered first. These agents are more comfortable for the patient, but they have a short duration of action and reduced penetration, so are inadequate on their own.
- Excess topical anaesthetic should be avoided as it is toxic to the cornea and can cause clouding, which will be problematic for the surgeon.

Side effects and complications

Local complications

Chemosis

- Chemosis is common particularly in novice hands. It is more common in peribulbar than retrobulbar block as the volume of LA is greater.
- Rapidly forming chemosis in STB may indicate misplacement of the cannula tip under the conjunctiva, not sub-Tenon's fascia.
- Small volumes of chemosis can be massaged peripherally with gentle digital pressure.

- Chemosis rarely presents a problem with the exception of in glaucoma surgery where chemosis disrupts the anatomy and the LA may interfere with re-modelling of the trabeculectomy flap.

Subconjunctival haemorrhage
- This is more common in patients taking anticoagulant or antiplatelet drugs (5–40%).
- It may be striking in appearance, but is seldom significant.
- Patients should be warned preoperatively that they are more likely to have a red eye after surgery.

Retrobulbar haemorrhage
- Retrobulbar haemorrhage (RBH) is uncommon (1% of retrobulbar blocks).
- Unlike subconjunctival haemorrhage, this may be sight threatening.
- RBH typically occurs with sharp needle techniques, but has been reported after STB.
- Sharp needle insertion in the supra-nasal quadrant should be avoided as it is particularly vessel-rich.
- Presentation is with proptosis and subconjunctival haemorrhage, followed by extensive bleeding around the orbit.
- If RBH occurs, the surgeon should assess retinal circulation. If the retina appears ischaemic, then measures must be taken to decompress the orbit. This may involve lateral canthotomy, and in rare instances may progress to dislocating the lateral rectus insertion to allow the globe to be displaced anteriorly within the orbit.

Globe perforation
- Globe damage is more common with sharp needle blocks, although it has been described in STB.
- The incidence of globe damage varies and has been reported to be as low as 1 in 12,000 blocks, although in patients with an axial length longer than 26mm it has been shown to occur in as many as 1 in 140 blocks.
- The needle may perforate the eye (through and through, tip outside the globe) or penetrate the eye (tip within the eye).
- Perforations may present with pain on injection, lack of a red reflex due to bleeding within the eye, and loss of vision.
- Visual loss results from bleeding into the eye or traction and detachment of the retina.
- Penetrations will present similarly to perforations, but pain may be severe.
- Interestingly, up to 50% of globe perforations may go unrecognized at the time.
- If globe penetration is not recognized and LA is injected into the globe, the intraocular pressure will rise rapidly and may result in expulsion of the contents of the globe anteriorly.

Extraocular muscle damage
- More common with sharp needle blocks (up to 1%).
- May lead to diplopia requiring surgical correction.
- Risks may be reduced by adding hyaluronidase and removing vasoconstrictors from LA solution.

Systemic complications

Brainstem anaesthesia

- It is possible for LA to be injected into the dural cuff which surrounds the optic nerve.
- The reported incidence is 1 in 350–500 retrobulbar injections.
- Symptoms (confusion, loss of consciousness, apnoea, and cardiovascular collapse) may start within 2 minutes, although they may be delayed for 10–20 minutes.
- Treatment is supportive with airway control, ventilation of the lungs, and maintenance of organ perfusion using fluids and vasopressors.

Systemic local anaesthetic toxicity

- LA toxicity may occur if an excess of LA is injected into the vessel-rich orbit, or an appropriate dose of LA is inadvertently injected directly into a blood vessel.
- A relatively small dose of LA may cause toxicity if it is injected at high pressure into an orbital artery with retrograde spread to the brain.
- Treatment is both supportive, with control of ventilation and maintenance of organ perfusion, and specific with treatment for convulsions and arrhythmias if they occur. Intralipid should be administered if the toxic effects of the LA are not controlled rapidly. See Chapter 4.

Techniques of ophthalmic block

Retrobulbar anaesthesia

- The retrobulbar anaesthetic (RBA) block was first described by Atkinson in 1936.
- A sharp 25mm 25G needle is used to place LA behind the globe, within the muscular cone.
- The needle is inserted, via the skin or conjunctiva, in the inferotemporal quadrant. The conjunctival route requires topical anaesthetic drops whereas the cutaneous route requires injection of a small bleb of LA at the injection site.
- Classically, the needle insertion site was described as being at the junction of the medial 2/3 and lateral 1/3 of the eye. However, using this insertion site the needle may pass through, and possibly damage, the belly of the inferior oblique muscle. Consequently, the most inferolateral position possible is now favoured. This places the needle in the fat-filled inferolateral quadrant where there are no major structures to damage.
- The needle should be advanced with the bevel facing the globe to reduce the chances of the needle snagging the sclera.
- Once past the equator, the needle is cautiously directed up and into the muscular cone.
- Originally, the patients were asked to look upwards and in. However, computed tomography studies have confirmed that this movement shifts the optic nerve and macula towards the advancing needle.
- Once the needle tip is in position, a small volume of LA (2–5mL) is slowly injected.
- The block of extraocular muscles is often rapid and profound. However, the facial muscles are not blocked so the patient will be able to squeeze their eye shut. This can be prevented by blockade of the facial nerve at the temple or immediately lateral to the lateral canthus. These injections are painful and associated with rare but significant adverse events.

Peribulbar anaesthesia

- Mandel and Davis described peribulbar anaesthetic (PBA) block in 1986.
- PBA differs from RBA in that LA is placed more peripherally in the orbit with the aim of reducing the risks of deep orbital retrobulbar injections.
- The greater distance to the target nerves means that larger volumes of LA (10–15mL) are required, usually using 2 or more injections.
- A 25mm 25G needle is required.
- Similarly to retrobulbar block, an inferotemporal transcutaneous or transconjunctival injection is performed first. See Fig. 16.1.
- Unlike retrobulbar block, the needle is passed posteriorly to a depth of 20–25mm from the conjunctiva and not directed up and into the muscular cone.
- A volume of 5mL of LA is injected and 5–10 minutes allowed to assess the effect on globe movement.
- If the eye has limited movement in each direction of gaze, then no further injections are required. However, more often than not, a 2nd injection is needed. Indeed some practitioners go on to a 2nd injection almost immediately after the 1st.

- The 2nd injection is normally performed at the medial canthus. See Fig. 16.2. The site of injection is the most medial corner of the medial canthus, carefully avoiding the lacrimal lacunae. The needle is directed straight back so the needle is parallel with the medial wall of the orbit. Care must be taken not to insert the needle >20mm as the trajectory of this injection is directly back towards the optic nerve where it exits the optic foramina. Resistance may be felt as the needle passes through the medial check ligament. A further 5mL of LA is injected and time allowed to assess the block.
- On the rare occasions that a 3rd injection is required, it should be directed to the deficiencies in the block, most commonly a repeat inferotemporal injection.

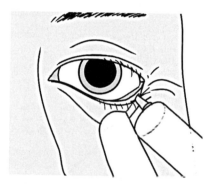

Fig. 16.1 An inferotemporal injection for a peribulbar block.

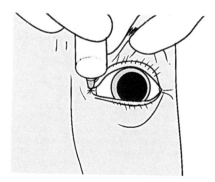

Fig. 16.2 A medial canthus injection for supplementation of a peribulbar block.

Sub-Tenon's anaesthesia

- The sub-Tenon's block (STB) was described Stevens in 1992.
- STB avoids the use of a sharp needle so should reduce risks.
- It may be performed in any quadrant, but the inferomedial quadrant is popular as the operator may steady their hands against the forehead and bridge of nose.
- Similarly to sharp needle blocks, the conjunctiva is first anaesthetized with topical anaesthetic drops followed by povidone iodine 5%, which is also used to clean the eyelids.
- Once the antiseptic solution has dried a speculum is inserted gently to keep the eyelids apart.
- A pair of non-toothed forceps is then used to grasp the conjunctiva 5–7mm away from the inferomedial limbus.
- The conjunctiva is tented up and a small incision is made through conjunctiva and adherent Tenon's facia, which provides access to the sub-Tenon's space.
- A blunt 19–20G cannula is then passed posteriorly until the tip lies beyond the equator of the globe.
- After aspiration, a small volume of LA 3–6mL is injected.
- The ciliary nerves lie within this space and are blocked rapidly, providing good analgesia almost immediately, although akinesia will develop more slowly over 5–10 minutes.
- See Fig. 16.3, Fig. 16.4, and Fig. 16.5.

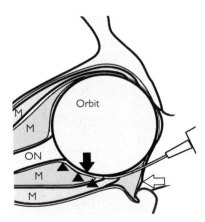

Fig. 16.3 Cross-section through the orbit showing the position of the needle during a sub-Tenon's block. ON, optic nerve; Black triangles, Tenon's fascia; Black arrow, sub-Tenon's space; M, extra ocular muscles; White arrow, conjunctiva.

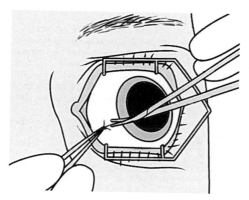

Fig. 16.4 Making the incision in the inferior nasal quadrant of the conjunctiva for a sub-Tenon's block.

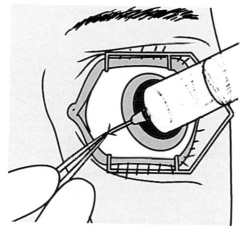

Fig. 16.5 Inserting a needle for a sub-Tenon's block.

Orbital compression

- Gentle orbital compression is often used after the injection, with the aim of improving distribution of LA solution and softening the eye.
- Ocular hypotony may reduce surgical complications for intraocular procedures.
- Care must be taken to avoid excessive pressure (>30mmHg) and prolonged compression (>20 minutes). This is particularly important for patients with compromised retinal circulation in whom it may be advisable to avoid ocular compression completely.
- Simple digital compression may be used, although there are devices which will do this (e.g. Honan balloon).

Local anaesthetic choices

- High concentrations of any of the currently available LAs will provide good conditions for surgery. However, prilocaine 3% and 4% have been associated with neuronal injury, although the mechanism is unclear, and are no longer licensed for ophthalmic blocks.
- Popular agents are lidocaine 2% and bupivacaine or levobupivacaine 0.5–0.75%. There are small differences in onset time between these agents and marked differences in duration.
- Other agents which may be used are ropivacaine 0.75–1% and articaine 2–4%, although there is less experience with the latter agent.

Adjuvants

Hyaluronidase

- Hyaluronidase may be added to improve the spread and depth of nerve block. Its action is thought to be mediated by hydrolysis of the hyaluronic acid component of intercellular ground substance, breaking down the intercellular glue and allowing more extensive distribution of LA around the orbit.
- The manufacturer recommends 15iu/mL, but the optimal dose is unknown. Doses from 1–300iu/mL have been documented.
- Improvements in onset time and quality of block for retrobulbar and sub-Tenon's anaesthesia have been demonstrated, although the data is less clear for peribulbar anaesthesia.
- The clinical advantage in terms of onset time is likely to be minimal. However, hyaluronidase has been shown to reduce the volume of LA solution required for sub-Tenon's anaesthesia, which may result in improved conditions for surgery.
- Observational studies where hyaluronidase has been unavailable have shown an increase in muscle injuries following ophthalmic block. This may be explained by hyaluronidase improving the block and reducing the need for additional injections, or by allowing rapid re-distribution of myotoxic LA away from the delicate extraocular muscles.
- Adverse effects of hyaluronidase are immune medicated and result in immediate allergic reactions, which have always been localized, or slower onset reactions causing pseudo-tumour formation (inflammation around the orbit).

Vasoconstrictors
- Epinephrine may be added to the LA solution to reduce washout of LA and prolong the duration of block.
- Epinephrine may have a modulating action on neuronal function which increases the density of block.
- Pre-mixed LA and epinephrine solutions contain stabilizers (e.g. sodium metabisulphite) which can cause allergic reactions.
- Freshly prepared epinephrine solutions reduce this risk, but introduce the possibility of mixing an incorrect concentration of epinephrine.
- Despite the claimed advantages and widespread use, there are no data to support the routine use of epinephrine.

Others

Other agents which have been added to LAs for ophthalmic surgery include bicarbonate, clonidine, and muscle relaxants. None has achieved wide-spread use in the UK.

Assessment of ophthalmic block

- The degree of akinesia is used to assess the block.
- The surgical requirements vary widely depending on the experience and confidence of the surgeon, and the procedure that is to be performed. Akinesia is rarely necessary for confident surgeons performing cataract surgery, but will need to be complete for less experienced surgeons performing corneal graft surgery or vitreo-retinal membrane peel surgery.

Specific considerations

The population undergoing ophthalmic surgery under LA are often elderly with significant comorbidity. Some conditions are common and may have a significant effect on the safety of a LA technique.

Hypertension

- Uncontrolled hypertension is associated with a small increase in the incidence of perioperative intraocular haemorrhage.
- It may also be a factor in systemic cardiovascular adverse events.
- The current Joint College Guidelines (2012) state that there is insufficient evidence to support a specific value above which surgery should be deferred, although many institutions would still use an upper limit of a systolic of 180mmHg or a diastolic of 100mmHg.

Anticoagulation

- Anticoagulant medication is common in this population. Antiplatelet agents should be continued as the risks of omitting therapy outweigh risks of bleeding around the eye.
- Patients taking warfarin should have their INR checked on the day of surgery.
- The Joint Colleges recommend that the INR should be within the therapeutic range. However, most anaesthetists will tolerate an INR of 3 for STB, but would want an INR of 1.5 or less for sharp needle blocks.

Diabetes

The Joint College document recommends that diabetes should be controlled prior to eye surgery under LA. However, this is not always possible. A pragmatic solution is to proceed if the patient feels well and is apyrexial, irrespective of an abnormal blood sugar.

Ultrasound-guided ophthalmic blocks

With the recent increase in use and enthusiasm for US-guided blocks, there have been descriptions of using US to guided orbital blocks. In many ways real-time US guidance is attractive in ophthalmic blocks; the ability to position the needle accurately, recognize and avoid sensitive structures, and watch the spread of LA.

However, US waves cause heating of the tissues they pass through as the energy is absorbed. Elsewhere in the body this causes no significant problems (and is used as an advantage in therapeutic US in physiotherapy). The delicate structures of the eye may be critically sensitive to the heating effects of US waves (and potentially from biomechanical effects of US waves). Most US machines used by anaesthetists are not appropriate (or in the USA, FDA approved) for use in ophthalmic settings. A recent animal study found a rise of >1.5°C (the recommended maximum) in the lens, cornea, and orbit of rabbits after a 10-minute US sound study using a Sonosite micromaxx®.

Therefore, unless an ophthalmic rated US machine is used, *the use of US cannot currently be recommended for orbital blocks.*

Further reading

Atkinson WS (1936). Retrobulbar injection of anesthetic within the muscular cone. *Arch Ophthalmol*, **16**(3), 494–503.

Davis DB II, Mandell MR (1986). Posterior peribulbar anesthesia: an alternative to retrobulbar anesthesia. *J Cataract Refract Surg*, **12**(2), 182–4.

Hamilton RC, Gimbel HV, Strunin L (1988). Regional anaesthesia for 12,000 cataract extraction and intraocular lens implantation procedures. *Can J Anaesth*, **35**(6), 615–23.

Stevens JD, Franks WA, Orr G, et al. (1992). Four-quadrant local anaestic technique for vitreoretinal surgery. *Eye (Lond)*, **6**(6), 583–6.

The Royal College of Anaesthetists and the Royal College of Ophthalmologists (2012). *Local anaesthesia for intraocular surgery*. London: The Royal College of Anaesthetists.

209

Maxillofacial blocks

Background

Landmarks:
US: N/A.

Introduction

Cutaneous sensory innervation of the face, eye, and part of the scalp is from branches of the trigeminal nerve (cranial nerve V). See Fig. 17.1. The neck, upper shoulders, and the posterior part of the scalp ('cape' distribution) have cutaneous sensory innervation from the superficial cervical plexus. Motor supply of the face is via the facial nerve (cranial nerve VII) and of the neck from the deep cervical plexus. Other blocks performed in the head and neck are glossopharyngeal nerve and stellate ganglion blocks.

Indications

Regional anaesthesia of the head and neck can be performed for the following:
- Chronic pain procedures
- Blocks for non-ocular ophthalmic surgery
- Dental blocks
- Perioperative blocks.

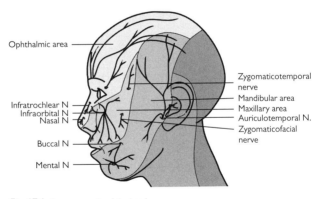

Ophthalmic area

Infratrochlear N
Infraorbital N
Nasal N

Buccal N

Mental N

Zygomaticotemporal nerve
Mandibular area
Maxillary area
Auriculotemporal N.
Zygomaticofacial nerve

Fig. 17.1 Sensory supply of the head.

Trigeminal nerve (V)

Anatomy

The rootlets of the trigeminal nerve arise from the brainstem and join to form a ganglion (trigeminal or Gasserian ganglion), that sits in a bony depression (Meckel's cave) in the petrous temporal bone. The posterior aspect is fully covered by dura mater and is in direct continuity with the CSF. It is sometimes necessary to block the ganglion itself, prior to the subdivision into its 3 main branches: the ophthalmic, maxillary, and the mandibular nerves.

Trigeminal ganglion nerve block

Indications

- For intractable pain from trigeminal neuralgia where 1 or more branches of cranial nerve V are involved. Typically, neurolytic injections (glycerol or alcohol) or radiofrequency rhizotomy is used for a more permanent effect.
- Intractable pain from malignancy.

Technique

- A technically very difficult block with significant complications, outside the scope of this book. It must be done in conjunction with radiological imaging techniques for correct location of the nerve and with the appropriate support available should the patient collapse. Specialist reference texts are advised and experienced mentored tuition is considered mandatory.

Complications

- Pain and bruising for a few days postoperatively is common.
- Corneal anaesthesia leading to ulceration is a significant problem.
- Subarachnoid injection can cause seizures or unconsciousness.

Trigeminal nerve: ophthalmic division (V1)

The ophthalmic nerve exits the skull through the superior orbital fissure as 3 sensory branches: the lacrimal nerve, frontal nerve, and nasociliary nerve. The frontal nerve divides into supraorbital and supratrochlear nerves.

Lacrimal nerve block

Indications
- Surgery involving the lacrimal gland or lateral canthus.

Anatomy
- The smallest of the ophthalmic branches runs along the lateral wall of the orbit, receiving a secretomotor branch from the zygomatic nerve that it gives to the lacrimal gland.
- It is sensory to a small area of skin at the lateral end of the upper eyelid and to both palpebral and ocular surfaces of the adjacent conjunctiva.

Technique
- Insert 25G needle through the upper eyelid at the lateral wall of the orbit.
- Advance it 1cm along the lateral wall until the orbital septum is penetrated and inject 1.5mL of LA.

Complications
- Bleeding from lacrimal artery.

Clinical notes
- If patient is supine, gravity will help distribute the local further posteriorly.

Frontal nerve block

Indications
- Frontalis suspensory surgery for ptosis repair. The motility of the upper eyelid and globe is retained whilst providing sensory anaesthesia to the upper eyelid and eyebrow and scalp.

Anatomy
- The nerve crosses the superior orbital fissure, runs forward above the levator palpebrae superioris and divides behind the superior orbital margin into supraorbital and supratrochlear branches.

Technique
- Insert a 22G, 4cm long needle through the middle of the upper eyelid just below the eyebrow and orbital margin.
- Advance the needle posteriorly in a stepwise manner along the roof of the orbit for 4cm. Then administer 0.5mL of solution. See Fig. 17.2.

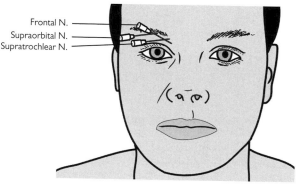

Frontal N. ————
Supraorbital N. ————
Supratrochlear N. ————

Fig. 17.2 Frontal nerve blocks.

Complications

- Retrobulbar haemorrhage (RBH).
  - If serious can produce blindness.
  - Features are:
    — pain
    — proptosis
    — afferent pupil defect
    — intraocular pressure >40mmHg.
  - Initial management:
    — acetazolamide 500mg bolus IV
    — mannitol 1–2g/kg (7.5–10mL/kg) of 20% solution over 30–60 minutes IV
    — methylprednisolone 1g IV
    — if this fails a surgical lateral canthotomy is urgently needed.
- blocking the distal branches—supraorbital and supratrochlear carries lower complications.

Clinical notes

- Stay on the roof of the orbit, as if lower may get motor anaesthesia of extraocular muscles.

Supraorbital nerve block (frontal nerve)

Indications

- Surgery of the upper eyelid, forehead, and anterior scalp.
- Pain—postoperative and neuralgic.

Anatomy

- Large branch of frontal nerve supplying the frontal sinus before it grooves or perforates the orbital margin to supply the upper eyelid (skin and conjunctiva,) all the forehead except a central strip and the frontal scalp up to the vertex (supplied by supratrochlear).

Technique
- Palpate the supraorbital foramen (lies in the mid-pupillary line 2.5cm lateral to the midline of the face along the supraorbital ridge). See Fig. 17.2.
- Insert short 27G needle, angle it medially (toward the nose) and parallel to brow to ensure you hit bony edge of foramen, avoiding neuropraxia.
- Inject 2mL of LA using a slow, aspirating technique.

Complications
- Neuropraxia.
- Intravascular injection (supraorbital artery) or puncture (treat with 20 minutes of pressure).

Clinical notes
- Slow injection minimizes discomfort.
- If patient reports paraesthesia—stop, withdraw 2mm, and continue if no further complaint.
- If block fails a 'field block' can be used—line of LA along the whole orbital rim, this blocks all ophthalmic branches.

Supratrochlear nerve block (frontal nerve)

Indications
- Surgery of the upper eyelid, forehead (above root of nose).

Functional anatomy
- This small branch of the frontal nerve leaves the orbit ~1cm medial to the supraorbital foramen.
- It supplies the upper eyelid, conjunctiva, and a narrow strip of forehead skin in the midline.

Technique
- Locate the nerve as it exits the orbit at the junction of the supraorbital rim and the medial wall of the orbit (1cm medial to the supraorbital foramen).
- Using a 26G needle inject 1mL superficial to the periosteum and continue injection as you withdraw. See Fig. 17.2.

Complications
- Trauma to the angular vein may obstruct surgical field.

Clinical notes
- Often used in conjunction with supraorbital block as much overlap in the areas innervated.
- To prevent swelling of eyelid apply gentle pressure to supraorbital ridge when injecting.

Nasociliary nerve block

Indications

• Surgery of the lacrimal sac (e.g. dacryocystorhinostomy) and nose.

Anatomy

• The nasociliary nerve enters the orbit via the superior orbital fissure.
• It gives rise to the communicating branch to the ciliary ganglion, the long ciliary nerves, the posterior and anterior ethmoidal nerves.
• It terminates as the infratrochlear and nasal branches, which supply the mucous membrane of the nose, the skin of the tip of the nose, and the conjunctiva.

Technique

• Insert 25G needle 1cm above the inner canthus, keeping in contact with bone.
• Advance 2cm posteriorly along the medial orbital wall and inject 2mL.
• If advanced a further 1cm can also block the anterior ethmoidal nerve.

Complications

• Trauma to ophthalmic artery or supraorbital vein.
• 2% risk of RBH. To manage this complication see ➲ Frontal nerve block, p. 212.

Clinical notes

• Very sensitive area so inject slowly, sometimes patients will need sedation.

Trigeminal nerve: maxillary division (V2)

The maxillary nerve exits the skull through the foramen rotundum and passes into the pterygopalatine fossa, where zygomatic, nasopalatine, palatine, and posterior superior alveolar branches come off. The main trunk continues into the infraorbital canal where it is renamed the infraorbital nerve.

Maxillary nerve block

Indications
- Acute or chronic herpetic neuralgia
- Pain from malignancy.

Technique
- With the patient's mouth slightly opened, an 8–10cm 22G needle is inserted extraorally between the zygomatic arch and the sigmoid notch of the mandible.
- After contact with the lateral pterygoid plate (about 4cm deep), the needle is slightly withdrawn and angled superiorly and anteriorly to pass into the pterygopalatine fossa.
- Deposit 2–5mL solution to anaesthetize both the maxillary nerve and the pterygopalatine (sphenopalatine) ganglion.

Complications
- Potential for significant haemorrhage and haematoma due to the presence of the pterygoid venous plexus.

Clinical notes
- A specialist nerve block, best first done under trained supervision.
- Aspiration essential.

Zygomaticotemporal nerve block

Indications
- Trauma and surgery over the temple.

Anatomy
- The zygomatic nerve arises from the maxillary nerve in the pterygopalatine fossa and passes into the orbit via the inferior orbital fissure.
- It branches first into the zygomatico*temporal* nerve and then the zygomatico*facial*.
- The zygomaticotemporal nerve courses laterally in the orbit to pass through a foramen into the anterior temporal fossa and rises beneath and posterior to the lateral orbital rim.
- It supplies sensation to a fan shaped area of skin posterior to the lateral orbital rim.

Technique

- Stand above the patient.
- Insert a 25G 25mm needle behind the lateral orbital rim at a point of insertion 1cm posterior and inferior to the palpable zygomaticofrontal suture (lateral end of the superior orbital ridge).
- Advance to a point 1cm below the lateral canthus.
- Inject 2mL of LA.

Complications

- None of significance.

Zygomaticofacial nerve block

Indications

- Surgery over the cheekbone.

Anatomy

- This 2nd, terminal, branch of the zygomatic nerve (see ➲ Zygomaticotemporal nerve block, p. 216) emerges from the orbit through a small foramen on the anterior surface of the zygoma, 3–5mm lateral to the inferior orbital rim.
- It supplies sensation over the cheek prominence.

Technique

- With the head slightly turned, palpate the junction between the lateral wall of the orbit and the inferior orbital rim (i.e. the most inferolateral point of the right orbit).
- Inject 1–2mL of LA subcutaneously just lateral to your finger.

Complications

- None of significance.

Clinical notes

- Usually undertaken in conjunction with a zygomaticotemporal block.

Infraorbital nerve block

Indications

- Regional anaesthesia of the cheek and ipsilateral side of the upper lip and nose.
- Relief of neuralgic pain.

Anatomy

- This nerve passes forwards through the infraorbital foramen exiting the front of the cheekbone to supply sensation to the lateral wall of the nose, cheek, ipsilateral half of the upper lip and lower eyelid.

Technique

The foramen lies 4–7mm below the inferior orbital rim on a vertical line dropped from the medial limbus of the iris.

There are 2 approaches: extraoral and intraoral:

- Extraoral approach:
  - with the patient staring straight forwards and palpating the inferior orbital rim, advance the needle to the position as described earlier, injecting up to 2mL solution.

- Intraoral approach (see Fig. 17.3):
  - palpating the inferior orbital rim with the index finger whilst retracting the upper lip with the thumb should give good access
  - insert the needle above the canine tooth, ~ 0.5–1cm above the root tip. Deposit up to 2mL of LA.

Complications
- Prolonged anaesthesia or potential nerve injury if injecting directly into the foramen.

Clinical notes
- The anterior superior alveolar nerve branches off and drops down from the infraorbital nerve anywhere from 5mm to 20mm proximal to the foramen. However, irrespective of its location, the incisor and canine teeth, and their gingivae on the labial side, will usually also be blocked.
- Bilateral injection allows for painless complete upper lip and nasal alar base surgery and treatment of dental trauma.

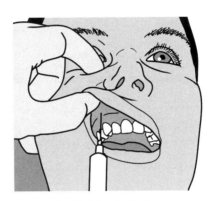

Fig. 17.3 Intraoral approach to block the infraorbital nerve.

Nasopalatine nerve block
Indications
- Dental procedures and trauma.

Anatomy
- This nerve drops down from the infraorbital nerve as it runs its course through the infraorbital canal.
- It passes through the incisive foramen below to supply sensation to the anterior 1/3 of the palate and the palatal gingiva of the incisor teeth.

Technique

- A short needle is inserted ~ 0.5cm posterior to the midline of the maxillary central incisor teeth, into a raised mucosal prominence called the incisive papilla, beneath which lies the foramen.
- The needle is angled 45° to the palate with the needle pointing towards the vertex of the scalp. See Fig. 17.4.
- Inject *only* 0.2mL LA.

Complications

- None of significance.

Clinical notes

- This is a painful injection due to the very adherent nature of the mucosa to the palate.
- Reduce discomfort by taking care not to penetrate the foramen and with the application of moderate pressure on the papilla for about 30 seconds prior to injecting. Topical anaesthetic also helps.

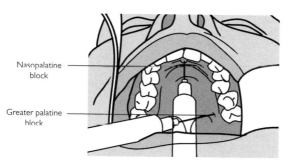

Nasopalatine block

Greater palatine block

Fig. 17.4 Nasopalatine and greater palatine nerve blocks.

Greater palatine nerve block

Indications

- Dental procedures and trauma.

Anatomy

- The greater palatine nerve, the anterior terminal branch of the palatine nerve, enters the oral cavity via the greater palatine foramen.
- This lies between the 2nd and 3rd molar teeth, ~ 1cm above the gingival margin on the hard palate.

Technique

- The head is extended 45° backwards.
- The tip of a short 27G needle is inserted 1cm above the gingival margin at the junction of the 2nd and 3rd molar teeth. See Fig. 17.4.
- Angle the needle at 90° to the curvature of the palate.
- Inject 0.3–0.5mL LA very slowly.

Complications
- Haemorrhage from the greater palatine artery. Prolonged digital pressure stops this.

Clinical notes
- A painful injection, so administer slowly. Blanching is common.
- Aspiration advised as intravascular injection common.
- The nerve sits with blood vessels in a channel of connective tissue, either side of which the mucosa is tightly bound on one side adjacent to the teeth and on the other to the hard palate. The nerve can therefore be palpated quite easily in a groove of slightly softer tissue.

Lesser palatine nerve block

Indications
- Trauma and postoperative pain relief following tonsillectomy.

Anatomy
- The lesser palatine nerve, the posterior terminal branch of the palatine nerve, enters the oral cavity via a foramen just 2–4mm posterior to the greater palatine foramen.
- Its branches however, pass in the opposite direction (posteriorly) providing sensory innervation to the soft palate and uvula.

Technique
- The technique is identical to that for the greater palatine injection, but the dental landmark is slightly more posterior, at the distal aspect of the 3rd molar tooth.
- Inject 0.2–0.5mL LA.

Complications
- Patients often experience a feeling of dysphagia or throat closure, which can be quite marked. Reassure as necessary.

Clinical notes
- Slightly less painful than the greater palatine block as the tissues are more lax, but still administer slowly.

Superior alveolar nerve block

Indications
- Dental procedures and trauma.

Anatomy
- The *posterior* superior alveolar nerve arises from the maxillary nerve in the pterygopalatine fossa and enters the posterior maxilla.
- It supplies the molar teeth, the gingiva, and the buccal mucosa above the level of the upper teeth.
- The *middle* and *anterior* branches arise from the infraorbital nerve and drop down through the floor of the infraorbital canal to supply teeth, the buccal gingivae, and buccal mucosa, further forwards.

- There is some cross innervation and anatomical variation, but the posterior nerve generally supplies the molars, the middle nerve supplies the premolar and canine region, and the anterior nerve supplies the incisors.

Technique

For the posterior superior alveolar nerve:
- Insert the tip of the non-dominant index finger between the maxillary molars and the cheek, palpating for the zygomatic process.
- Rotate the finger 180° upwards with the pad inside the patient's cheek, applying an outwards pressure at the same time to retract it.
- Aim the needle along the middle of the nail plate of the index finger, posteriorly, superiorly, and medially in direction.
- Advance 2.5cm and inject 3mL LA.
- If bone is contacted, retract the needle and reposition more laterally.

For the middle and anterior superior alveolar nerves:
- These nerves travel within the maxillary bone and it is not possible to block them.
- The infiltration of 0.5mL is advised, high in the buccal sulcus adjacent to the tooth apex where anaesthesia is required.

Complications

- Haematoma if injecting too far distal when attempting to block the posterior superior alveolar nerve.

Clinical notes

- It is only possible to truly block the posterior branch before it enters the maxilla.
- For dental anaesthesia, best to infiltrate adjacent to the required teeth rather than attempt blocks.

Trigeminal nerve: mandibular division (V3)

The mandibular nerve exits the skull through the foramen ovale and passes into the pterygopalatine fossa where it splits into an anterior, predominantly motor trunk (muscles of mastication) and a posterior trunk. The anterior trunk gives rise to the long buccal nerve and the posterior trunk to 3 sensory branches; the inferior alveolar nerve, lingual nerve, and auriculotemporal nerve.

Mandibular nerve block
Indications
- Pain relief for trigeminal neuralgia.
- Intractable pain from malignancy and postoperative pain relief.

Technique
- With the patient's mouth slightly opened, an 8–10cm 22G needle is inserted extraorally between the zygomatic arch and the sigmoid notch of the mandible.
- After contact with the lateral pterygoid plate (about 4cm deep), the needle is slightly withdrawn and angled superiorly and posteriorly towards the ear.
- Inject 2–5mL of LA.

Complications
- Haemorrhage. Transient facial palsy (if injected into the parotid capsule). If caused, manage by reassuring the patient, taping down the eyelid and applying an eye patch until the effects have worn off.

Inferior alveolar (dental) nerve block
Indications
- The most commonly administered nerve block in dentistry. Used to anaesthetize the teeth in the lower jaw.
- Occasionally given for relief of neuralgic pain.

Anatomy
- The nerve enters the lower jaw via the mandibular foramen, on the medial aspect of the ramus ~ 2cm behind its anterior border and 1cm above the occlusal plane of the molar teeth.
- It travels forwards through the bone to the mental foramen where it divides into 2 branches.
- The larger branch exits the jaw bone to the side of the chin via this foramen and becomes the mental nerve.
- The smaller branch, renamed the incisive nerve, continues within the bone to innervate the canine and incisor teeth.
- An inferior alveolar nerve block (ID block) affects sensation to
  - all the teeth
  - vermilion border
  - skin of the lip and chin
  - the lateral gum margins of the teeth *anterior* to the premolar teeth.

Technique

Direct method—this is the main technique used by dentists:
- The index finger retracts the cheek at the level of the occlusal plane, with the tip being placed on the external oblique ridge of the mandible.
- A long, 35mm 27G needle is inserted 1cm above the midpoint of the last adult molar tooth just medial to the external oblique ridge, with the syringe directed from the premolar teeth on the opposite side. See Fig. 17.5.
- Advance the needle ~ 2cm to the mid section of the medial ramus until bone is identified.
- Withdraw 2mm, aspirate, and slowly inject 1.5mL LA.

Indirect 'closed mouth' (Akinosi) method:
- With the mouth closed, a long, 35mm 27G needle is inserted parallel to the maxillary occlusal plane at the level of the gingival/tooth margins, medial to the anterior border of the ramus and buccal to the maxillary alveolus.
- The needle is advanced until the hub is level with the distal aspect of the 2nd maxillary molar tooth.
- Aspirate and inject 1.5mL LA.

Complications
- Transient facial palsy (if injected into the parotid capsule). If caused, manage by reassuring the patient, taping down the eyelid and applying an eye patch until the effects have worn off.
- Haematoma leading to trismus. It is important to identify this within 2 weeks and commence progressive jaw opening exercises to prevent a permanent limitation of mouth opening.
- Direct nerve injury.

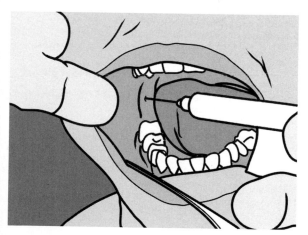

Fig. 17.5 Inferior alveolar nerve block.

Special contraindications
- Severe coagulopathies.
- Severe dento-facial infection at the injection site.

Clinical notes
- Whilst simple buccal infiltrations in the maxilla will anaesthetize individual teeth, the bone in the mandible and multiple teeth require an inferior alveolar block. In children the bone is less dense and buccal infiltrations suffice. In adults, articaine hydrochloride (4% with 1:100,000 epinephrine) has good bone penetrative properties and is being used more now as a simple infiltration technique in adults. There are, however, concerns about its potential for tissue necrosis and persistent nerve paraesthesia.
- If the 'direct' method is used for dental extraction purposes, remember that neither the lateral gum margins distal to the mental foramen nor any of the lingual gum will be anaesthetized. Additional lingual and long buccal blocks would therefore be required.
- The 'Akinosi' method is particularly useful in patients with limited mouth opening. However, no bony landmark is present and there is a risk of penetrating the vessels of the pterygoid plexus.
- Cross innervation from the contralateral lateral side occurs in the incisor region, so often a supplementary block is necessary on the opposite side when treating the lower incisor teeth. This is usually achieved with a mental nerve block.

Mental nerve block

Indications
- Soft tissue surgery of the lower lip or chin.
- Supplemental contralateral anaesthesia for incisor teeth.
- Pain relief for, or diagnostic confirmation of, trigeminal neuralgia.

Anatomy
- A large nerve arising from the inferior alveolar nerve as it exits the mental foramen.
- Provides sensation to the lower lip, chin, vermillion, and teeth and lateral gums anterior to the foramen.

Technique
- Standing over the patient, direct a 27G needle vertically downwards in the buccal sulcus between the 2 premolar teeth, aiming 2mm below the midpoint between the 2 root apices. See Fig. 17.6.
- Make contact with bone, withdraw 1mm and inject 1mL of LA.

Complications
- None of significance.

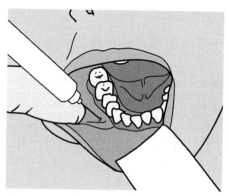

Fig. 17.6 Mental nerve block.

Clinical notes
- Can be used for dental procedures on teeth anterior to the premolars on the ipsilateral side to avoid the need for an inferior alveolar block. However, it relies upon solution entering the mental foramen and reaching the incisive nerve, so accuracy is paramount. If used for this purpose, remember the inner (lingual) gingivae will not be anaesthetized and will need local infiltration.

Lingual nerve block

Indications
- Soft tissue surgery to the anterior 2/3 of the tongue.
- Typically in conjunction with an inferior alveolar/dental nerve block.

Anatomy
- A nerve with a convoluted path, passing posteriorly between medial pterygoid and the ramus of the mandible and traversing forwards and medially over the submandibular duct in the floor of the mouth to the inferolateral aspect of the tongue, innervating it along its length as it passes.

Technique
- Similar approach as that of the 'direct' inferior alveolar nerve block, but stopping short of the ramus and injecting 0.5mL LA 5mm medially and 5mm ventrally to the lingula.

Complications
- As for inferior alveolar nerve.

Buccal (long buccal) nerve block

Indications
- To anaesthetize the gum and cheek mucosa lateral to the molar teeth, below the level of the occlusal place.

Anatomy
- Arising from the anterior division of the mandibular nerve, the buccal nerve emerges between the 2 heads of the lateral pterygoid muscle.
- It courses inferiorly along the deep surface of temporalis and then superficially to buccinator, which it pierces.
- It gives branches to the skin of the outer cheek before doing so and thereafter, to the inner mucous membrane and lateral gum margins of the back teeth (i.e. behind the mental nerve).

Complications
- None of significance.

Clinical notes
- A short 32G needle is inserted just above the buccal fold near the 3rd molar (wisdom tooth) and advanced towards the mandibular ramus. See Fig. 17.7.
- Inject 0.5mL LA.
- Typically undertaken in conjunction with an inferior alveolar block.
- Remember, it does not anaesthetize the lateral gum anterior to the mental foramen.

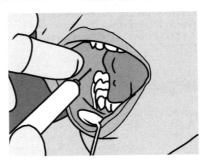

Fig. 17.7 Buccal (long buccal) nerve block.

Auriculotemporal nerve block

Indications
- To help distinguish between temporomandibular joint (TMJ) pain of arthrogenous and myogenous origin.
- Relief of TMJ pain.
- Temporal artery biopsy and temporal skin surgery.
- Surgery to the pinna (above the level of the ear lobe).
- Diagnostic parotid gland salivary assay.

Functional anatomy

- The nerve passes laterally behind the TMJ and ascends over the posterior root of the zygomatic arch superiorly to supply the skin of the temporal region. See Fig. 17.9.
- Small associated branches innervate the upper pinna, the ear drum, and the TMJ.
- Secretomotor fibres from cranial nerve IX accompany the nerve to the parotid gland.

Technique

- Administered extraorally in front of the ear, a short 32G needle is inserted ~ 0.5cm anterior to the mid-point of the ear lobe, slightly behind the condylar neck and angled forward towards it. See Fig. 17.8.
- Advance the needle to touch the bone of the condylar neck.
- Withdraw 3–5mm and inject 0.5mL LA.

Complications

- Transient facial palsy (if injected into the parotid capsule). If caused, manage by reassuring the patient, taping down the eyelid, and applying an eye patch until the effects have worn off.

Clinical notes

- Ask the patient to open and close the mouth a few times to feel if the needle is against movable bone. If not, reposition the needle until it is, before withdrawing and injecting.
- Withdrawing the needle is essential to avoid intracapsular TMJ infiltration, thereby reducing the effectiveness of the block.
- For complete anaesthesia of the TMJ, it is sometimes necessary to complement the deeper block with a more superficial block in front of the capsule.

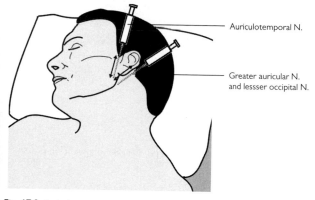

Auriculotemporal N.

Greater auricular N. and lessser occipital N.

Fig. 17.8 Auriculotemporal, greater auricular, and lesser occipital nerve blocks.

Facial nerve (VII)

A purely motor nerve supplying the muscles of facial expression.

Facial nerve block

Indications
- Occasionally to relieve spastic contraction of the facial muscles.
- For symptomatic relief of herpes zoster affecting this nerve.
- Some surgical procedures on the eye.

Anatomy
- It accompanies cranial nerve VIII into the internal acoustic meatus, travelling through the petrous temporal bone into the middle ear.
- It exits posteriorly and inferiorly through the stylomastoid foramen and emerges deep, close to the mastoid process.
- From here it passes forwards, rising superficially as it does so, across the face, temple, forehead, and neck, classically described as 5 branches (temporal, zygomatic, buccal, mandibular, and cervical) but in reality more.

Technique
- Injection point is at the midpoint of the mandibular ramus, just anterior to the mastoid process and beneath the external auditory meatus.
- It lies 1–2cm deep.
- After careful aspiration inject 2–3mL of LA.

Complications
- If inserted too deeply, the glossopharyngeal and vagal nerves may also be blocked. Moderate risk of intravascular injection due to the close proximity of the carotid artery and internal jugular vein.
-

Glossopharyngeal nerve (IX)

A complex, predominantly sensory nerve joined by many branches along its course.

Glossopharyngeal nerve block

Indications

- Pain relief from malignant growths at the tongue base, epiglottis, and palatine tonsils.
- To distinguish glossopharyngeal, from trigeminal and geniculate neuralgias.

Anatomy

- The main trunk exits the skull through the jugular foramen passing between internal and external carotid arteries and medially to the stylomastoid process.
- It supplies sensation to the pharynx, tonsil, and posterior 1/3 tongue and motor fibres to the stylopharyngeus muscle (facilitates swallowing through larynx and pharynx elevation).
- It also supplies special sensory (taste) sensation to the posterior 1/3 tongue and secretomotor fibres helping to release saliva from the parotid gland.

Technique

- Insert a 5cm 22G needle just posterior to the angle of the mandible.
- Inject 2mL of LA, 3–4cm deep in conjunction with a nerve stimulator to confirm accurate positioning.
- An alternative approach is positioning the needle midway between the mastoid process and the angle of the mandible, over the styloid process.
- The nerve is located just anterior to the styloid process.

Complications

- Dysphagia and vagal blockade resulting in ipsilateral vocal cord paralysis and tachycardia.
- Accessory and hypoglossal blocks cause paralysis of the trapezius muscle and the tongue respectively.

Clinical notes

- Careful aspiration and nerve stimulator strongly recommended.

Cervical plexus of nerves (C1–C4)

This is a plexus of the ventral rami of the first 4 cervical spinal nerves. C1 is purely motor with C2, C3, and C4 being both motor and sensory.

There are 4 terminal sensory branches from the plexus:
- The lesser occipital (C2)
- The greater auricular (C2 & C3)
- The transverse cervical (C2 & C3)
- The supraclavicular (C3 & C4).

The motor supply is to the muscles of the neck:
- Straps—ansa cervicalis (C1–C3)
- Scalenes—segmental branches (C1–C4)
- Diaphragm (C3–C5).

For blockade of the entire plexus see Chapter 18. Descriptions of blocks of the terminal nerves follow.

Lesser occipital nerve block

Indications
- Surgery of the auricle and adjacent lateral scalp
- Chronic pain
- Occipital neuralgia.

Anatomy
- It arises from the lateral branch of the ventral ramus of the 2nd cervical nerve, sometimes also from the 3rd.
- It curves around and ascends along the posterior border of the sternocleidomastoid. See Fig. 17.9.
- Near the cranium it perforates the deep fascia and is continued upward along the side of the head behind the auricle, supplying the skin and communicating with the greater occipital, the great auricular. and the post-auricular branch of the facial nerve.
- It gives off an auricular branch, which supplies the skin of the upper and posterior part of the auricle, communicating with the mastoid branch of the great auricular.

Technique
- Insert a 24G needle behind the ear at a level corresponding to the middle of the occipital scalp.
- Advance it superiorly and inject 4mL of LA. See Fig. 17.8.

Complications
- Bleeding (rare).

Clinical notes
- Very sensitive area so inject slowly.

Great auricular nerve block

Indications
- Surgery of the external ear.
- Postoperative analgesia following mastoidectomy and otoplasty.

Anatomy

- It arises from the 2nd and 3rd cervical nerves and winds around the posterior border of the sternocleidomastoid (SCM). See Fig. 17.9.
- After perforating the deep fascia, it ascends upon SCM beneath the platysma to the parotid gland, where it divides into an anterior and a posterior branch.
- The anterior branch is distributed to the skin of the face over the parotid gland and communicates in the substance of the gland with the facial nerve.
- The posterior branch supplies the skin over the mastoid process and on the back of the auricle, except at its upper part.
- A filament pierces the auricle to reach its lateral surface, where it is distributed to the lobe and lower part of the concha.
- The posterior branch communicates with the lesser occipital, the auricular branch of the vagus, and the post-auricular branch of the facial nerve.

Technique

- Palpate the cricoid cartilage and draw a line from its superior margin laterally to the posterior border of SCM.
- Inject 2–3mL of LA superficial to SCM muscle at this point.

Complications

- If too deep you will get a cervical plexus block with possible Horner's syndrome and block of the phrenic nerve.

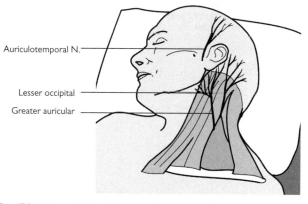

Auriculotemporal N.

Lesser occipital

Greater auricular

Fig. 17.9 Anatomy of the auriculotemporal, greater auricular and lesser occipital nerves.

Greater occipital nerve block

Indications
- Acute occipital pain
- Posterior fossa surgery
- Chronic occipital pain
- 2° to occipital neuralgia.

Anatomy
- The medial branch of the dorsal 1° ramus of the 2nd cervical nerve.
- It arises from between the 1st and 2nd cervical vertebrae along with the lesser occipital nerve.
- After emerging from the subocciptal triangle, it ascends obliquely between the inferior oblique and semispinalis capitis muscle.
- It then passes through the trapezius muscle and ascends to innervate the skin along the posterior part of the scalp to the vertex.
- It also innervates the scalp at the top of the head, above the ear and overlying the parotid glands.

Technique
- With the patient's head on the side, palpate the occipital artery at the level of the superior nuchal line.
- The nerve is medial to the artery and 2mL of LA is injected.

Complications
- Intravascular injection is rare.

Clinical notes
- The use of US to identify both the occipital artery and greater occipital nerve have been described.

Further reading

Christ S, Kaviani R, Rindfleisch F, *et al*. (2012). Brief report: identification of the great auricular nerve by ultrasound imaging and transcutaneous nerve stimulation. *Anesth Analg*, **114**(5), 1128–30.

Greher M, Moriggl B, Curatolo M, *et al*. (2010). Sonographic visualization and ultrasound-guided blockade of the greater occipital nerve: a comparison of two selective techniques confirmed by anatomical dissection. *Br J Anaesth*, **104**(5), 637–42.

Cervical plexus blocks

Background

Indications

Anaesthesia
- Carotid endarterectomy
- Lymph node biopsy
- Internal jugular cannulation.

Analgesia
- Carotid surgery
- Thyroid surgery
- Mastoid and ear surgery
- Supplement to brachial plexus block for open shoulder surgery.

Chronic pain intervention
- Cervical radiculopathy
- Cervicogenic headache.

Introduction

Traditionally cervical plexus blocks have been divided into superficial and deep blocks. Superficial blocks were described as subcutaneous injections and deep blocks as deep to the deep cervical fascia into the prevertebral space. More recent cadaveric and US studies have suggested an *intermediate* cervical plexus block; that is, deep to the investing fascia of the neck but superficial to the deep fascia. Some evidence exists that fluid deep to the investing fascia will diffuse into the prevertebral space.

This chapter will therefore describe blocks (based on a recent proposal) as:
- *Superficial* or *subcutaneous* cervical plexus block.
- *Intermediate* or *'subfascial'* cervical plexus block: an injection deep to the investing fascia of the neck.
- *Deep* cervical plexus block: an injection beneath the deep cervical fascia close to transverse process of vertebra.

For carotid endarterectomy, superficial, intermediate, and deep cervical plexus blocks (and a combination of these) have been used. However, deep cervical plexus blocks are more than twice as likely to yield a serious life-threatening complication as superficial blocks, although absolute incidence is low in both. Deep cervical plexus blocks are ~ 5 times more likely to need conversion to GA. *Therefore deep block should not be routinely used for carotid endarterectomies*. Superficial cervical plexus blocks alone do not provide any motor block but this does not seem to be a problem surgically. Subcutaneous and 'intermediate' blocks appear to be equally effective.

For descriptions of blocks of the individual terminal nerves see Cervical plexus of nerves (C1–C4), p. 230.

Anatomy
- The cervical plexus is formed from the ventral rami of C1–C4.
- After exiting neural foramen they pass posterior to the vertebral artery and C2–C4 roots divide into ascending and descending branches which loop and unite to form a plexus superficial to scalenus medius and levator scapulae.

- This then divides into 4 superficial terminal branches:
  - lesser occipital nerve (C2) ascends along the posterior border of SCM to supply the upper neck and the scalp
  - great auricular nerve (C2, C3) ascends across SCM and reach to supply the skin over the parotid gland and posterior auricle
  - transverse cervical nerve (C2, C3) crosses SCM horizontally, deep to platysma, to supply the skin of the anterior triangle of the neck
  - supraclavicular nerves (C3, C4) descend behind SCM and branch out to supply the skin over the shoulder and upper pectoral region.
- Superficial branches are pure sensory while deep are purely motor and supply muscles of neck and upper back. C1 is motor and gives a communicating branch to hypoglossal nerve.
- Phrenic nerve (C3, C4, C5) conveys sensory, motor, and sympathetic fibres to diaphragm and lies on scalenus anterior.
- At the midpoint of SCM or the apex of interscalene groove, the superficial branches lie posterior to SCM and underneath investing fascia. They emerge at the lateral edge of SCM muscle. See Fig. 18.1.

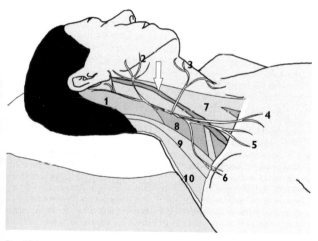

Fig. 18.1 The superficial cervical plexus as it emerges from the lateral edge of sternocleidomastoid. **1** lesser occipital nerve; **2** greater auricular nerve; **3** transverse cervical nerve; **4** medial supraclavicular nerve; **5** intermediate supraclavicular nerve; **6** lateral supraclavicular nerve; **7** sternocleidomastoid muscle; **8** scalene muscles; **9** levator scapulae muscle; **10** trapezius muscle; Arrow, external jugular vein.

Specific contraindications
- Contralateral phrenic nerve palsy
- Contralateral recurrent laryngeal nerve palsy
- Severe respiratory disease (relative).

Side effects and complications
Side effects
- Hemi-diaphragmatic paralysis due to phrenic nerve block (deep and intermediate block).
- Horner's syndrome due to stellate ganglion blockade (deep).
- Hoarse voice due to recurrent laryngeal nerve blockade (deep).
- Haematoma from external jugular vein puncture.
- Partial brachial plexus block leading to paraesthesia or numbness/heavy arm. More common in shoulder/upper arm region.

Complications
- *Intrathecal*, *epidural*, and *intracord injection* from deep blocks.
- Vertebral artery puncture and intra-arterial injection. Seizures may occur immediately—inject 1mL of LA and pause before injecting remainder in fractionated doses.
- Neurological injury.

Clinical notes
- For carotid surgery, continue infiltration along SCM right up to the mastoid process. Trigeminal contribution along the angle of jaw and facial nerve supply to muscles can be addressed by submandibular infiltration for discomfort from proximal wound retraction.
- The carotid sheath is not always well anaesthetized (although intermediate cervical plexus blocks may surround the sheath with LA) and therefore surgical infiltration or US-guided perivascular infiltration of the sheath is needed.
- Carotid endarterectomy patients may have atheromatous plaques that could be dislodged with head hyperextension or cause cerebral ischaemia with head rotation.
- A low-concentration LA (a combination of 1% lidocaine and epinephrine 1:200,000 with 0.25% bupivacaine) is usually sufficient as there is no motor component in the superficial block.

Superficial or subcutaneous block of the cervical plexus: landmark technique

Landmarks: ▬▬▬◆▬

There is no motor innervation from the superficial branches of the cervical plexus so a PNS is of no use.

Landmarks

- The posterior border of the clavicular head of the SCM muscle (this can be made easier by asking the patient to lift their head off the pillow).
- Cricoid cartilage (C6) or midpoint of SCM.

Technique

- The patient is positioned supine with the head turned away from the side to be blocked.
- Prepare the skin with 0.5% chlorhexidine in 70% alcohol. Wait until the skin is dry.
- Anaesthetize the skin with a subcutaneous injection of 1% lidocaine at the point of needle insertion.
- A 25mm 21–25G needle is inserted perpendicular to the skin. See Fig. 18.2.
- After careful aspiration (watch out for the external jugular vein!) 10mL of LA is injected subcutaneously.
- If in the correct place this should be sufficient, but most practitioners would infiltrate (subcutaneously) cranially and caudally along the lateral/posterior boarder of SCM.
- For an intermediate cervical plexus block, insert the needle a little deeper until a 'pop' is felt as the needle passes through the investing fascia of the neck. After negative aspiration 10mL LA is injected.

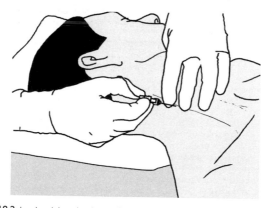

Fig. 18.2 Landmark-based technique for superficial cervical plexus block. Needle insertion is at the mid point of the lateral border of sternocleidomastoid muscle.

Intermediate or subfascial block of the cervical plexus: ultrasound technique

US:

Preliminary scan

- Position the patient supine with head turned 45° to the contralateral side or in lateral position. (Lateral is especially helpful if critical stenosis in carotids make the patient symptomatic on turning head.)
- Place the probe in a transverse (axial) plane at the middle of SCM (level of cricoid cartilage).
- Identify the lateral tapering border of SCM, deep to this are scalenus anterior and scalenus medius with the *brachial plexus* roots between them.
- The nerves of the plexus may be visible as small hypoechoic nodules between SCM and scalenus medius. The greater auricular nerve is the largest and may be visible. However, they are small nerves and may not be easily seen. See Fig. 18.3.
- The hyperechoic deep fascia overlying the brachial plexus roots and scalene muscle may also be seen.
- The carotid artery and internal jugular vein should be visible medially.

US settings

- Probe: high-frequency (>10MHz) linear L38 broadband probe.
- Settings: MB—resolution.
- Depth: 0.5–2cm.
- Orientation: transverse (axial).
- Needle: 25–50mm short bevel.

Technique

- Position the patient as for preliminary scan.
- Prepare the skin with 0.5% chlorhexidine in 70% alcohol. Wait until the skin is dry.
- Anaesthetize the skin with a subcutaneous injection of 1% lidocaine at the point of needle insertion.
- In-plane approach is advocated with needle coming from lateral to medial (shorter track and does not go through SCM muscle)—see Fig. 18.4. A medial to lateral approach can also be used.
- Needle is passed through skin and investing fascia and the tip is positioned adjacent to the plexus deep to SCM.
- Inject 1–2mL LA to confirm needle position. 10–15mL of LA is injected after negative aspiration. It should spread down towards carotid sheath and ideally surround it.
- If the plexus is not visualized the injection can be placed under the posterior border of SCM below the investing fascia at the level of cricoid cartilage.

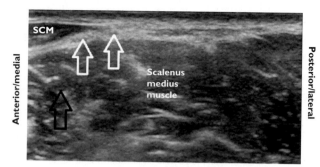

Fig. 18.3 Ultrasound of neck showing the location of the superficial cervical plexus. SCM, lateral edge of sternocleidomastoid muscle; White arrows, nerves of the superficial cervical plexus; Black arrow, C5 nerve root in interscalene groove.

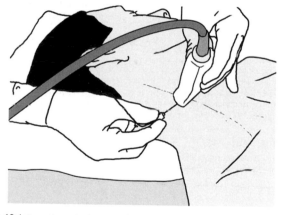

Fig. 18.4 Set up for an in-plane superficial cervical plexus block.

Deep block of the cervical plexus: peripheral nerve stimulator technique

PNS:

Landmarks
- Chassaignac tubercle (anterior tubercle of transverse process C6).
- Mastoid process.

Technique
- The patient is positioned supine with the head turned away from the side to be blocked.
- Draw a line between Chassaignac tubercle and mastoid process.
- Draw a parallel line 1cm posterior.
- The transverse process of C2 is 1.5cm caudad to the mastoid process, C3 1.5cm further caudad, C4 1.5cm further caudad, etc.
- Injections can be at each vertebral level, or a single injection at C4 (level of thyroid cartilage).
- Prepare the skin with 0.5% chlorhexidine in 70% alcohol. Wait until the skin is dry.
- Anaesthetize the skin with a subcutaneous injection of 1% lidocaine at the point of needle insertion.
- A 50mm 25G needle is inserted perpendicular to the skin, with a slight caudad angulation.
- Bony contact with the transverse process is an acceptable endpoint, (or traditionally paraesthesia), at C3 scalenus medius may be stimulated and at C4 scalenus anterior.
- After careful aspiration (watch out for the vertebral artery!), 4mL of LA is injected at each level, or 10–15mL as a single C4 injection.

Clinical notes
- This is not generally needed for anaesthesia of the neck region and should be used with caution, if at all.

Deep block of the cervical plexus: ultrasound techniques

US:

Preliminary scan

- Patient is best placed in a lateral decubitus position.
- The US probe is placed in a transverse (axial) plane anterolaterally across the neck at level of cricoid cartilage for C6 level.
- Brachial plexus roots can be seen as round hypoechoic structures going from a deep to a superficial position in the interscalene groove.
- A hypoechoic shadow of bone can be appreciated as a double hump which represents the anterior and posterior tubercle of the transverse process.
- C7 level is identified by a prominent posterior tubercle and absence of anterior tubercle. This can help to identify the correct level.
- The probe is moved cephalad while counting the levels and C4 transverse process and its anterior and posterior tubercle is identified. The nerve root can be visualized entering between the 2 humps as a hypoechoic structure.
- Vertebral artery must be identified with colour Doppler and its position relative to nerve root ascertained (usually anterior).

US settings

- Probe: high frequency (>10MHz) linear L38 broadband probe.
- Settings: MB—resolution.
- Depth: 3–6cm.
- Orientation: transverse, anterolaterally across neck.
- Needle: 50mm short bevelled.

Technique

- Position the patient lateral with neck exposed.
- Prepare the skin with 0.5% chlorhexidine in 70% alcohol. Wait until the skin is dry.
- Anaesthetize the skin with a subcutaneous injection of 1% lidocaine at the point of needle insertion.
- After identifying C4 nerve root entering the foramen in the preliminary scan, the needle is advanced in-plane from posterior to anterior. It is absolutely essential to keep the tip in view at all times.
- Once the tip approaches the posterior tubercle bony contact can be made or the tip gradually moved closer to nerve root and a 5–10mL single LA injection made after negative aspiration. (Visualizing C2 or C3 is difficult in this way and a different approach is used.)

Clinical notes

- This is not generally needed for anaesthesia of the neck region and should be used with caution, if at all.

Further reading

Guay J (2008). Regional anesthesia for carotid surgery. *Curr Opin Anaesthesiol*, **21**(5), 638–44.

Narouze SN, Vydyanathan A, Kapural L, et al. (2009). Ultrasound-guided cervical selective nerve root block. *Reg Anesth Pain Med*, **34**(4), 343–8.

Pandit JJ, Dutta D, Morris JF (2003). Spread of injectate with superficial cervical plexus block in humans: an anatomical study. *Br J Anaesth*, **91**(5), 733–5.

Pandit JJ, Satya-Krishna R, Gration P (2007). Superficial or deep cervical plexus block for carotid endarterectomy: a systematic review of complications. *Br J Anaesth*, **99**(2), 159–69.

Ramachandran SK, Picton P, Shanks A, et al. (2011). Comparison of intermediate vs subcutaneous cervical plexus block for carotid endarterectomy. *Br J Anaesth*, **107**(2), 157–63.

Stellate ganglion (cervical sympathetic trunk) block

Background

Landmarks:

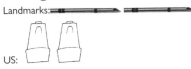

US:

Indications
- Sympathetic blockade of the upper limb.
- Analgesia in chronic pain states (herpes zoster of the upper limb, refractory angina).
- Improve blood supply (Raynaud's, scleroderma).

Anatomy
- The stellate ganglion is formed from the fusion of the inferior cervical ganglion and the 1st thoracic ganglion at the level of the 7th cervical vertebrae.
- It lies on the anterolateral border of longus colli muscle, which separates it from the transverse processes of the cervical vertebrae. See Fig. 19.1.
- The carotid artery is just anterolateral, the vertebral artery just deep, and inferior thyroid artery just superior-medial to the stellate ganglion.
- The oesophagus is just medial and the dome of the pleura just caudad to the stellate ganglion.

Specific contraindications
- Coagulopathy.
- Infection over the site of injection.
- Patient refusal.

Relative contraindications
- Bradycardia.
- Severe respiratory distress.

Side effects and complications

Side effects
- Horner's syndrome.
- Recurrent laryngeal nerve palsy.

Complications
- Intravascular injection—arterial or venous.
- Intrathecal spread of LA.
- Perforation of oesophagus leading to mediastinitis.
- Pneumothorax.

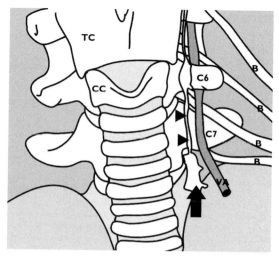

Fig.19.1 Anatomy of the stellate ganglion. TC, thyroid cartilage; B, brachial plexus nerve roots; CC, cricoid cartilage; C6, transverse process C6; Black triangles, sympathetic chain; VA, vertebral artery; C7, transverse process C7; Black arrow, stellate ganglion.

Landmark technique

Traditionally blocks were done blind, with no X-ray or US assistance. This would not be a common technique now. The blocks tend to be done at the level of C6 and rely on spread down to the stellate ganglion at C7.

Landmarks
- Cricoid cartilage.
- Anterior tubercle of transverse process of C6 (Chassaignac tubercle).

Technique
- Position the patient supine (or occasionally in the lateral decubitus position).
- The patient's neck is slightly extended and rotated away from the side of the procedure.
- The cricoid cartilage is identified and marked.
- Palpate the neck, finding the carotid at the level of C6 (cricoid cartilage).
- Gently palpate medial to the carotid until the transverse process of C6 is identified (the anterior tubercle of the transverse process is called the Chassaignac tubercle). Pressure on this tubercle is uncomfortable.
- Prepare the skin with 0.5% chlorhexidine in 70% alcohol. Wait until the skin is dry.
- Anaesthetize the skin with a subcutaneous injection of 1% lidocaine.
- Use the fingers to displace the carotid laterally.
- Insert a 22G needle in the anterior-posterior plane down onto the transverse process of C6. See Fig. 19.2.
- Take care to ensure contact with bone immediately deep to the palpating fingers. As the transverse process is relatively narrow (caudad to cephalad) it is easy to miss it and pass the needle deep to the process and into the nerve root or epidural sheath.
- Withdraw the needle off bone ~ 2mm.
- Inject a small volume of radio-opaque dye whilst screening with image intensification. The dye should spread both caudad and cephalad. This ensures that then needle is not intravascular. Many people add epinephrine to any LA for further reassurance.
- Inject LA with radio-opaque dye slowly with X-ray screening to ensure adequate spread. Inject small increments of 2–3mL. A total of 15mL can be injected.

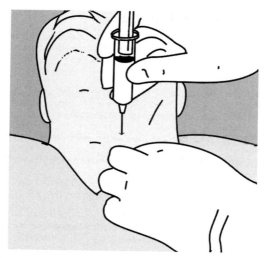

Fig. 19.2 Landmark technique for stellate ganglion block showing the fingers displacing the carotid artery laterally and the needle being inserted at the level of C6.

Ultrasound technique

Ultrasound allows continuous visualization of the major structures that you wish to avoid, such as arteries, veins, oesophagus. It also does not require the use of X-ray screening at its attendant problems.

Preliminary scan

- Position the patient supine (or occasionally in the lateral decubitus position.
- The patient's neck is slightly extended and rotated away from the side of the procedure.
- Place the probe in a transverse plane on the anterolateral aspect of the neck.
- Identify the transverse process of C6 (there is a prominent anterior process).
- Scan medially identifying the carotid, the anterior aspect of the transverse process, and the longus colli muscle. See Fig. 19.3.

US settings

- Probe: high-frequency (>10MHz) linear L38 broadband probe.
- Settings: MB—resolution.
- Depth: 3–4cm.
- Orientation: transverse (axial).
- Needle: 25–50mm of choice.

Technique

- Depending on the anatomy an out-of-plane or a lateral to medial in-plane approach is acceptable.
- Prepare the skin with 0.5% chlorhexidine in 70% alcohol. Wait until the skin is dry.
- Anaesthetize the skin with a subcutaneous injection of 1% lidocaine.
- The needle tips should be directed to the anterior part of longus colli muscle, deep to the prevertebral fascia.
- After careful aspiration, inject 5mL of LA slowly, ensuring that the LA is visible on the US screen.

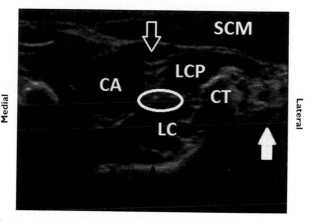

Fig. 19.3 Ultrasound showing the longus colli muscle just anterior to the transverse process of C6. SCM, sternocleidomastoid muscle; LC, longus colli muscle; LCP, longus capitus muscle; CA, carotid artery; CT, Chassaignac's tubercle; Black triangles, transverse process C6; White arrow, C6 nerve root; Black arrow, internal jugular vein; White oval, position of stellate ganglion.

Further reading

Boas RA (1998). Sympathetic nerve blocks: in search of a role. *Reg Anesth Pain Med*, **23**(3), 292–305.

Bhatia A, Flamer D, Peng PW (2012). Evaluation of sonoanatomy relevant to performing stellate ganglion blocks using anterior and lateral simulated approaches: an observational study. *Can J Anaesth*, **59**(11), 1040–7.

Cepeda MS, Carr DB, Lau J (2005). Local anaesthetic sympathetic blockade for complex regional pain syndrome. *Cochrane Database Syst Rev*, **4**, CD004598. doi:10.1002/14651858.CD004598.pub2.

Kapral S, Krafft P, Gosch M, et al. (1995). Ultrasound imaging for stellate ganglion block: direct visualisation of the puncture site and anaesthetic spread. A pilot study. *Reg Anesth*, **20**(4), 323–8.

Menon R, Swanepoel A (2010). Sympathetic blocks. *Contin Educ Anaesth Crit Care Pain*, **10**(3), 88–92.

Topical and regional anaesthesia of the upper airways

Background

Landmarks: ██████▶ ██████▶

Indications

Awake fibreoptic intubation (FOI).

Introduction

Anaesthesia of the airway, principally for awake FOI, can be achieved by either topical application of LA, nerve blocks, or a combination of the 2.

Anatomy

The upper airways are innervated by 3 major cranial nerves:
- Trigeminal
- Glossopharyngeal
- Vagus.

Nasal cavity and nasopharynx

This is supplied by the *greater and lesser palatine nerves* and the *anterior ethmoidal nerve*. The palatine nerves arise from *the maxillary branch of the trigeminal nerve* via the pterygopalatine ganglion and supply the nasal turbinates and the posterior 2/3 of the nasal septum. The anterior ethmoidal nerve arises from the *olfactory nerve* and supplies the anterior nares and the anterior 1/3 of the nasal septum (see Fig. 20.1).

Tongue and oropharynx

Sensory innervation of the anterior 2/3 of the tongue is by the *lingual branch of the mandibular nerve*. The oropharynx and the posterior 1/3 of the tongue are supplied by branches of the *glossopharyngeal nerve*. They travel along the lateral surface of the pharynx and also supply the vallecula and anterior surface of the epiglottis (*lingual branch*), walls of the pharynx (*pharyngeal branch*) and tonsils (*tonsillar branch*).

Larynx and the trachea

These are supplied by branches of the *vagus nerve*. The superior laryngeal nerve (SLN) supplies sensory fibres to the base of the tongue, posterior epiglottis, aryepiglottic folds and arytenoids. The recurrent laryngeal nerve (RLN) supplies sensory innervation to the vocal cords and trachea, and motor innervation to all the laryngeal muscles except cricothyroid muscle. The right RLN loops around the innominate artery and the left RLN loops around the aortic arch (see Fig. 20.2).

Patient preparation

- Obtain IV access.
- Establish full monitoring.
- Sedation is recommended with fentanyl (100–200 micrograms) or remifentanil (3ng/mL target-controlled infusion or 50ng/kg/min) and perhaps also small doses of midazolam 1–2mg.
- Administer antisialogogues (glycopyrronium bromide 0.4mg IV) as early as is practical.

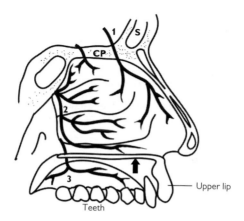

Fig. 20.1 Nerve supply of lateral wall of nose. CP, cribriform plate; S, frontal sinus; 1 anterior ethmoidal nerve; 2 greater palatine nerve; 3 lesser palatine nerve; Black arrow, hard palate.

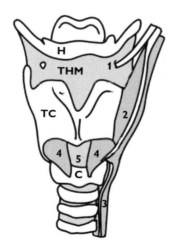

Fig. 20.2 Nerve supply of larynx. 1 internal branch of the superior laryngeal nerve; 2 external branch of the superior laryngeal nerve; 3 recurrent laryngeal nerve; 4 cricothyroid muscle; 5 cricothyroid membrane; C, cricoid cartilage; THM, thyrohyoid membrane; TC, thyroid cartilage; H, hyoid bone.

Topical techniques

This is the spreading of LA over a region of mucosa to achieve terminal nerve blockade. This can be accomplished by the following methods:

Direct application with spray

Using a fine-bore multi-perforated catheter, 2–4% lidocaine is sprayed onto the mucosal surface of nose, mouth, tongue, and naso- and oropharynx. Lidocaine 10% is used to spray the tonsillar pillars and posterior pharynx.

Local anaesthetic reservoirs

Viscous or aqueous solutions of LA-soaked cotton pledgets or ribbon gauzes are applied to the nasal mucosal for 5–15 minutes to produce a dense block. Cocaine paste (4%, 10%, 25%) or lidocaine with epinephrine (1:200,000) or phenylephrine (0.5%) can be used for this purpose. This also results in vasoconstriction and a dry mucosa.

Atomizer device

Syringe-powered atomizer devices deliver lidocaine as an aerosol using the Venturi principle. They are more efficient when used with side-stream air/oxygen flow. This achieves anaesthesia of the nasal passages and nasopharynx.

Nebulizers

Inhalation of nebulized lidocaine (2–4%) for 15–30 minutes using a standard nebulizer with a face mask achieves oropharyngeal and tracheal anaesthesia. Anaesthesia is improved by asking the patient to inhale the vapours deeply.

'Spray as you go technique'

This method achieves anaesthesia of the airways by spraying lignocaine (2–4%) through a 16G epidural catheter via the working channel of the fibre-optic bronchoscope.

> **Clinical notes**
> - Before spraying LA to the nasal passages use vasoconstrictors, such as phenylephrine or xylometazoline, to decrease the blood supply. This prolongs the effect of the LA as well as reducing the risk of bleeding when performing the intubation.
> - Often more than one of these techniques are used together, but take care with the total dose of LA.

Nerve block techniques

Superior laryngeal nerve block

Injections are required bilaterally at the level of the greater cornu of the hyoid bone.

Landmarks
* Thyroid cartilage
* Cornu of hyoid bone
* Angle of mandible.

Technique
* Patient is placed supine with the neck extended.
* Identify the thyroid notch and follow the superior margin of the thyroid cartilage posteriorly to find the superior cornu.
* The greater cornu of the hyoid bone lies just above the superior cornu of the thyroid cartilage and is identified as a rounded structure below the angle of the mandible.
* Prepare the skin with 0.5% chlorhexidine in 70% alcohol. Wait until the skin is dry.
* Anaesthetize the skin with a subcutaneous injection of 1% lidocaine.
* A 25mm 25G needle is inserted anteromedially to make contact with the greater cornu of the hyoid bone (Fig. 20.3).
* The needle is 'walked off' the inferior border of the greater cornu to just pierce the thyrohyoid membrane.
* The needle is aspirated to check for air or blood and 2mL of lidocaine 4% with or without epinephrine 1:200,000 is injected.
* If air is aspirated, the needle tip lies in the larynx and hence must be withdrawn. If blood is aspirated, the needle is removed and the procedure is repeated.

Contraindications
* Patient refusal.
* Therapeutic anticoagulation.
* Distorted anatomy due to tumours, arteriovenous malformations and surgical reconstruction.

Side effects and complications
* Puncture of the carotid artery.
* Blockade of the external laryngeal nerve resulting in weakness of cricothyroid muscle and hence alteration of the airway diameter.

Clinical notes
* Always perform the blocks bilaterally to achieve adequate anaesthesia.
* Firmly displace the hyoid bone towards the side to be blocked.
* Do not insert the needle into the thyroid cartilage, since injection of LA at the level of vocal cords may cause oedema and airway obstruction.
* As well as this injection technique the SLN can also be blocked by placing LA soaked cotton-pledgets onto the pyriform fossa on both sides, via the mouth.

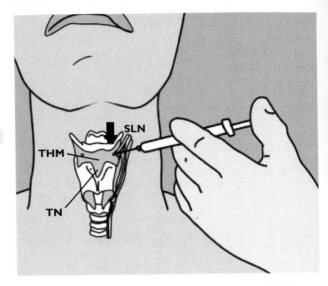

Fig. 20.3 Superior laryngeal nerve block. Black arrow, greater cornu of hyoid bone; SLN, superior laryngeal nerve; THM, thyrohyoid membrane; TN, thyroid notch.

Glossopharyngeal nerve block

This abolishes gag reflex and permits direct laryngoscopy and passage of nasotracheal tube through the posterior pharynx. The nerve can be blocked by topical spray, direct mucosal contact using cotton pledgets, and by injection. The injection can be done intra- and extraorally.

Landmarks
- Angle of mandible
- Mastoid process
- Styloid process
- Palatoglossal fold.

Technique

Extraoral (peristyloid approach):
- Patient is placed supine with the neck turned to the opposite side.
- A line is drawn between the angle of mandible and mastoid process. The styloid process is located by deep palpation on this line.
- Prepare the skin with 0.5% chlorhexidine in 70% alcohol. Wait until the skin is dry.
- Anaesthetize the skin with a subcutaneous injection of 1% lidocaine.

- A 25mm, 25G needle is used to contact the styloid process. The needle is then withdrawn slightly and directed posteriorly off the styloid process.
- After negative aspiration, 5–7mL of lidocaine 2%, with or without epinephrine (1:200,000), is injected.

Intraoral

After topical anaesthesia of the oropharynx, a 10cm 22G needle is used to inject submucosally at the base of palatoglossal fold, after negative aspiration, with 2–5mL of lidocaine 2%, with or without epinephrine (1:200,000). See Fig. 20.4.

Contraindications
- Patient refusal
- Therapeutic anticoagulation.

Side effects and complications
- Carotid artery puncture.

Clinical notes
- Careful aspiration is vital to avoid intra-arterial injection.
- Always perform the blocks bilaterally to achieve adequate anaesthesia.

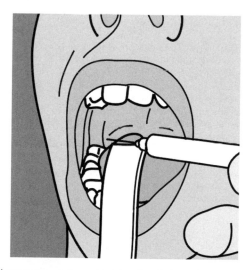

Fig 20.4 Glossopharyngeal nerve block (needle at the base of palatoglossal fold).

Recurrent laryngeal nerve block (cricothyroid puncture, translaryngeal injection)

Translaryngeal injection of LA through the cricothyroid membrane provides topical anaesthesia for both vagal branches (SLN and RLN). It results in the spread of LA both above and below the cords.

Landmarks
- Thyroid cartilage
- Cricoid cartilage.

Technique
- Patient is placed supine, with the neck hyperextended.
- Identify the cricothyroid membrane between the thyroid and cricoid cartilages.
- Prepare the skin with 0.5% chlorhexidine in 70% alcohol. Wait until the skin is dry.
- The trachea is held in place with the thumb and index finger on either side of the thyroid cartilage.
- After identifying the midline anaesthetize the skin with a subcutaneous injection of 1% lidocaine.
- The cricothyroid membrane is punctured using a 5mL syringe containing 4% lignocaine mounted on a 22G IV cannula. The cannula is introduced into the lumen of the trachea. The direction of the cannula should be at an angle of 45° caudally. See Fig. 20.5.
- A loss of resistance is felt and air is aspirated to confirm the cannula in the trachea and the needle is removed from the cannula leaving only the plastic catheter.
- The patient is instructed to take a deep breath and exhale forcefully. At the end of the expiration, 3–4mL of lidocaine is rapidly injected into the trachea, spreading over the tracheal mucosa.

Contraindications
- Patient refusal.
- Therapeutic anticoagulation.
- Patients with an unstable neck, as the injection induces coughing.

Side effects and complications
- Coughing.
- Structural injuries: the posterior tracheal wall, vocal cords, and major vessels can be damaged, if the cannula is not stabilized during injection.
- Intravascular injection.
- Subcutaneous emphysema.

Clinical notes
- The catheter should be left in place until intubation is performed to inject more LA if needed and to decrease the likelihood of subcutaneous emphysema.

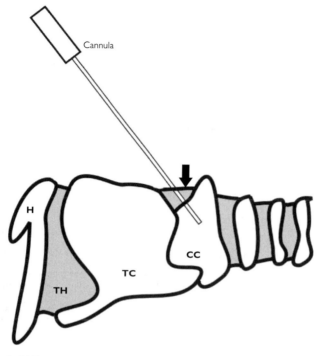

Fig 20.5 Cricothyroid puncture. CC, cricoid cartilage; Arrow, cricothyroid membrane; TC, thyroid cartilage; TH, thyrohyoid membrane; H, hyoid bone.

Blocks for palatine and anterior ethmoidal nerves

This block helps in achieving anaesthesia of the nasal passages for awake nasal FOI. As discussed earlier, topical application of the nasal mucosa is sufficient to block these nerves. However, if the blockade is not fully established, anaesthesia can be achieved by blocking the sphenopalatine ganglion using a cotton-tipped applicator soaked with lignocaine 4% and passing it along the upper border of the middle turbinate up to the posterior wall of nasopharynx. This is left for 5–15 minutes. Oral and percutaneous approaches are also described but due to technical difficulty and high rate of complications, their routine use is not justified.

Along with topical LA application, the anterior ethmoidal nerve can be selectively blocked by using a cotton applicator soaked in LA and passed along the dorsal surface of the nose up to the cribriform plate. It is left for 5–15 minutes.

Further reading

Hadzic A (2007). *Textbook of Regional Anesthesia and Acute Pain Management*. New York: McGraw-Hill Professional.
Popat M (2009). *Difficult Airway Management*. Oxford: Oxford University Press.
Sudheer P, Stacey MR (2003). Anaesthesia for awake intubation. *Br J Anaesth CEPD Rev*, **3**(4),120–3.

Part 3

Upper Limb

Interscalene brachial plexus block

Background

PNS: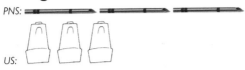

US:

Indications

- Anaesthesia: shoulder and/or proximal upper arm surgery. The superficial cervical plexus may also need to be blocked for skin anaesthesia over the shoulder (see ➔ Superficial or subcutaneous block of the cervical plexus: landmark technique, p. 239).
- Analgesia: postoperative pain relief for shoulder or proximal upper arm surgery. Physiotherapy and/or mobilization (e.g. frozen shoulder) in the shoulder region.

Introduction

The interscalene approach to the brachial plexus is principally indicated for surgery on the shoulder as it is the only approach to the brachial plexus that reliably blocks the suprascapular nerve, which provides sensory innervation to 70% of the shoulder joint. It has a large number of side effects and potential complications, which makes it one of the more dangerous blocks to perform.

The modern approach was described by Winnie in 1970, as a medially directed, single-injection technique at the level of C6. However, this approach has been criticized as it can be associated with the risk of intraforaminal needle passage and subsequent epidural/intrathecal injection, as well as vertebral artery injection. More recently described techniques have popularized a more lateral or parasagittal needle direction (Meier, Borgeat), which avoids the central neuraxis and facilitates both single injection and catheter techniques.

This block is *not* suitable for hand or distal arm surgery as it will not achieve reliable blockade of the C7–T1 nerve roots even with excessive volumes of LA (>40mL). There are other more reliable and safer brachial plexus blocks for this (see Chapters 23, 24, 25, and 26).

Anatomy

- The brachial plexus is formed from the anterior rami of the spinal nerves of C5, C6, C7, C8, and T1 (occasionally from C4='prefixed', or T2='postfixed').
- The interscalene approach blocks the plexus at the level of the roots/ upper and middle trunks of the plexus.
- The roots emerge from between the anterior and posterior tubercles of the transverse processes of the cervical vertebrae and descend sandwiched between the anterior and middle scalene muscles forming the superior trunk (C5/6), middle trunk (C7) and inferior trunk (C8, T1). See Fig. 21.1.
- Anatomical variation is extremely common in the interscalene region; one or more nerve roots may pass *through* the anterior or middle

scalene muscles, or even anterior to them. The formation of the trunks also may occur at the any level even close to the cervical foramina.
- The vertebral artery lies anterior-medial to the plexus and is vulnerable to intravascular injection depending upon the approach used.
- The upper and middle trunks lie superior to the subclavian artery, and the lower trunk postero-lateral to the subclavian artery, close to the 1st rib.
- Relevant branches of the plexus include the suprascapular nerve (C5/6—motor supply to supraspinatus and infraspinatus and sensory innervation of ~70% of posterior shoulder joint), and the dorsal scapular nerve (C5—motor innervation to rhomboid muscles).
- Cutaneous innervation over the clavicle and anterior/superior aspect of the shoulder is from the lateral and intermediate supraclavicular nerves (C4) from the superficial cervical plexus.

Specific contraindications
- Contralateral phrenic nerve palsy
- Contralateral recurrent laryngeal nerve palsy
- Severe respiratory disease (relative).

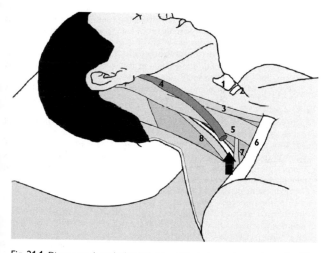

Fig. 21.1 Diagram to show the brachial plexus sitting between the anterior and middle scalene muscles, posterior to the clavicular head of the sternoclavicular muscle.
1 thyroid cartilage; **2** cricoid cartilage; **3** sternal head of sternocleidomastoid muscle; **4** external jugular vein; **5** clavicular head of sternocleidomastoid muscle; **6** clavicle; **7** anterior scalene muscle; **8** middle scalene muscle; Black arrow, brachial plexus.

Side effects and complications

Side effects

- Hemidiaphragmatic paralysis due to phrenic nerve block is almost universal and is accompanied by a 25–30% reduction in pulmonary function. Caution in patients with limited respiratory reserve. The incidence of block of the phrenic nerve may be reduced by use of low-volume injections (<10mL), but may fail to block the superficial cervical plexus.
- Horner's syndrome due to stellate ganglion blockade.
- Recurrent laryngeal nerve blockade (hoarse voice).

Complications

Complications of interscalene block depend to some extent on the approach used:

- *Intrathecal, epidural, and intracord injection* have all been described and are potentially devastating.
- Vertebral artery puncture and intra-arterial injection. Seizures may occur immediately—inject 1mL of LA and pause before injecting remainder in fractionated doses.
- Neurological injury. Permanent injury is rare (0.2%), but temporary paraesthesia, dysaesthesia, and/or pain unrelated to surgery are more common: 8–14% incidence at 10 days, reducing to 3.7% at 1 month, and 0.6–0.9% at 6 months. Comorbidities such as carpal tunnel syndrome, complex regional pain syndrome, or sulcus ulnaris syndrome are accountable for the majority of these symptoms.
- Pneumothorax (0.2%).

Clinical notes

Awake or asleep?

All the case reports of serious complications relating to injection of LA into the central neuraxis have occurred when patients were asleep for their block. This led to ASRA making an advisory statement that all inter-scalene brachial plexus blocks be performed in awake or lightly sedated patients and should not be performed in anaesthetized patients. However, the fault may have been in the technique, and not necessarily prevented by the patient being awake (although it may have been recognized at the time). In the event of a permanent neurological complication, it may be a difficult position to defend medicolegally if the block was performed in an anaesthetized patient. For these reason it is recommended to only perform interscalene brachial plexus blocks on awake or lightly sedated patients, or to document good reasons why the block was performed on an anaesthetized patient.

Peripheral nerve stimulator technique: Winnie's approach

Landmarks

- Identify the posterior border of the clavicular head of the SCM muscle (this can be made easier by asking the patient to lift their head off the pillow).
- Immediately behind is the belly of the anterior scalene muscle.
- Moving the fingers laterally/posteriorly allows the interscalene groove to be palpated between the anterior and middle scalene muscles.
- The groove can be made more prominent by turning the neck away from the side of the block and asking the patient to take deep slow breaths or sniff.
- The needle insertion point is in the interscalene groove at the level of the cricoid cartilage (C6). Commonly the external jugular vein crosses the interscalene groove at this level, but this is not a constant landmark.

Technique

- The patient is positioned supine with the head turned away from the side to be blocked.
- Prepare the skin with 0.5% chlorhexidine in 70% alcohol. Wait until the skin is dry.
- Anaesthetize the skin with a subcutaneous injection of 1% lidocaine at the point of needle insertion.
- A 25–50mm 22G stimulating needle is inserted perpendicular to the skin: this gives a medial, ~45° caudad and slight dorsal angulation (towards the contralateral elbow, when the arm lies at the patient's side). See Fig. 21.2.
- The plexus is a very superficial structure and is rarely >20mm deep at this level. (The original description indicates continuing on the same trajectory, if the plexus is not encountered, until contact with the transverse process—*this practice cannot be recommended and the needle should not be inserted >25mm*.)
- Once appropriate response to nerve stimulation is achieved (see ➔ Endpoints for nerve stimulation techniques, p. 271), aspirate and disconnect to minimize risk of intravascular needle placement and inject 25–30mL of LA in 5mL aliquots. A cylindrical, 'sausage shape' fullness can often be felt between the anterior and middle scalene muscles.
- Note that the needle direction is towards the midline and the central-neuraxis. The minimum distance to the intervertebral foramen is 25mm—intrathecal and intracord injections have been described with this approach.
- The perpendicular angle of approach to the plexus makes this technique less suited to catheter insertion.

Peripheral nerve stimulator technique: Meier's approach

In this approach the needle is directed laterally, away from the midline, thus reducing the chance of damage to the central neuraxis or vertebral artery injection. In addition the tangential approach to the plexus facilitates catheter insertion.

Landmarks

- The needle insertion site is at the level of C4, marked by the thyroid notch (~2 cm above the level of the cricoid cartilage) at the posterior edge of the SCM muscle.
- Subclavian artery in the supraclavicular fossa.

Technique

- Prepare the skin with 0.5% chlorhexidine in 70% alcohol. Wait until the skin is dry.
- Anaesthetize the skin with a subcutaneous injection of 1% lidocaine at the point of needle insertion.
- A 50mm 22G stimulating needle is directed along the interscalene groove, with a 30° angle to the skin, in a caudad and lateral direction towards a point just lateral to the subclavian artery pulsation. (The subclavian artery may only be palpable in 50% of patients—in this case use the mid-clavicular point as the lower landmark, or a Doppler probe.)
- The plexus should be found at a depth of 3–4cm.
- Once appropriate response to nerve stimulation is achieved (see ➜ Endpoints for nerve stimulation techniques, p. 271), aspirate and disconnect to minimize risk of intravascular needle placement and inject 25–30mL of LA in 5mL aliquots. A cylindrical, 'sausage shape' fullness can often be felt between the anterior and middle scalene muscles.

Endpoints for nerve stimulation techniques

For shoulder surgery the following motor responses are acceptable with a stimulating current of between 0.2mA and 0.5mA:

- Biceps
- Triceps
- Deltoid.

Other motor responses may be obtained and can be used as cues for needle redirection:

- *Phrenic nerve*: diaphragm contraction. The phrenic nerve lies on the anterior surface of the anterior scalene muscle, and indicates too anterior needle position—redirect more posteriorly.
- *Dorsal scapular nerve*: rhomboid muscle contraction—shoulder and scapular movement. This lies posterior to the middle scalene muscle and indicates the need for more anterior needle redirection.
- *Nerve to levator scapulae*: scapular and shoulder movement—anterior and more caudad needle redirection required.
- *Accessory nerve*: trapezius muscle contraction—needle too cephalad and too posterior—redirect caudad and anteriorly.

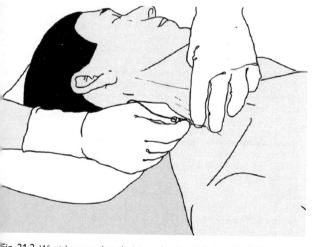

Fig. 21.2 Winnie's approach to the interscalene brachial plexus block. The fingers of the left hand are palpating the interscalene groove and the needle is inserted at the level of C6, aiming towards the contralateral elbow.

Ultrasound techniques

Preliminary scan

- Well-defined landmarks. The plexus being so superficial and the sensitive surrounding anatomy make this an attractive block to perform with US. However, a systematic approach to identifying the plexus and surrounding structures is important. This can be done scanning from the midline postero-laterally, or scanning proximally, up the neck from the supraclavicular fossa.
- Scanning from medial to lateral; identify the trachea, thyroid gland, carotid artery, and internal jugular vein. The SCM muscle is seen superficial to the artery and vein. Moving the probe posteriorly the first muscle seen deep to the flattened lateral tail of SCM is the anterior scalene muscle. The brachial plexus can be identified posterior to this between the anterior and middle scalene muscles.
- Scanning from the supraclavicular fossa cephalad; place the probe parallel to and behind the clavicle in the supraclavicular fossa. Identify the subclavian artery (pulsatile, anechoic) and the trunks / divisions of the brachial plexus superior/posterior/lateral to the artery ('bunch of grapes' appearance). Then scan cephalad to follow the nerves proximally, with the anterior and middle scalene muscles becoming visible on either side.
- At this level the nerves of the plexus appear as hypoechoic, round, or oval structures (see Fig. 21.3). It is important to angle the probe slightly caudad as the nerves are passing laterally towards the 1st rib following the scalene muscles.
- Usually the more superficial roots are the more proximal ones. If the lower nerve roots (C8, T1) are visible, then scan more proximally.
- The phrenic nerve can also be seen close to the C5 nerve root, lying on the anterior scalene beneath the prevertebral fascia that encloses both the muscle and the interscalene groove. The suprascapular artery also can be seen crossing the anterior scalene at this level.
- It is useful to identify the deeper structures; the transverse processess of the vertebrae, and observe the nerve roots entering/exiting their respective intervertebral foramina. Also identifty the vertebral artery on the lateral aspect of the vertebral bodies anterior to the emerging nerve roots inbetween the transerve foramina of the upper 6 cervical verabrae.

US settings

- Probe: high-frequency (>10MHz) linear L38 broadband probe.
- Settings: MB—resolution.
- Depth: 2–3cm.
- Orientation: axial with caudad angulation.
- Needle: 25–50mm of choice.

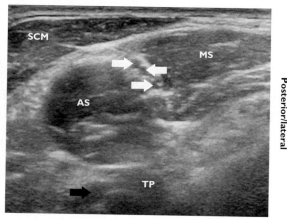

Anterior/medial

Posterior/lateral

Fig. 21.3 Ultrasound of the brachial plexus in the interscalene groove. SCM, sternocleidomastoid muscle; MS, middle scalene muscle; White arrows, nerve roots of the brachial plexus; AS, anterior scalene muscle; Black arrow, vertebral artery; TP, tip of transverse process.

Technique

- Position the patient supine with the head turned 45° to the contralateral side. A lateral position (block side up) can be used, which can facilitate an in-plane lateral approach (machine in front of patient and operator behind).
- Either an in-plane or out-of-plane approach may be used. The in-plane approach can be performed either from medially (passing through anterior scalene) or laterally (passing through middle scalene), see Fig. 21.4. The out-of-plane approach mimics the Meier's insertion and facilitates both familiarity and catheter placement.
- Prepare the skin with 0.5% chlorhexidine in 70% alcohol. Wait until the skin is dry.
- Anaesthetize the skin with a subcutaneous injection of 1% lidocaine at the point of needle insertion.
- Insert needle to the side of the plexus alongside C5 or C6.
- For shoulder surgery only the C5 and C6 nerve roots need to be blocked and performing the block proximally should ensure blockade of the suprascapular nerve (and dorsal scapular nerve) before they leave the plexus.
- After negative aspiration inject LA in small (1–2mL) aliquots and observe spread. The needle may need to be repositioned to the other side of the plexus.
- With US, small volumes of LA (5–10mL) targeted around the C5 and C6 nerve roots appear sufficient for postoperative pain relief, but may not spread to adequately block the superficial cervical plexus that innervates the skin over the shoulder and this may need to be blocked separately (see ➲ Superficial or subcutaneous block of the cervical plexus: landmark technique, p. 239).

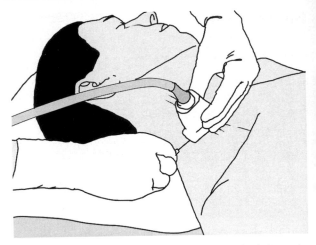

Fig. 21.4 Set up for a lateral in-plane approach for an ultrasound-guided interscalene brachial plexus block.

Further reading

Benumof JL (2000). Permanent loss of cervical spinal cord function associated with interscalene block performed under general anesthesia. *Anesthesiology*, **93**(6), 1541–4.

Fredrickson MJ, Kilfoyle DH (2009). Neurological complication analysis of 1000 ultrasound guided peripheral nerve blocks for elective orthopaedic surgery: a prospective study. *Anaesthesia*, **64**(8), 836–44.

Gautier P, Vandepitte C, Ramquet C, *et al.* (2011). The minimum effective anesthetic volume of 0.75% ropivacaine in ultrasound-guided interscalene brachial plexus block. *Anesth Analg*, **113**(4), 951–5.

Riazi S, Carmichael N, Awad I, *et al.* (2008). Effect of local anaesthetic volume (20 vs 5 mL) on the efficacy and respiratory consequences of ultrasound-guided interscalene brachial plexus block. *Br J Anaesth*, **101**(4), 549–56.

Sardesai, AM, Patel R, Denny NM, *et al.* (2006). Interscalene brachial plexus block: can the risk of entering the spinal canal be reduced? A study of needle angles in volunteers undergoing magnetic resonance imaging. *Anesthesiology*, **105**(1), 9–13.

Suprascapular
nerve block

Background

PNS:

US:

Indications
- Analgesia for shoulder surgery (where an interscalene brachial plexus block is unsuccessful or inadvisable).

Anatomy
- The suprascapular nerve arises from the upper trunk of the brachial plexus (C5, C6).
- It crosses the posterior triangle of the neck deep and parallel to the inferior belly of omohyoid then passes under trapezius muscle.
- It passes through the scapular notch, below the suprascapular ligament into the supraspinatous fossa.
- It supplies supraspinatous, infraspinatous and sensation to the shoulder and acromioclavicular joints.
- The suprascapular artery enters the suprascapular fossa by passing over the suprascapular ligament.

Side effects and complicatios

Complications
- Rarely pneumothorax.

Peripheral nerve stimulator technique

Landmarks
- Midpoint of the spine of the scapula.
- Inferior angle of the scapula.

Technique
- Position the patient sitting or lateral (operative side uppermost), with hand on the opposite shoulder.
- Mark the midpoint of the spine of the scapula.
- Draw a line from the inferior angle of the scapula to the midpoint of the spine and then mark a point 1cm more cranially. This is the needle insertion point. See Fig. 22.1.
- Prepare the skin with 0.5% chlorhexidine in 70% alcohol. Wait until the skin is dry.
- Anaesthetize the skin with a subcutaneous injection of 1% lidocaine at the point of needle insertion.
- Insert a 22G 50mm stimulating needle perpendicular to the skin in all planes (transverse, with caudad and slight medial angulation).
- Advance anteriorly looking for abduction or external rotation of the shoulder.
- The needle is cautiously repositioned to achieve a threshold current of 0.3–0.5mA and after negative aspiration 10–15mL of LA are injected in fractionated doses.

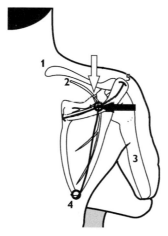

Fig. 22.1 Landmarks for suprascapular nerve block. 1 clavicle; 2 suprascapular nerve; 3 humerus; 4 inferior angle of scapula; 5 spine of scapula; White arrow, suprascapular notch; Black arrow, midpoint of spine of scapula.

Ultrasound technique

Preliminary scan

- Position the patient sitting or lateral (operative side uppermost), with hand on the opposite shoulder.
- Place the transducer above the midpoint and parallel to the spine of the scapula. Angle the probe markedly caudally, almost in a coronal plane. See Fig. 22.2.
- Identify the trapezius muscle and deep to this the supraspinatous muscle, sitting on the scapula.
- The scapular notch can be identified as a depression in the contour of the scapular cortex. See Fig. 22.3.
- The suprascapular ligament can often be seen covering over this depression.
- The nerve can sometime be visualized beneath the ligament in the scapular notch. As it is travelling in an oblique direction it can be hard to get a good image of the nerve and gentle rotational and tilting movements may be needed.
- Try to identify the suprascapular artery (anechoic, pulsatile) with the Doppler. This is usually lateral to the nerve and above the suprascapular ligament.

US settings

- Probe: medium/high-frequency linear L38 broadband probe.
- Settings: MB—general/resolution.
- Depth: 3–6cm.
- Orientation: coronal/transverse with marked caudal angulation.
- Needle: 50–80mm short bevelled.

Technique

- Identify the structures described earlier.
- Prepare the skin with 0.5% chlorhexidine in 70% alcohol. Wait until the skin is dry.
- Anaesthetize the skin with a subcutaneous injection of 1% lidocaine at the point of needle insertion.
- Use an in-plane approach from medial to lateral.
- After careful aspiration inject 5mL of LA around the nerve.
- If the nerve is not clearly seen, inject the LA below supraspinatus muscle on the floor of the suprascapular fossa. LA will spread to block the nerve.

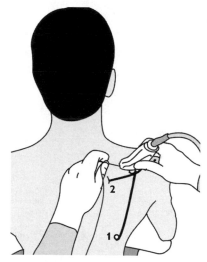

Fig. 22.2 Set up for a suprascapular ultrasound-guided nerve block. 1 inferior angle of scapula; 2 spine of scapula.

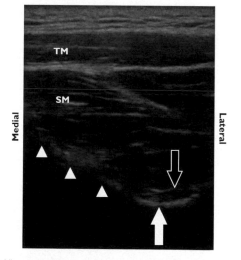

Fig. 22.3 Ultrasound of the suprascapular notch. TM, trapezius muscle; SM, supraspinatous muscle; White triangles, scapula; Black arrow, suprascapular ligament; White arrow, scapular notch.

Further reading

Harmon D, Hearty C (2007). Ultrasound-guided suprascapular nerve block technique. *Pain Physician*, **10**(6), 743–6.

Chapter 23

Supraclavicular brachial plexus block

Background

PNS: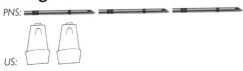

US:

Indications
- Anaesthesia: any surgery of the upper limb and hand.
- Analgesia: postoperative analgesia for surgery of the upper limb or hand.

Introduction
The supraclavicular block approaches the brachial plexus at about the same level as the vertical infraclavicular approach. As such, LA is injected around the narrowest part of the plexus and has the fastest onset of brachial plexus blocks. This has led to it being described as the 'spinal of the arm'.

Kulenkampff is said to have carried out the first percutaneous supraclavicular block on himself in 1911 (Hirschel had published a surgical approach prior to this). Kulenkampff's technique described inserting a needle above the midpoint of the clavicle where the subclavian pulse could be felt and the needle aimed at the spinous process of T2. This allowed LA to be deposited on the brachial plexus at the level of the trunks with fast onset of a dense and widespread block. However, it carried an unacceptable risk of pneumothorax. Brown published the 'plumb-bob' technique in 1993.

Anatomy
- The subclavian artery arches over the 1st rib immediately posterior to the insertion of anterior scalene muscle to the 1st rib.
- The brachial plexus, just above the 1st rib, lies postero-lateral to the subclavian artery. The middle scalene muscles lie further posterior, also inserting onto the 1st rib. See Fig. 23.1.
- The roots of C5 through to T1 join together to form the trunks and divide into anterior and posterior divisions. These changes produce a US picture similar to a 'bunch of grapes' sitting on the 1st rib.
- At this point the suprascapular nerve and the long thoracic nerve have often already left the perivascular sheath. Therefore this is not an ideal approach for shoulder surgery.

Side effects and complications
Side effects
- Horner's syndrome and recurrent laryngeal nerve palsy. These side effects are less likely than with interscalene approaches.

Complications
- Pneumothorax is the most feared complication from this procedure. The rate should be <1:1000 (0.1%) in experienced hands for landmark techniques.
- Arterial puncture (20% for landmark techniques).
- Intravascular injection.
- Haematoma.

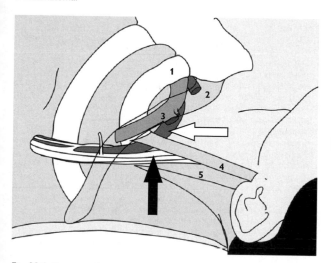

Fig. 23.1 Illustration of the brachial plexus emerging from between the scalene muscle to join the subclavian artery resting on the 1st rib, behind the clavicle. **1** 1st rib; **2** clavicle; **3** subclavian vein; **4** anterior scalene muscle; **5** middle scalene muscle; White arrow, subclavian artery; Black arrow, brachial plexus.

Peripheral nerve stimulator technique

The commonest current technique is a modification of Brown's, described by Winnie. Also known as the subclavian perivascular block.

Landmarks

- Interscalene groove
- Subclavian artery.

Technique

- The patient lies supine with the head turned slightly to the opposite side to that being blocked.
- The interscalene groove is palpated as for an interscalene block at the level of C6 (cricoids cartilage). The lateral border of sternocleidomastoid is palpated. As the operator's finger slides off the posterior border, the anterior scalene muscle is found.
- The operator's finger is slid down the interscalene groove till the supraclavicular area flattens out and the subclavian pulse can be palpated.
- Prepare the skin with 0.5% chlorhexidine in 70% alcohol. Wait until the skin is dry.
- Anaesthetize the skin with a subcutaneous injection of 1% lidocaine at the point of needle insertion.
- The interscalene groove may be lost by the traversing omohyoid muscle.
- The subclavian pulse is also not palpable in all patients.
- At the lowest point that the interscalene groove is palpated, a short-bevelled needle is inserted posterior and medial to the palpating finger in a caudad direction towards the ipsilateral great toe. See Fig. 23.2.
- The needle should *never* be directed medially (keep the hub of the needle against the side of the neck).
- Stimulation of the plexus should give wrist or finger flexion/extension. If no stimulation is found, carefully redirect the needle in the same caudal direction, but from a more anterior, then posterior starting point. If the artery is punctured move more posteriorly.
- Manipulate the needle until stimulation is produced between 0.3mA and 0.5mA. Disconnect syringe before injection to exclude passive reflux of blood and inject 5mL aliquots of LA, aspirating regularly to exclude intravascular injection.
- Use about 0.5mL/kg up to 40mL.

Clinical notes

- As the lower trunk of the plexus tends to sit close to the subclavian artery on the 1st rib it is less reliably blocked. This results in sparing of C8/T1 nerve roots /ulnar nerve (the medial side of the hand and forearm).

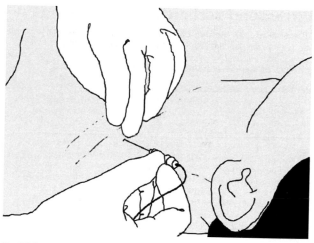

Fig. 23.2 Winnie's subclavian perivascular approach. The middle finger of the left hand is on the subclavian artery.

Ultrasound technique

The ability to easily visualize the brachial plexus, subclavian artery, 1st rib, and pleural with US (Fig. 23.3), make this an attractive block to perform and should reduce the feared risk of pneumothorax. However the close proximity of sensitive anatomy requires excellent needling skills.

Preliminary scan

- The patient should be supine or semi-recumbent with the head turned about 45° away from the side being blocked and the neck muscles should be relaxed.
- The US probe is placed in the supraclavicular fossa, posterior and ~ parallel to the clavicle.
- The subclavian artery is identified as a round (rather than oval), pulsatile, anechoic structure.
- The plexus should be visible immediately posterior or slightly superior and posterior to the artery.
- The plexus often has the appearance of 'a bunch of grapes' and it is difficult to determine individual roots, trunks, divisions, or cords.
- It is *essential* that the probe lies in a plane to see the 1st rib deep to the artery and plexus. This affords some protection if the needle is advanced too far.
- It is *essential* to use colour Doppler to scan the plexus and artery, as branches of the subclavian artery often run through the plexus at this level (see Fig. 23.4). The suprascapular artery and vein, and the transverse cervical artery can also run over the top of the plexus.

US settings

- Probe: high-frequency (>10MHz) linear L38 broadband probe.
- Settings: MB—resolution.
- Depth: 3–4 cm.
- Orientation: sagittal oblique, behind and parallel to clavicle.
- Needle: 50–80mm of choice.

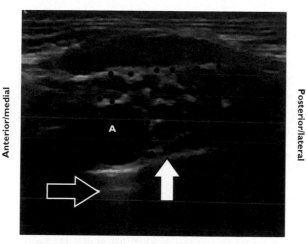

Fig. 23.3 Ultrasound images of the brachial plexus in the supraclavicular fossa. Also shows the 1st rib, pleura, and subclavian artery. Black dots, outline of brachial plexus; A, subclavian artery; White arrow, 1st rib; Black arrow, acoustic shadow.

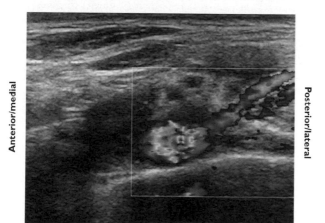

Fig. 23.4 Ultrasound of the supraclavicular fossa showing an artery traversing the brachial plexus.

Technique

- Position patient supine or semi recumbent, with the head turned 30–45° to the opposite side.
- This block should only be performed as an *in-plane* technique to maximize needle visibility.
- Both the medial (anterior) and lateral (posterior) approaches are used (see Fig. 23.5 and Fig. 23.6). The medial approach may be easier ergonomically with the patient supine, although with the patient semi recumbent and the operator standing behind the shoulder (with the US machine on the contralateral side of the patient) the lateral approach is also comfortable.
- It is important to select a plane where the 1st rib is below the plexus and subclavian artery as this gives added protection against pneumothorax if the needle is inadvertently advanced too deep.
- Prepare the skin with 0.5% chlorhexidine in 70% alcohol. Wait until the skin is dry.
- Anaesthetize the skin with a subcutaneous injection of 1% lidocaine at the point of needle insertion.
- Coming from the lateral side, initially direct the needle underneath the plexus and inject small aliquots of LA to lift the plexus off the 1st rib. Then carefully advance the needle tip to the junction of the lower part of the plexus and the subclavian artery and inject some LA at this point. Ideally hydro-dissect the plexus off the artery, then redirect the needle over the top of the plexus, surrounding it with LA. Injection of LA within the plexus is often also done (avoiding nerve structures).
- Coming from the medial/anterior direction, aim to hydro-dissect the plexus off the artery and slide the needle tip over the top and down the posterior side of the artery to reach the lower part of the plexus and inject LA underneath it. Surround the plexus and inject within it as needed.
- The minimum effective volume has been calculated as 32mL, but as always with US, observe the spread of the LA and adjust as needed.
- As always frequent aspiration and fractionated injections are advised, especially when near the artery.
- This block appears easy, but the needle tip must be visible at all times to avoid accidental pneumothorax or arterial puncture.

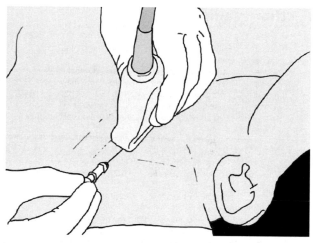

Fig. 23.5 Lateral approach for ultrasound-guided supraclavicular brachial plexus block.

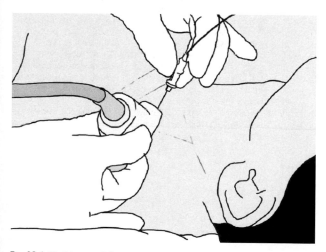

Fig. 23.6 Medial approach for ultrasound-guided supraclavicular brachial plexus block.

Further reading

Brown DL, Cahill DR, Bridenbaugh LD (1993). Supraclavicular nerve block: anatomic analysis of a method to prevent pneumothorax. *Anesth Analg*, **76**(3), 530–4.

Chan VW, Perlas A, Rawson R, *et al.* (2003). Ultrasound-guided supraclavicular brachial plexus block. *Anesth Analg*, **97**(5), 1514–17.

Murata H, Sakai A, Hadzic A, *et al.* (2012). The presence of transverse cervical and dorsal scapular arteries at three ultrasound probe positions commonly used in supraclavicular brachial plexus blockade. *Anesth Analg*, **115**(2), 470–3.

Soares LG, Brull R, Lai J, *et al.* (2007). Eight ball, corner pocket: the optimal needle position for ultrasound-guided supraclavicular block. *Reg Anesth Pain Med*, **32**(1), 94–5.

Tran de QH, Dugani S, Correa JA, *et al.* (2011). Minimum effective volume of lidocaine for ultrasound-guided supraclavicular block. *Reg Anesth Pain Med*, **36**(5), 466–9.

Supraclavicular vs. Interscalene Brachial Plexus Block for Shoulder Surgery ℞ http://www.asra.com/display_spring_2010.php?id=314.Subclaviam

Infraclavicular brachial plexus block

Background

PNS: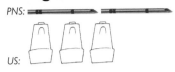

US:

Indications
- Anaesthesia and analgesia of the elbow, distal arm, and hand.

Introduction
A number of approaches to the plexus at this level have been described along the course of the plexus from the middle clavicle point to the axilla, including the vertical infraclavicular block (VIB—Kilka), the coracoid block (Whiffler), the subcoracoid block, the lateral infraclavicular block, and more recently US-guided approaches.

Anatomy
- The cords of the brachial plexus are formed from the divisions of the plexus, which re-unite and enter the infraclavicular region lateral to the axillary artery at the midpoint of the clavicle. See Fig. 24.1.
- The cords are enclosed within a sheath together with the axillary vein and artery.
- The 3 cords are named lateral, medial, and posterior with respect to their orientation to the 2nd part of the axillary artery (behind pectoralis minor).
- Below pectoralis minor the cords give off their terminal branches, which maintain the same relation to the artery as the cords. See Table 24.1.
- As the cords innervate several terminal nerves, patterns of muscle stimulation can be more difficult to determine.

Specific contraindications
- Previous clavicle fracture that has healed with deformity (VIB)—anatomy may be distorted.
- Severe respiratory disease.
- Patients with bullous lung disease—↑ risk of pneumothroax.
- Coagulopathy—the close relationship of the plexus to uncompressible major vessels makes these approaches unwise in the coagulopathic patient.
- Bilateral block.

Complications
- Pneumothorax, although rare (0.2–0.7%), may occur with the VIB, and is usually associated with either too deep or too medial needle placement. There is some evidence this risk may be higher in women. Pneumothorax has also been described for subcoracoid block, but the risk is much lower and may be due to incorrect identification of the coracoid with too medial needle insertion.
- Vascular puncture (subclavian vein or artery) after VIB is associated with too medial needle angulation, and is associated with ↑ risk of pneumothorax. The subclavian vein puncture rate is up to 30%.

- Horner's syndrome, recurrent laryngeal nerve block and phrenic nerve block have been all been reported and are more frequent with the VIB than the subcoracoid approach.

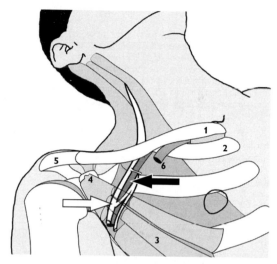

Fig. 24.1 Diagram to show the relationship of the brachial plexus to the axillary artery as they emerge behind the clavicle. **1** clavicle; **2** 1st Rib, **3** pectoralis minor; **4** coracoid process; **5** acromion; **6** axillary vein; Black arrow, axillary artery; White arrow, brachial plexus.

Table 24.1 Brachial plexus cords and their terminal nerves

Lateral cord	Musculocutaneous nerve
	Lateral root of median nerve
	Lateral pectoral nerve
Posterior cord	Radial nerve
	Axillary nerve
	Upper and lower subscapular nerves
	Thoracodorsal nerve
Medial cord	Ulnar nerve
	Medial root of median nerve
	Medial cutaneous nerve of arm
	Medial cutaneous nerve of forearm
	Medial pectoral nerve

Peripheral nerve stimulator technique: vertical infraclavicular block (Kilka)

Landmarks
- Jugular notch.
- Ventral process (most anterior part) of the acromion.
- The needle insertion point is half way along the line between the jugular notch and the ventral process of the acromion.
- A modification has been described to further refine the puncture point—the length of the line joining the ventral process of the acromion and the jugular notch is measured. If this length is <22cm then move the needle insertion point 2mm laterally for every cm less than 22cm. If the length is >22cm, move the insertion point 2mm medially for every cm longer.

Technique
- The patient is positioned supine with no pillow.
- Prior to needle insertion the subclavian pulse is palpated above the clavicle—the insertion point should be lateral to the artery—if not recheck the landmarks.
- Using a Doppler probe, mark the axillary artery, immediately below the clavicle. This marks the most medial place that the plexus can be situated. All 3 cords of the plexus lie lateral to the artery.
- Prepare the skin with 0.5% chlorhexidine in 70% alcohol. Wait until the skin is dry.
- Anaesthetize the skin with a subcutaneous injection of 1% lidocaine at the point of needle insertion.
- Insert a 22G 50mm stimulating needle perpendicular to the skin in all planes, immediately below the inferior surface of the clavicle. See Fig. 24.2.
- The needle is slowly advanced until a suitable motor response (posterior cord–wrist/finger extension) is obtained.
- The plexus is normally found between 2cm to 5cm. The needle is cautiously repositioned to achieve a threshold current of 0.3–0.5mA and after negative aspiration 30–40mL of LA are injected in fractionated doses.
- If no motor response is obtained, first re-insert the needle more laterally (do not angle needle—remove and re-insert). If this is unsuccessful then recheck landmarks, and re-insert slightly medial to the original puncture site.
- Posterior cord stimulation is associated with higher success rates. Note that paradoxically at this point the posterior cord lies lateral relative to the subclavian artery. Lateral cord stimulation (biceps/elbow flexion) should not be accepted as this may be the MCN which can leave the plexus quite proximally and be outside the fascial sheath.
- Onset time should be fast—mean 13.5 minutes.

Clinical notes

• The acromion may be difficult to identify in some patients, and
  following the spine of the scapula anteriorly may help. Do not confuse
  with the humerus—the acromion does not move when the arm is
  rotated.

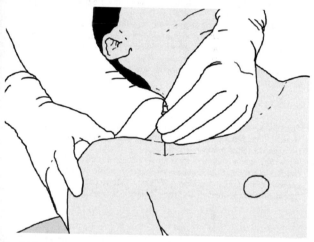

Fig. 24.2 Landmark vertical infraclavicular block. The needle insertion is at the mid
point between anterior acromion and jugular notch, just lateral to the subclavian/
axillary artery Doppler pulse.

Peripheral nerve stimulator technique: subcoracoid

Landmarks
- Midpoint of coracoid process
- Insertion point is 2cm caudad and 1cm medial to the coracoid process.

Technique
- The patient is positioned supine with no pillow, with the arm to be blocked flexed and resting on the abdomen.
- Prepare the skin with 0.5% chlorhexidine in 70% alcohol. Wait until the skin is dry.
- Anaesthetize the skin with a subcutaneous injection of 1% lidocaine at the point of needle insertion.
- A 50–80mm (50mm may be too short in large patients) stimulating needle is inserted in a vertical direction—strictly perpendicular in all planes.
- The needle is advanced until posterior cord stimulation is elicited with a threshold current of 0.3–0.5mA. After negative aspiration 30–40mL of LA are injected in fractionated doses.
- If no stimulation is elicited then the needle is withdrawn and reinserted caudad and then, if no response cephalad from the insertion point.
- Lateral cord stimulation (elbow flexion) is not accepted and the needle is reinserted first deeper, and then if still unsuccessful more cephalad.

Clinical notes
- The coracoid process may be easily found by facing the patient, and grasping the shoulder with an outstretched hand (patient's left shoulder, operator's right hand)—the operator's thumb will naturally tend to fall on the coracoid process, which is often tender to palpation.

Endpoints for nerve stimulation techniques

- The optimum endpoint is posterior cord stimulation (wrist/finger extension).
- Medial cord stimulation (wrist/finger flexion) is also acceptable, particularly if surgery is in ulnar nerve territory.
- Lateral cord stimulation (elbow flexion/wrist pronation) increases the risk of failure—the musculocutaneous nerve may have left the plexus already.

Ultrasound technique

Preliminary scan

- The patient is positioned supine with the arm abducted to 90° (or resting by their side if unable to do so).
- The probe is placed immediately medial to the coracoid process in the parasagittal plane. See Fig. 24.4.
- Identify the pectoralis major and minor muscles superficially and the axillary artery and vein(s) deep to this. The vein is usually caudad relative to the artery.
- The cords of the brachial plexus are seen as either hypoechoic or hyperechoic structures positioned around the axillary artery. The lateral cord is lateral (cephalad) to the artery, the medial cord medial (caudad), and the posterior cord posterior (deep). They can be difficult to visualize but are usually positioned closely to the artery. See Fig. 24.3.

US settings

- Probe: high-frequency (>10MHz) linear L38 broadband probe.
- Settings: MB—resolution/general.
- Depth: 3–6cm.
- Orientation: parasagittal.
- Needle: 50–100mm depending on depth of plexus.

Technique

- An in-plane approach is recommended, inserted from the cephalad end of the transducer. See Fig. 24.4.
- Needle tip visualization may be challenging as the needle angle can be quite steep.
- As the nerves can be difficult to identify a nerve stimulator can be used to confirm that these structures seen are indeed components of the brachial plexus (although this does not necessarily improve success rates).
- Prepare the skin with 0.5% chlorhexidine in 70% alcohol. Wait until the skin is dry.
- Anaesthetize the skin with a subcutaneous injection of 1% lidocaine at the point of needle insertion.
- The needle is first advanced posterolateral to the artery to deposit LA around the posterior cord, 5 o'clock position on artery, Fig. 24.3.
- After careful aspiration LA is injected in small aliquots, observing the spread of the LA which ideally occurs behind and up both sides of the artery forming a 'U' shape around the artery, 1–9 o'clock on Fig. 24.3.
- If medial (caudad) spread is not observed then reinsertion of the needle between the axillary artery and vein, adjacent to the medial cord may be required.
- Volumes of 25mL are satisfactory if appropriate spread is confirmed, although up to 30mL can be used.

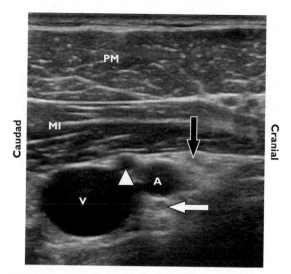

Fig. 24.3 Ultrasound showing the brachial plexus around the axillary artery in the infraclavicular area. PM, pectoralis major muscle; MI, pectoralis minor muscle; A, axillary artery; V, axillary vein; Black arrow, lateral cord; White arrow, posterior cord; White triangle, medial cord.

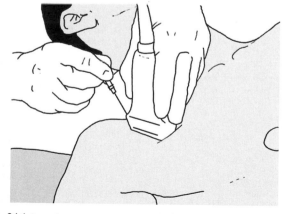

Fig. 24.4 Set up for an in-plane ultrasound-guided infraclavicular brachial plexus block.

Further reading

Borene SC, Edwards JN, Boezaart AP (2004). At the cords, the pinkie towards: Interpreting infracla-vicular motor responses to neurostimulation. *Reg Anesth Pain Med*, **29**(2), 125–9.

Crews JC, Gerancher JC, Weller RS (2007). Pneumothorax after coracoid infraclavicular brachial plexus block. *Anesth Analg*, **105**(1), 275–7.

Dingemans E, Williams S, Arcand G, et al. (2007). Neurostimulation in ultrasound-guided infraclav-icular block: a prospective randomized trial. *Anesth Analg*, **104**(5), 1275–80.

Greher M, Retzl G, Niel P, et al. (2002). Ultrasonographic assessment of topographic anatomy in volunteers suggests a modification of the infraclavicular vertical brachial plexus block. *Br J Anaesth*, **88**(5), 632–6.

Kilka HG, Geiger P, Mehrkens HH (1995). Infraclavicular vertical brachial plexus blockade. A new method for anesthesia of the upper extremity. An anatomical and clinical study. *Der Anaesthesist*, **44**(5), 339–44.

Background

PNS: ▬▬▬▬▬

US:

Indications

- Anaesthesia or analgesia for hand and arm surgery. Virtually any procedure about or below the elbow is suitable.

Introduction

The axillary block is a very safe technique, which does not carry with it the risk of pneumothorax, or phrenic nerve blockade, making it especially suitable for patients with severe respiratory disease. The ability to easily compress the puncture site means that it is the approach to the brachial plexus most suitable for patients with mildly prolonged coagulation.

Descriptions of the relative anatomy can get confusing in the axilla as the 'anatomical position' differs to that in which the block is performed. In the anatomical position the median nerve is described as lateral to the artery but with the shoulder abducted and slightly external rotated, to give access to the axilla, it would now be described as superior to the artery. Similarly, the ulnar nerve on the medial side of the artery, is described as inferior to the artery.

Anatomy

- This approach blocks the brachial plexus at the level of the terminal branches.
- At the level of the axilla the musculocutaneous, median, ulnar, and radial nerve commonly lie in 4 quadrants around the axillary artery (see Fig. 25.1), although this arrangement is subject to interindividual variability.
- In the most common arrangement the musculocutaneous nerve is superior and posterior to the artery, the median nerve superior and anterior, the ulnar nerve inferior and anterior, and the radial nerve inferior and posterior.
- US examination has shown that the nerves are grouped closest together at the proximal edge of the axilla (lateral edge of pectoralis minor) and steadily diverge from the artery as they run distally.
- The median, ulnar, and radial nerves are enclosed together with the axillary artery within a connective tissue sheath derived from the prevertebral fascia. The exact nature of the axillary sheath is contentious—current works suggests it is filled with loose connective tissue with perineural cleavage planes surrounding individual nerves within the sheath. LA spread often occurs better longitudinally than circumferentially within the sheath, explaining the improved success rate of multiple nerve stimulation techniques.
- The musculocutaneous nerve leaves the brachial plexus early and at the level of the axilla is usually located within the coracobrachialis muscle.
- There are often multiple veins accompanying the artery, especially posteriorly and medially.

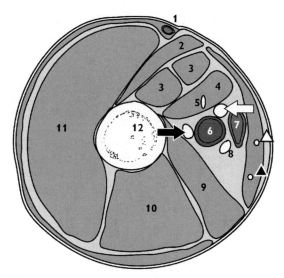

Fig. 25.1 Cross section of the axilla showing the 'usual' position of the nerves around the axillary artery. **1** cephalic vein; **2** pectoris major muscle/tendon; **3** biceps muscle; **4** coracobrachialis muscle; **5** musculocutaneous nerve; **6** axillary artery; **7** axillary vein; **8** ulnar nerve; **9** conjoint tendon latissimus dorsi and teres major muscles; **10** triceps muscle; **11** deltoid muscle; **12** humerus; White arrow, median nerve; Black arrow, radial nerve; White triangle, medial cutaneous nerve of the arm; Black triangle, intercostobrachial nerve.

Side effects and complications

Complications

• Vascular puncture and intravascular injection may lead to systemic LA toxicity.
• Haematoma is rare (0.2% even using a transarterial technique) but may cause vascular insufficiency and compressive nerve injury. The compressible nature of the axillary vessels means that the axillary block is the approach to the brachial plexus most suitable for use in patients with mild coagulation abnormalities.
• Neurological injury—1.2% in 607 patients undergoing repeated axillary block—all resolved within 20 weeks.

Peripheral nerve stimulation: multiple nerve technique

Landmarks
- The axillary artery high in the axilla.
- A good working knowledge of the usual orientation of the 4 main nerves around the axillary artery is essential to accurately target needle placement (subject to interindividual variability).

Technique
- The patient is positioned supine with the shoulder abducted to 90°, externally rotated and the elbow flexed to 90°.
- Prepare the skin with 0.5% chlorhexidine in 70% alcohol. Wait until the skin is dry.
- The axillary artery is palpated high in the axilla and fixed between the index and middle finger. See Fig. 25.2.
- Anaesthetize the skin with a subcutaneous injection of 1% lidocaine at the point of needle insertion.
- Insert a short-bevelled, 50mm 22G stimulating needle immediately above the axillary artery looking for median nerve stimulation (finger and wrist flexion) which should be no more than 1–2cm deep. Carefully manipulate the needle until stimulating current is between 0.3mA and 0.5mA. After careful aspiration, 15mL of LA is injected in 5mL aliquots.
- The needle is then withdrawn, angled slightly superiorly and advanced deeper, into the substance of the coracobrachialis muscle. Biceps contraction confirms musculocutaneous stimulation. Carefully manipulate the needle until stimulating current is between 0.3mA and 0.5mA. After careful aspiration, 6mL of LA are injected.

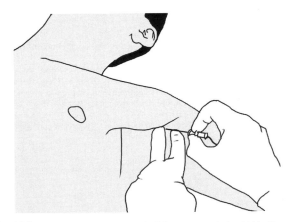

Fig. 25.2 Axillary brachial plexus block. Both fingers are on the brachial/axillary artery.

- Finally the needle is redirected underneath and slightly posterior to the axillary artery and radial nerve stimulation (wrist and finger extension) is elicited. (A transarterial approach, deliberately passing through the artery has been described but is not recommended.) Carefully manipulate the needle until stimulating current is between 0.3mA and 0.5mA. After careful aspiration, 15mL of LA is injected in 5mL aliquots. Triceps contraction alone should not be accepted as this may reflect direct stimulation of the branch of the radial nerve to the triceps muscle and may lead to inadequate block.
- Unless surgery is being performed on the ulnar territory, there is little to be gained by selectively blocking the ulnar nerve, as ulnar nerve blockade is usually accomplished either by spread of LA from the radial and/or median nerve injections. However, the ulnar nerve can be located inferior and superficial to the artery, with stimulation producing finger flexion and ulnar flexion of the wrist.

Clinical notes

- Some anaesthetists also like to block the intercostobrachial nerve (T2) and medial cutaneous nerve of the arm in an attempt to limit tourniquet pain. This is accomplished by subcutaneous infiltration of LA across the width of the proximal arm. However, tourniquet pain is multifactorial and predominantly influenced by muscle ischaemia, and it is questionable whether this cutaneous anaesthesia offers any benefit.
- Acceptance of stimulation of the musculocutaneous nerve (biceps twitch) in a single injection technique will result in a high incidence of block failure because it lies outside the fascial sheath. Conversely, failure to block musculocutaneous nerve is common with axillary blocks, and if required blockade of the musculocutaneous nerve is best achieved by separate injection into the coracobrachialis muscle.
- Numerous studies have shown that the success rate and speed of block onset can be improved by stimulating more than 1 of the nerves of the plexus and splitting administration of the anaesthetic dose between the sites. The optimum sequence appears to be blockade of 3 nerves (median, radial, and musculocutaneous). Omission of ulnar nerve block does not affect the latency of block onset or extent of block, but reduces block performance time, and pain during block. If a single injection technique is to be performed, the highest success rates are associated with a radial nerve response.
- In some patients the artery may be difficult to identify and either US, or observation of the disappearance of the pulse oximeter waveform in response to digital pressure, may be helpful in pinpointing the exact location.
- Over abduction of the arm may cause the axillary pulse to disappear.
- With either a multiple nerve stimulation technique or US, as little as 5mL of LA per nerve may be required. For single injection techniques volumes of 30–40mL are usually used.
- The multiple stimulation technique allows long-acting LA to be placed on the nerves supplying the principal area of surgery, with short-acting LA used elsewhere.
- LA additive agents are not routinely required, but clonidine in doses up to 150 micrograms, has been shown to prolong the duration of analgesia.

Ultrasound technique

Preliminary scan

- The relatively superficial nature of the brachial plexus around the axillary artery, and the absence of bony structures to impair the image make high-resolution US imaging of this block possible.
- A further rotation to the orientation occurs as the probe is placed transversely in the axialla. This changes superior and inferior to left and right on the screen.
- Identify the axillary artery as a pulsatile anechoic circular structure and confirm with colour flow. Multiple axillary veins may be seen in some individuals, but beware that these are easily compressed by the probe and may not be visible. Reduce probe pressure to locate the veins.
- The wedge-shaped conjoint tendon of latissimus dorsi and teres major, inserting into the humerus deep to the plexus and artery, indicates the inferior (medial) side.
- The radial, median, and ulnar nerves may be identified in cross section around the axillary artery as hypoechic round/oval shaped structures (Fig. 25.3). There is often a speckled or fibrillar pattern within the nerves.
- Scanning distally helps to identify the nerves.
- The ulnar nerve moves more inferiorly (medially) and runs superficially down to the cubital tunnel at the elbow.
- The median nerve stays adjacent to the artery, but will pass from the lateral to medial side where it sits in the antecubical fossa. It will usually cross superficially, but it can pass deep to the artery.
- The musculocutaneous nerve is usually easily visible as a bright hyperechoic (flattened) structure within the coracobrachialis muscle a bit more distally, which then passes between coracobrachialis muscle and biceps muscle.
- The radial nerve can sometimes be difficult to visualize; avoid mistaking the postcystic enhancement of the axillary artery as the radial nerve. It must sit superficial to the conjoint tendon of latissimus dorsi and teres major, and scanning distally it descends deep towards the humerus accompanied by the profunda brachii artery.

US settings

- Probe: high-frequency (>10MHz) linear L38 broadband probe.
- Settings: MB—resolution.
- Depth: 2–3cm.
- Orientation: transverse in axilla (parallel to axillary crease).
- Needle: 50mm of choice.

Technique

- An in-plane approach from the superior aspect is recommended, although both an out-of-plane approach and an in-plane inferior approach have been used.

- A 50mm 22G needle is advanced in line with the US beam adjacent to each of the nerves, and 5–10mL of LA deposited around each nerve to achieve good circumferential spread.
- Nerve stimulation may be used to confirm that the structures blocked are indeed the expected nerves.
- If necessary, reposition the needle to ensure LA spread around both sides of the nerve.

Benefits of ultrasound

Whether US guidance can increase the success rate and reduce complications of axillary block compared to multiple nerve stimulation techniques is still not clearly established. Chan demonstrated ↑ success using US, but their success rates for conventional stimulator-guided block were lower than reported in other papers. Casati failed to demonstrate any difference between US and multiple nerve stimulation in terms of success rates and complications (see ➔ Further reading, p. 310).

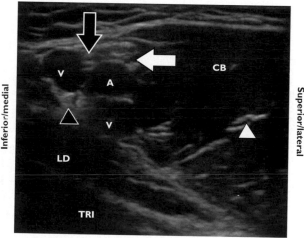

Fig. 25.3 Ultrasound of the axilla showing the typical arrangement of the nerves around the axillary artery. Black arrow, ulnar nerve; White arrow, median nerve; V, axillary veins; A, axillary artery; Black triangle, radial nerve; CB, coracobrachialis muscle; White arrow, musculocutaneous nerve; LD, conjoint tendon latissimus dorsi and teres major muscles; TRI, triceps muscle.

Further reading

Casati A, Danelli G, Baciarello M, *et al.* (2007). A prospective, randomized comparison between ultrasound and nerve stimulation guidance for multiple injection axillary brachial plexus block. *Anesthesiology*, **106**(5), 992–6.

Chan VW, Perlas A, McCartney CJ, *et al.* (2007). Ultrasound guidance improves success rate of axillary brachial plexus block. *Can J Anaesth*, **54**(3), 176–82.

Franco CD, Rahman A, Voronov G, *et al.* (2008). Gross anatomy of the brachial plexus sheath in human cadavers. *Reg Anesth Pain Med*, **33**(1), 64–9.

Horlocker TT, Kufner RP, Bishop AT, *et al.* (1999). The risk of persistent paresthesia is not increased with repeated axillary block. *Anesth Analg*, **88**(2), 382–7.

Retzl G, Kapral S, Greher M, *et al.* (2001). Ultrasonographic findings of the axillary part of the brachial plexus. *Anesth Analg*, **92**(5), 1271–5.

Rodríguez J, Taboada M, Del Río S, *et al.* (2005). A comparison of four stimulation patterns in axillary block. *Reg Anesth Pain Med*, **30**(4), 324–8.

Mid-humeral block

Background

PNS:

US:

Introduction

- This approach to the brachial plexus was first described by Dupré in 1994. Described as the humeral canal block.
- This block is carried out at the junction of the middle and upper thirds of the humerus. This point corresponds to the insertion of deltoid into the humerus.
- This is a technically more difficult block than the axillary, as the nerves are further apart and diffusion of LA from one nerve to the other is less likely.

Anatomy

As the major nerves of the brachial plexus leave the axilla, they separate from the brachial artery (see Fig. 26.1):

- The median nerve starts to move from a lateral position becoming superficial to the artery and by the antecubital fossa it becomes medial.
- The musculocutaneous nerve moves more lateral as it moves distal in the arm, lying between biceps and coracobrachialis.
- The ulnar nerve moves more medially towards the cubital tunnel as it moves distally in the arm.
- The radial nerve moves deep towards the spiral groove of the humerus. It runs posteriorly and emerges on the lateral aspect of the arm.

Side effects and complications

Complications

- Vascular puncture. This is no more likely than any other upper arm block.

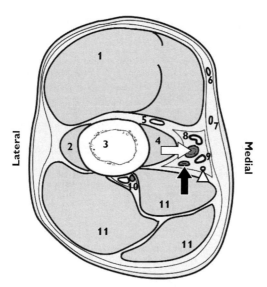

Fig. 26.1 Cross-sectional anatomy. 1 biceps muscle; 2 deltoid muscle; 3 humerus;
4 coracobrachialis muscle; 5 musculocutaneous nerve; 6 intercostal brachial nerve;
7 medial cutaneous nerve of arm; 8 median nerve; 9 ulnar nerve; White arrow,
brachial artery; Black arrow, cephalic vein; White triangle, medial cutaneous nerve of
forearm; 10 radial nerve with profunda brachii artery; 11 triceps.

Peripheral stimulator technique

Landmarks

- Divide the humerus into thirds, marking the junction of the upper and middle thirds. This point corresponds to the insertion of deltoid into the humerus. See Fig. 26.2.
- Palpate the brachial artery at this point.

Technique

- With the patient supine, abduct the shoulder to 90°. It is helpful to also have the elbow flexed.
- Prepare the skin with 0.5% chlorhexidine in 70% alcohol. Wait until the skin is dry.
- Anaesthetize the skin with a subcutaneous injection of 1% lidocaine superficial to the brachial artery. All the 4 nerves should be able to be blocked from the same skin puncture.
- Use a 5mm short-bevel stimulating needle.

Median nerve

Angle the needle proximally towards the axilla and, initially, to the lateral border of the artery. The nerve is frequently adherent to the artery at this level. If appropriate motor stimulation is not found, then angle the needle to lie superficial to the artery and then slightly medial to it. Once appropriate motor response is found—flexion of wrist and fingers/pronation of wrist—carefully manipulate the needle until stimulating current is between 0.3mA and 0.5mA. After careful aspiration, 8–10mL of LA is injected in 4–5mL aliquots.

Ulnar nerve

Direct the needle medial to the artery. The ulnar nerve almost always lies just medial to the artery as it moves towards the cubital tunnel. Once appropriate motor response is found—flexion of fingers and wrist (look for contraction of flexor carpi ulnaris)—carefully manipulate the needle until stimulating current is between 0.3mA and 0.5mA. After careful aspiration, 8–10mL of LA is injected in 4–5mL aliquots.

Radial nerve

Redirect the needle medial to the artery to the medial aspect of the humerus. Once appropriate motor response is found—extension of wrist and fingers—carefully manipulate the needle until stimulating current is between 0.3mA and 0.5mA. After careful aspiration, 8–10mL of LA is injected in 4–5mL aliquots.

Musculocutaneous nerve

Bring the needle back to skin. Redirect the needle to lateral to the artery aiming just lateral to the humerus. Once appropriate motor response is found—flexion of elbow—carefully manipulate the needle until stimulating current is between 0.3mA and 0.5mA. After careful aspiration, 8–10mL of LA is injected in 4–5mL aliquots.

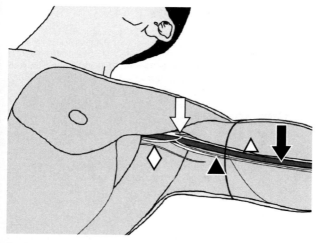

Fig. 26.2 Landmarks for the mid-humeral block. Black circle, insertion of deltoid muscle; Black arrow, brachial artery; White arrow, musculocutaneous nerve; White triangle, median nerve; Black triangle, ulnar nerve; White diamond, intercostal brachial nerve.

Ultrasound technique

As this block is a distal axillary block the US technique will be similar as for an US-guided axillary block. Although one of the benefits of US is the ability to block a nerve anywhere along its course, at this point however, the nerves with be separated and the radial nerve will be much more difficult to visualize. For those reasons it is not a common block performed under US.

Further reading

Dupré LJ (1994). Bloc du plexus brachial au canal huméral. *Can Anesthesiol*, **42**(6), 767–9.

Elbow and forearm blocks

General background

PNS:

US:

Introduction

- Blockade of the terminal branches of the plexus may be achieved at or below the elbow.
- Variations in the innervation of the distal arm, overlap of areas of innervation and the lack of tourniquet coverage, mean that these blocks are best suited to providing postoperative analgesia. It is unwise to rely on selective blockade of one nerve for surgical anaesthesia alone.
- The combination of a proximal brachial plexus block with a short-acting LA agent together with distal blocks with longer-acting LAs to provide postoperative analgesia is popular with some anaesthetists.
- Elbow/forearm blocks are also useful for supplementing incomplete proximal brachial plexus blocks.
- The use of US has revolutionized the ease and reliability with which these blocks may be performed.

Cutaneous nerves

- Medial cutaneous nerve of the forearm (from medial cord).
- Lateral cutaneous nerve of the forearm (from musculocutaneous nerve).
- Posterior cutaneous nerve of the forearm (from redial nerve).
- These can all be blocked by subcutaneous infiltration in the appropriate areas around the elbow.

Side effects and complications

Complications

- Nil specific.
- Vascular puncture and injection, especially median nerve at the elbow.
- Nerve damage.

Background: radial nerve block

Indications

- Postoperative analgesia in radial nerve territory in association with GA or more proximal short-acting plexus block.
- Supplementation of incomplete proximal plexus block.

Anatomy

The radial nerve descends down the upper arm in the spiral groove accompanied by the profunda brachii vessel. After emerging from the spiral groove, the nerve pierces the lateral intermuscular septum and enters the anterior compartment of the arm, running between brachialis and brachioradialis. The nerve passes in front of the lateral epicondyle of the humerus to enter the forearm where it bifurcates into a superficial (sensory) and deep branch (mainly motor).

The superficial radial nerve travels along the lateral aspect of the forearm beneath the brachioradialis muscle, and lies lateral to the adjacent radial artery, before splitting into lateral and medial branches, which are sensory to the base of the thumb, the dorsum of the hand, and the dorsum of the index, middle, and ring fingers.

The deep branch of the radial nerve enters the extensor compartment through the supinator muscle and becomes the posterior interosseous nerve, supplying the extensors of the wrist, thumb, and fingers. The posterior interosseous nerve also has sensory branches to the interosseous membrane and the articulation between the radius and ulna.

Peripheral nerve stimulator technique

Landmarks

- Brachioradialis and biceps tendon.

Technique

- With the arm supinated, palpate the groove between brachioradialis and biceps tendon 1.5–2cm proximal to the elbow crease.
- Prepare the skin with 0.5% chlorhexidine in 70% alcohol. Wait until the skin is dry.
- Anaesthetize the skin with a subcutaneous injection of 1% lidocaine at the point of needle insertion.
- Insert a 22G 50mm stimulating needle and advanced towards the lateral epicondyle of the humerus.
- The nerve is usually found at a depth of 2–4cm. The needle is re-positioned to achieve optimal motor stimulation at 0.3–0.5mA. Thumb extension is essential.
- 5mL of LA is usually sufficient.

Ultrasound technique: radial nerve

- The radial nerve may be blocked either proximal to the elbow after it has emerged from the spiral groove of the humerus, or just distal to the elbow as it splits into its deep and superficial branches. The proximal approach is recommended.

Preliminary scan
- The US probe is placed on the lateral aspect of the arm 3–5cm proximal to the lateral epicondyle. See Fig. 27.1.
- Identify the radial nerve which can be seen as a round/oval hypoechoic structure ~1–2cm deep. See Fig. 27.2.
- Follow the nerve as it wraps around to the anterior side of the elbow to sit between brachialis and brachioradialis.
- Use colour Doppler to identify any accompanying blood vessels.

US settings
- Probe: high-frequency (>10MHz) linear L38 broadband probe
- Settings: MB—resolution
- Depth: 2–3cm
- Orientation: transverse
- Needle: 50mm of choice.

Technique
- Prepare the skin with 0.5% chlorhexidine in 70% alcohol. Wait until the skin is dry.
- Anaesthetize the skin with a subcutaneous injection of 1% lidocaine at the point of needle insertion.
- An in-plane approach allows maximal visualization of the needle tip.
- 5mL of LA is placed around the nerve under US guidance.

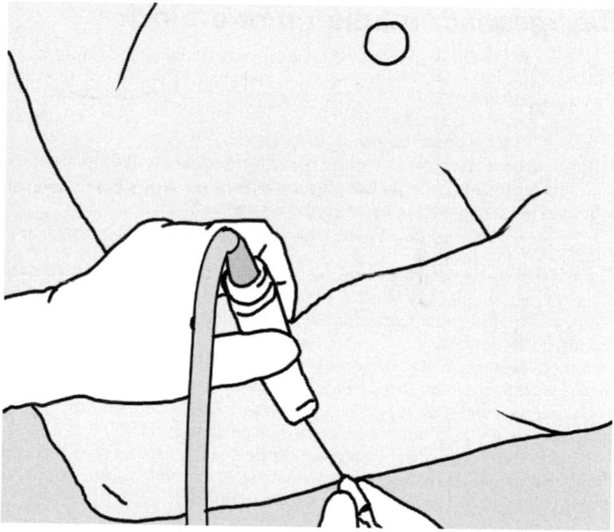

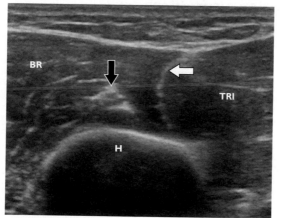

Fig. 27.1 Set up for ultrasound-guided radial nerve block just proximal to the elbow.

Fig. 27.2 Ultrasound image of the radial nerve just proximal to the elbow. BR, brachioradialis muscle; TRI, triceps muscle; Black arrow, radial nerve; H, humerus; White arrow, lateral intermuscular septum.

Background: median nerve block

Indications
- Anaesthesia for surgery on lateral aspect of palm and palmar surface of thumb, index, and middle fingers.
- Anaesthesia for carpel tunnel decompression.
- Postoperative analgesia in median nerve territory in association with GA or more proximal short-acting plexus block.
- Supplementation of incomplete proximal plexus block.

Anatomy
The median nerve lies lateral to the artery in the axilla but then crosses (usually) the anterior surface of the artery to lie medial to the brachial artery in the distal upper arm medial to the biceps brachii tendon and on the brachialis muscles.

In the antecubital fossa the nerve is immediately medial to the artery, and then descends between the 2 heads of pronator teres.

The nerve continues in the forearm sandwiched between flexor digitorum superficialis (FDS) and flexor digitorum profundus (FDP).

A palmar cutaneous branch is given off before the nerve passes through the carpal tunnel. At this point the median nerve lies deep to, and lateral to Palmaris Longus and medial to Flexor Carpi Radialis.

Peripheral nerve stimulator technique: median nerve block

Landmarks
- Brachial artery at the elbow.

Technique
- Prepare the skin with 0.5% chlorhexidine in 70% alcohol. Wait until the skin is dry.
- Anaesthetize the skin with a subcutaneous injection of 1% lidocaine at the point of needle insertion.
- With the arm supinated, a 22G 25–50mm stimulating needle is inserted at a point just medial to the brachial artery, at the elbow crease and angled cephalad with a 45° angle to the skin.
- Median nerve stimulation (finger flexion) at 0.3–0.5mA is sought. Alternatively paraesthesiae in the thumb or index finger is an acceptable endpoint.
- 5mL of LA is adequate.

Ultrasound technique: median nerve

Preliminary scan

- The median nerve is most easily identified below the elbow crease as an oval hyperechoic structure medial to the brachial artery.
- Following it down the forearm, it initially descends deep to the flexor muscles and can be difficult to see with US.
- In the middle 1/3 of the forearm it can be readily identified as an oval/round hyperechoic structure with a fascicular pattern between the muscle bellies of FDS and FDP. This is a good place to block the nerve as there are no immediately adjacent vascular structures. See Fig. 27.3.
- The nerve displays a significant degree of anisotropy here so careful tilting of the probe may be required to get a good image.

US settings

- Probe: high-frequency (>10MHz) linear L38 broadband probe.
- Settings: MB—resolution.
- Depth: 2–3cm.
- Orientation: transverse.
- Needle: 50mm of choice.

Technique

- Prepare the skin with 0.5% chlorhexidine in 70% alcohol. Wait until the skin is dry.
- Anaesthetize the skin with a subcutaneous injection of 1% lidocaine at the point of needle insertion.
- An in-plane approach allows maximal visualization of the needle tip.
- 5mL of LA is placed around the nerve under US guidance.

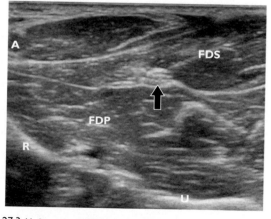

Fig. 27.3 Median nerve mid forearm. FDS, flexor digitorum superficialis muscle; A, radial artery; Black arrow, median nerve; FDP, flexor digitorum profundus muscle; R, radius; U, ulna.

Background: ulnar nerve block

Indications
- Anaesthesia for surgery on little finger, or 5th ray.
- Postoperative analgesia in ulnar nerve territory in association with GA or more proximal short-acting plexus block.
- Supplementation of incomplete proximal plexus block.

Anatomy
The ulnar nerve runs superficially along the medial/posterior aspect of the arm, then passes behind the medial epicondyle, through the cubital tunnel.

It then enters the anterior compartment of the forearm between the heads of flexor carpi ulnaris and runs alongside the ulnar aspect of the forearm. It soon joins with the ulnar artery, and the two travel distally together, deep to the flexor carpi ulnaris muscle on the medial edge of FDP.

The ulnar nerve and artery pass superficial to the flexor retinaculum via Guyon's canal before entering the palm of the hand. Sensory innervation is to the medial 1½ digits.

Peripheral nerve stimulator technique: ulnar nerve

- The ulnar nerve is most conveniently blocked just 2cm proximal to the ulnar groove.
- The arm is flexed to facilitate identification of the ulnar groove. A 22G 50mm stimulating needle is inserted at a 45° angle along the line joining the ulnar groove and the axilla.
- Injection at the level of the ulnar groove is not recommended due to the theoretical risk of a compressive neuropathy (although this is unsubstantiated by case reports).
- The nerve will usually be encountered at a depth of 1–3cm, and needle position is adjusted until ulnar nerve response (4th + 5th digit flexion, and thumb adduction) is obtained at 0.3–0.5mA.
- Again 5mL of LA is sufficient.

Ultrasound-guided technique: ulnar nerve

- The ulnar nerve may be blocked anywhere along its course, but is most conveniently blocked in the proximal forearm, before it joins with the ulnar artery.

Preliminary scan

- Abduct the arm and externally rotate as tolerated.
- Place the probe transversely on the anterior-medial side of the forearm.
- Identify the round/oval hyperechoic structure often with a fascicular pattern.
- Scanning distally the ulna artery should join it from the lateral side.
- Return more proximally until the artery has moved away from the nerve. See Fig. 27.4.
- Alternatively, identify the nerve and artery more distally, under the tendon of flexor carpi ulnaris and follow them back more proximally.

US setting

- Probe: high-frequency (>10MHz) linear L38 broadband probe
- Settings: MB—resolution
- Depth: 2–3cm
- Orientation: transverse
- Needle: 50mm of choice.

Technique

- Prepare the skin with 0.5% chlorhexidine in 70% alcohol. Wait until the skin is dry.
- Anaesthetize the skin with a subcutaneous injection of 1% lidocaine at the point of needle insertion.
- An in-plane approach allows maximal visualization of the needle tip, ideally from the medial side (so as not to pass near the artery), if this is ergonomic.
- 5mL of LA is placed around the nerve under US guidance.

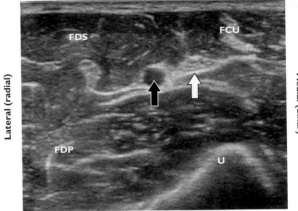

Fig. 27.4 Ulnar nerve mid forearm. FDS, flexor digitorum superficialis muscle; FCU, flexor carpi ulnaris muscle; FDP, flexor digitorum profundus muscle; White arrow, ulnar nerve; Black arrow, ulnar artery; U, ulna.

Further reading

McCartney C, Xu D, Constantinescu C, *et al.* (2007). Ultrasound examination of peripheral nerves in the forearm. *Reg Anesth Pain Med*, **32**(9), 434–9.

Wrist, hand, and finger blocks

Background

Landmarks/PNS: ━━━━━ ━━━━

US:

Indications

- Sensory block of the hand for surgery, especially useful when movement is desirable during surgery, such as tenolysis.
- Post-op analgesia. Patients generally dislike prolonged motor block after hand surgery. A proximal short-acting block, with distal (wrist) block of operative dermatome can be useful.
- Top-up of partial proximal block (failed block).

Introduction

- Distal arm blocks are useful for providing analgesia with minimal motor loss.
- Surgery of the hand can be successfully carried out with wrist blocks, but if a tourniquet is required, it will need to be distal—either at the wrist or on individual fingers.
- Median, ulnar, and radial nerves all innervate part of the hand.

Anatomy

The median nerve

- It enters the forearm lying on the medial side of the brachial artery. It passes through the 2 heads of pronator teres, it then passes deep to the superficial flexors. As the nerve approaches the distal forearm it becomes superficial travelling between the superficial flexors and flexor carpi radialis.
- After passing through pronator teres the anterior interosseous nerve separates from the median nerve supplying forearm flexor muscles.
- At the palmar crease it lies between the palmaris longis and flexor carpi radialis tendons. See Fig. 28.1.
- The median nerve gives off a small palmar cutaneous branch that travels over the flexor retinaculum, supplying the skin of the thenar eminence.
- The median nerve traverses the carpal tunnel, with the cutaneous supply to the palm and palmar surface of thumb, and the radial 2½ fingers and the dorsal aspect of the same digits from tip to approximately the distal interphalangeal joints.

The ulnar nerve

- It passes through the cubital tunnel, posterior to the medial epicondyle of the humerus. It passes between the heads of flexor carpi ulnaris (FCU), travelling deep to FCU and superficial to flexor digitorum profundus.
- At the wrist it lies medial (ulnar) to the ulnar artery, underneath the tendon of FCU. See Fig. 28.1.

- The dorsal branch arises about 5cm proximal to the wrist, which supplies the dorsum of the medial 1½ fingers.
- Cutaneous supply is to the ulnar border of the hand and ulnar 1½ fingers.

The radial nerve

- It enters the anterior compartment of the forearm crossing the anterior aspect of the lateral epicondyle of the humerus piercing supinator.
- The posterior cutaneous branch descends along the posterior aspect of the forearm to the wrist supplying the skin along its course.
- The superficial radial nerve descends under brachioradialis, emerging in the distal part of the forearm to cross the anatomical snuff box, supplying the dorsal aspect of the hand not supplied by the median and ulnar nerves, although there is considerable overlap.
- The deep branch of the radial nerve is the direct continuation of the radial nerve. After piercing supinator muscle it winds around the neck of the radius entering the posterior compartment supplying the extensor muscle of the hand.
- The posterior interosseous nerve is the terminal branch of the deep branch and ends on the interosseous membrane.

Side effects and complications

Complications

- Intravascular injection
- Nerve damage
- Finger ischaemia.

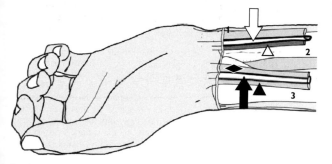

Fig. 28.1 Anatomy of the wrist, showing the median and ulnar nerves. **1** flexor carpi ulnaris tendon; White arrow, ulnar nerve; White triangle, ulnar artery; **2** ulna; Black diamond, palmaris longus tendon; Black arrow, median nerve; Black triangle, flexor carpi radialis tendon; **3** radius.

Landmark techniques

Median nerve

- Measure 5cm proximal to the wrist crease, between the palmaris longus and flexor carpi radialis tendons.
- Prepare the skin with 0.5% chlorhexidine in 70% alcohol. Wait until the skin is dry.
- Anaesthetize the skin with a subcutaneous injection of 1% lidocaine at the point of needle insertion.
- Insert a 25–50mm short-bevel needle on the lateral side of palmaris longus tendon (or medial to flexor carpi radialis tendon if absent).
- Insert by ~ 5mm avoiding paraesthesia.
- Nerve stimulation will cause finger flexion and thumb opposition.

Ulnar nerve

- The approach is 5cm proximal to the wrist crease on the ulnar side of the wrist, to block the dorsal branch.
- Prepare the skin with 0.5% chlorhexidine in 70% alcohol. Wait until the skin is dry.
- Anaesthetize the skin with a subcutaneous injection of 1% lidocaine at the point of needle insertion.
- Insert the block needle immediately lateral to the FCU tendon. See Fig. 28.2.
- Look for flexion of the little finger with stimulation.

Radial nerve

- There is no motor component to the superficial radial nerve—nerve stimulation is not normally used.
- Inject about 3mL of LA subcutaneously in a sausage across the lateral aspect of the distal forearm 5cm proximal to the anatomical snuff box. See Fig. 28.3.

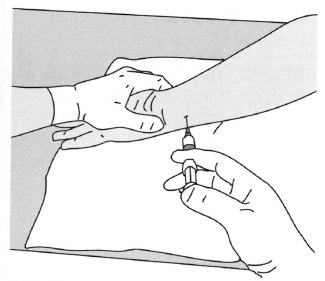

Fig. 28.2 Performance of an ulnar nerve block at the left wrist. The thumb of the left hand is palpating the edge of the flexor carpi ulnaris tendon.

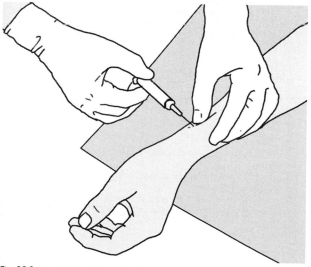

Fig. 28.3 Superficial radial nerve block.

Ultrasound technique

Preliminary scan

Median nerve

- Identify the nerve in the middle 1/3 of the forearm where it can be readily identified as an oval/round hyperechoic structure with a fascicular pattern between the muscle bellies of flexor digitorum superficialis and flexor digitorum profunda. The nerve displays a significant degree of anisotropy here so careful tilting of the probe may be required to get a good image.
- Follow it distally until it lies about 5cm proximal to the wrist crease, before the cutaneous branch separates. See Fig. 28.4.
- More distally, under the flexor retinaculum, the nerve is more difficult to distinguish from the flexor tendons. See Fig. 28.5.

Ulnar nerve

- Place the probe on the medial aspect of the forearm.
- Identify the ulnar artery. The nerve is a triangular-shaped hyperechoic structure on the medial aspect of the artery, underneath the tendon of FCU. See Fig. 28.6.

Superficial radial nerve

- Track the radial nerve distally from the elbow—see ➲ Ultrasound technique: radial nerve, p. 320.
- The superficial and deep branches split in the antecubital fossa. The superficial redial nerve then joins the lateral side of the radial artery continuing distally under brachioradialis muscle.
- It emerges from below brachioradialis about 2.5cm proximal to the anatomical snuff-box.
- The nerve can be seen as a bundle of 3–4 'bubbles' sitting subcutaneously. See Fig. 28.7.

US settings

- Probe: high-frequency (>10MHz) linear L38 broadband probe
- Settings: MB—resolution
- Depth: 2–3cm
- Orientation: transverse
- Needle: 25–50mm of choice.

Technique

- Prepare the skin with 0.5% chlorhexidine in 70% alcohol. Wait until the skin is dry.
- Anaesthetize the skin with a subcutaneous injection of 1% lidocaine at the point of needle insertion.
- Either an in-plane or out-of-plane approach can be used.
- 1–3mL of LA should be sufficient for each nerve.

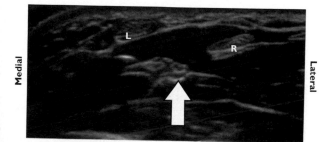

Fig. 28.4 Ultrasound of median nerve. L, palmaris longus tendon; R, flexor carpi radialis tendon; White arrow, median nerve.

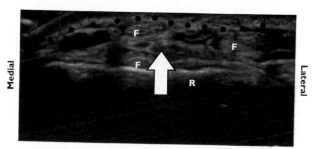

Fig. 28.5 Ultrasound of median nerve under the flexor retinaculum. Black dots, flexor retinaculum; White arrow, median nerve; F, flexor tendons; R, radial head.

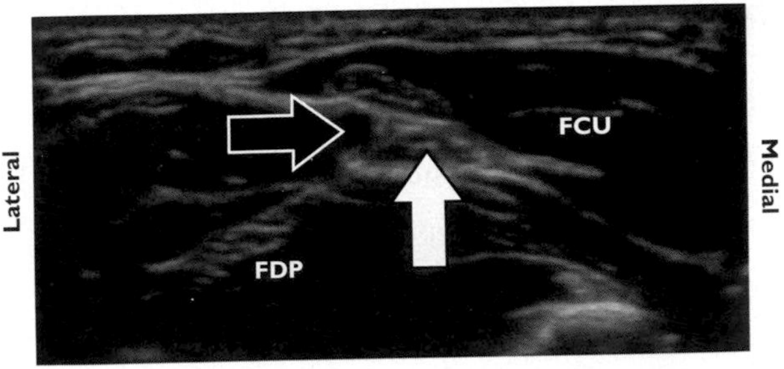

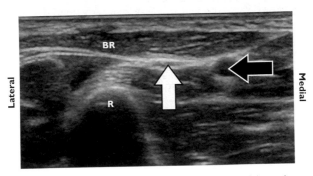

Fig. 28.6 Ultrasound of the ulnar nerve at the wrist. FCU, flexor carpi ulnaris muscle/tendon; Black arrow, ulnar artery; White arrow, ulnar nerve; FDP, flexor digitorum profundus muscle.

Fig. 28.7 Ultrasound of the superficial radial nerve. BR, brachio-radialis muscle; White arrow, superficial radial nerve; Black arrow, radial artery; R, radius.

Digital block

Anatomy

- The fingers are innervated by the palmar digital branches of the median and ulnar nerves.
- They run down both sides of each finger, along the palmar aspect, alongside the digital arteries.
- The skin of the dorsum of the fingers is also supplied by cutaneous branches of the ulnar and radial nerves via the dorsum of the hand.

Ring blocks

- Are generally painful, but work effectively.
- Place the hand palmar surface down.
- Prepare the skin with 0.5% chlorhexidine in 70% alcohol. Wait until the skin is dry.
- Insert a 27G needle vertically down the side of the base of the proximal phalanx, almost to the palmar surface.
- Aspirate to exclude intravascular needle position and inject 0.5–1mL of LA.
- Repeat on the other side of the finger.
- Continue to inject LA as you withdraw the needle and complete the 'ring' by injecting subcutaneously along the dorsum of the finger.

Web-space blocks

- Can be less painful than ring blocks.
- Place the hand palmar surface down, with your non-dominant index finger on the palm just proximal to the metacarpal heads.
- Prepare the skin with 0.5% chlorhexidine in 70% alcohol. Wait until the skin is dry.
- Insert a 27G needle distally into the web space between the fingers with the needle pointing towards the palm (the tip of your finger) injecting LA as you insert the needle.
- When you feel the LA filling the space just deep to the palmar surface, stop advancing the needle.
- Inject 2–3mL of LA. This will anaesthetize the digital nerve as it separates to the 2 fingers either side of the needle.
- A partial ring block is required for the outer surface of the little and index fingers.

Clinical notes

Avoiding epinephrine for extremity blocks is weakly supported by limited numbers of case reports involving unknown concentrations of epinephrine and other confounding variables (e.g. infection). No case reports of digital gangrene exist following the use of commercial preparations of lidocaine with epinephrine and there are case series and RCTs to support its routine use. As always, a balance of risk should be struck between the risks of epinephrine in LAs and the potential advantages it may bring (the avoidance of mechanical tourniquets and prolonged analgesia).

Further reading

Denkler K (2001). A comprehensive review of epinephrine in the finger: to do or not to do. *Plast Reconstr Surg*, **108**(1), 114–24.

Knoop K, Trott A, Syverud S (1994). Comparison of digital versus metacarpal block for repair of finger injuries. *Ann Emerg Med*, **23**(6) 1296–300.

McCartney C, Xu D, Constantinescu C, *et al.* (2007). Ultrasound examination of peripheral nerves in the forearm. *Reg Anesth Pain Med*, **32**(5), 434–9.

Thomson CJ, Lalonde DH (2006). Randomised double-blind comparison of duration of anaesthesia among three commonly used agents in digital nerve block. *Plast Reconstr Surg*, **118**(2), 429–32.

Intravenous regional anaesthesia (Bier's block)

Background

Indications
- Surgery on the limb distal to the cuff, such as fracture manipulation, minor hand surgery.
- Up to 40 minutes' duration.
- Note that the anaesthesia rapidly diminishes when the cuffs are deflated. Therefore supplemental LA (infiltration or nerve block) may need to be used.

Introduction
- August Bier is credited with being the first physician to use this technique, in 1908.
- Bier used procaine 0.25% to 0.5%.
- In the UK prilocaine is now almost exclusively used, and in the USA lignocaine.

Anatomy
The local anaesthetic appears to work by 2 mechanisms:
- Firstly by direct action on the tissues in the exsanguinated limb.
- Secondly by action on the nerves running through these tissues.

Specific contraindications
- Patient refusal.
- Severe vascular disease/ischaemia, crush injury.

Relative contraindication
- Sickle cell disease.
- Uncontrolled hypertension as it is difficult to get the tourniquet pressure sufficiently above the blood pressure.
- Obesity—the tourniquet often simply acts as a venous tourniquet causing a swollen bruised limb.

Technique

- It is important to give the patient a good explanation of the technique as initially the tourniquet and ischaemia can be uncomfortable or painful, before the LA takes effect.
- For simple procedures, where there is no risk of needing to convert to a GA, there is no need to fast. If there is potential need for sedation or GA then normal fasting precautions should be followed.
- Insert an IV cannula in a non-operative limb for the administration of essential drugs. A cannula is also inserted into a vein on the operative limb. Ideally, but not essentially, place distal to the operative area.
- Place a double-cuff tourniquet proximally on the operative limb. Exsanguinate the limb either with elevation, compression of the supplying artery, Eschmarch bandage, or a combination, depending on the nature of the injury or surgery.
- Inflate the distal cuff first to 100mgHg above the systolic blood pressure. This tests the function of this cuff. Then inflate the proximal cuff to the same pressure. When both cuffs are shown to be effective, the distal cuff is deflated.
- LA is injected slowly intravenously, avoiding high pressures that will exceed the tourniquet pressure.
- A usual volume is 40mL, although in a small arm 30mL should be sufficient and in a large arm 50 to 60mL may be needed.
- Prilocaine is the drug of choice in the UK, used as 0.5–1%. The maximum dose is 6mg/kg. Lidocaine is used in other countries. Bupivacaine and ropivacaine are contraindicated.
- Additional distal pressure is advocated by some clinicians to limit the spread of the LA to the area of surgery.
- When all the LA is injected, the IV cannula is removed. Pressure is placed over the cannula site, but oozing of blood and LA is inevitable and rarely causes any postoperative bruises of significance.
- The distal cuff is inflated after 10 minutes or when the patient finds the tourniquet pressure is becoming intolerable, whichever is later.
- As the distal cuff lies over an area where the LA has taken effect, this cuff should be much less distressing.
- Deflating the tourniquet should *not* be done before 20 minutes have passed from injection of the LA. The patient should be monitored for signs of LA toxicity.

Further reading

Casey WF (1992). Intravenous regional anaesthesia (Bier's block). *Update Anaesth*, **1**, 2–3.
Mohr B (2006). Safety and effectiveness of intravenous regional anaesthesia (Bier block) for outpatient management of forearm trauma. *CJEM*, **8**(4), 247–50.

Part 4
Trunk Blocks

Intercostal and interpleural blocks

Background

Landmarks: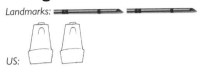

US:

Indications

Anaesthesia
Rarely used as a sole anaesthetic.

Analgesia
- Fractured ribs
- Neuralgia
- Postoperative for breast surgery, thoracic surgery, cholecystectomy, renal surgery.

Introduction
Intercostal and interpleural blocks can be used to provide good analgesia in a variety of settings but are rarely used as a sole anaesthetic technique. Systemic LA absorption and the risk of pneumothorax perhaps limits their use. Interpleural blocks work due to spread of LA into the paravertebral gutter, blocking the sympathetic chain as well.

Anatomy
- The intercostal nerves leave the paravertebral space (PVS) laterally between the innermost intercostal membrane anteriorly and the posterior (internal) intercostal membrane posteriorly (PIM).
- They remain in this plane, near the caudal aspect of the rib in the subcostal groove, as they pass around the thorax accompanied by the intercostal vessels.
- Near the mid-axillary line, the intercostal nerves divide into lateral and anterior cutaneous branches. See Fig. 30.1.
- The lateral branches pass through the intercostal muscles, dividing into anterior and posterior divisions, to supply most of the thorax and abdominal wall.
- The anterior thoracic branches continue in the subcostal groove and supply a small area on the anteromedial surface of the chest and also cross the midline to a small extent.
- In order to ensure blockade of the lateral cutaneous branches, the injection should be performed posterior to the mid-axillary line.

Side effects and complications

Complications
Intercostal block
- Failure is ~1% in expert hands.
- Clinically significant pneumothorax occurs with a frequency of <0.1%.

- Haemothorax is rare.
- LA toxicity is a significant risk.
- Intercostal neuralgia is rare.
- Total spinal anaesthesia has been reported.

Interpleural block

- Failure is <1% in expert hands.
- Clinically significant pneumothorax may occur at a rate of 1:50, but is less than this in expert hands.
- Haemothorax is rare.
- LA toxicity is a significant risk, which is not reduced by epinephrine.
- Intercostal neuralgia is rare.

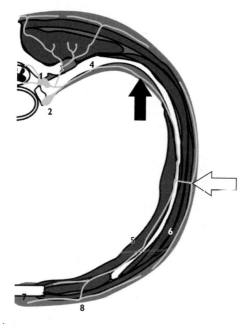

Fig. 30.1 Cross-section of the chest showing the course of the intercostal nerve. **1** spinal ganglion; **2** sympathetic ganglion; **3** posterior primary ramus of spinal nerve; Black arrow, intercostal nerve; White arrow, lateral cutaneous branch; **4** rib; **5** innermost intercostal muscle; **6** internal and external intercostal muscles; **7** sternum; **8** anterior cutaneous branch.

Landmark technique: intercostal block

Landmarks
- Midline (spinous processes)
- Paraspinal muscles
- Ribs.

Technique
- If the patient is awake, the upright or prone position is ideal. Otherwise, the patient should be positioned laterally, with the side to be blocked uppermost.
- The arm should be abducted and flexed to retract the scapula.
- Palpate the appropriate vertebral level(s).
- Mark an insertion point 40–80mm lateral to the midline, just lateral to the paraspinal muscles, over the caudal end of the corresponding rib angle. (In the upper thoracic area use a more medial insertion point than for the lower thoracic ribs.)
- Prepare the skin with 0.5% chlorhexidine in 70% alcohol. Wait until the skin is dry.
- The skin is retracted cranially and dilute LA is injected down to the periosteum of the rib for awake patients.
- A 50mm needle attached to a syringe containing the chosen LA is introduced to contact bone.
- The skin pressure is relaxed, allowing caudal direction of the needle, which is then advanced 3mm below the rib contact point, with 20° of cranial angulation.
- The needle should not be advanced >8mm deep to bone contact. As the intercostal vessels are in close proximity, careful aspiration should be performed to avoid intravascular injection.
- After aspiration, 3–5mL of LA plus epinephrine is injected. 4–8 hours of analgesia can be expected with 0.5% levobupivacaine or ropivacaine.
- Epinephrine should be added to limit absorption, as this block is associated with high blood levels of LA.
- Although the intercostal space is continuous with the paravertebral space, spread to adjacent intercostal nerves is minimal, unless a catheter is inserted in a medial direction.
- If >4 intercostal nerves need to be blocked, an alternative technique should be chosen or a catheter inserted.
- To insert a catheter, select an injection site as medial as possible. Using an 18G Tuohy needle, direct this medially and insert the catheter 5cm. Continuous infusion of 0.1mL/kg/hour of 0.1–0.2% levobupivacaine or ropivacaine will prolong analgesia.

Landmark technique: interpleural block

LA placed between the visceral and parietal pleura can be encouraged to pool in the paravertebral gutter under the influence of gravity. It also diffuses across the parietal pleura and the thin innermost intercostal membrane, to block the intercostal nerves. However, the pleura has a rich blood supply and a large surface area, so that LA is rapidly absorbed into the circulation, resulting in low intensity, brief blockade, unless a continuous infusion is used. High blood levels of LA may result and epinephrine does not reduce this.

Landmarks

- Midline (spinous processes)
- Paraspinal muscles
- Ribs.

Technique

- The patient should be in the lateral position, with the affected side uppermost.
- The arm should be abducted and flexed to retract the scapula.
- Palpate the appropriate vertebral level.
- Mark an insertion point 40–80mm lateral to the midline, just lateral to the paraspinal muscles, over the caudal end of the corresponding rib angle. (In the upper thoracic area use a more medial insertion point than for the lower thoracic ribs.)
- For a catheter technique, full aseptic precautions should be employed, including skin preparation with 0.5% chlorhexidine in 70% alcohol, drapes, hat, mask, gown, and gloves.
- Dilute LA is injected down to periosteum for awake patients.
- An 18G Tuohy needle is attached to a 3-way tap. A saline infusion is attached to the side-limb.
- The patient should be breathing spontaneously, or if paralysed, should be disconnected briefly from the ventilator.
- The Tuohy needle is inserted to contact the rib and then advanced slowly in a craniomedial direction, over the rib.
- The infusion is adjusted to allow a slow drip rate, as the needle tip enters the intercostal muscles.
- The needle is slowly advanced, noting an increase in the drip rate on entering the intercostal space, a slowing as the pleura is indented and a rapid increase when the pleura is penetrated.
- The 3-way tap is then opened to the exterior and the infusion adjusted to allow an external fluid leak.
- A catheter is then inserted through the 3-way tap to a depth of 5–7cm.
- A bolus of dilute LA, *without* epinephrine, should be injected. 20mL 0.25% levobupivacaine or ropivacaine will provide analgesia for 4–8 hours.
- Position the patient to encourage spread, assisted by gravity. To assist block in the higher thoracic dermatomes, tip the patient head-down.
- Continuous infusion will prolong analgesia, e.g. 0.1mL/kg/hour of 0.1–0.2% levobupivacaine or ropivacaine. However, intermittent bolus injection in the lateral position may be preferable.

Ultrasound techniques

US can be used to guide intercostal and interpleural block, under direct vision.

Preliminary scan

- The probe is aligned in the sagittal plane (craniocaudal direction), but in order to be perpendicular to the rib, slight rotation is required, as the ribs are angled slightly caudally.
- Identify the rib, pleura, and PIM. See Fig. 30.2.

Ultrasound settings

- Probe: high-frequency linear L38 broadband probe
- Settings: MB—resolution/general
- Depth: 3–8cm
- Needle: 50mm
- US plane: parasagittal.

Technique

- The probe is aligned in the parasagittal plane (craniocaudal direction), but in order to be perpendicular to the rib, slight rotation is required, as the ribs are angled slightly caudally.
- Prepare the skin with 0.5% chlorhexidine in 70% alcohol. Wait until the skin is dry.
- For a catheter technique, full aseptic precautions should be employed, including skin preparation with 0.5% chlorhexidine in 70% alcohol, drapes, hat, mask, gown, and gloves.
- Dilute LA is injected down to periosteum for awake patients.
- The needle can be introduced in-plane or out-of-plane.
- For intercostal block, the needle tip should be placed deep to the PIM, so that the parietal pleura is reflected anteriorly with LA injection. It is rarely possible to see the innermost intercostal muscle or membrane.
- For interpleural block, the pleura should be indented and then penetrated, splitting the parietal and visceral pleura with LA injection.

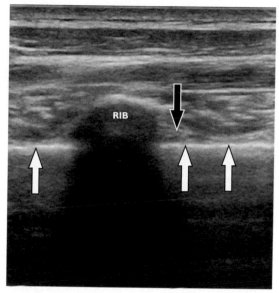

Fig. 30.2 Ultrasound image 5cm from the mid-line. The internal intercostal muscle has become membranous and the innermost intercostal membrane/muscle is not visible. The image shows the 5th rib, pleura, and the posterior (internal) intercostal membrane (PIM). The intercostal nerves run anterior to the PIM. Black arrow, posterior intercostal membrane (PIM); White arrows, pleura.

Further reading

Dravid RM, Paul RE (2007). Interpleural block – part 1. *Anaesthesia*, **62**(10), 1039–49.

Dravid RM, Paul RE (2007). Interpleural block – part 2. *Anaesthesia*, **62**(11), 1143–53.

Moore D, Bridenbaugh L (1962). Pneumothorax: its incidence following intercostal nerve block. *JAMA*, **182**(10), 1005–8.

Nunn J, Slavin C (1980). Posterior intercostal nerve block for pain relief after cholecystectomy. *Br J Anaesth*, **52**(3), 253–60.

Stromskag KE, Minor B, Steen PA (1990). Side effects and complications related to interpleural analgesia: an update. *Acta Anesthesiol Scand*, **34**(6), 473–7.

Van Kleef J, Burm A, Vletter AA (1990). Single-dose interpleural vs, intercostal blockade: nerve block characteristics and plasma concentration profiles after administration of 0.5% bupivacaine with epinephrine. *Anesth Analg*, **70**(5), 484–8.

Paravertebral block

Background

PNS: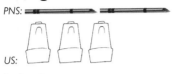

US:

Indications

Anaesthesia
- Breast surgery, thoracic surgery, cholecystectomy, renal surgery, appendicectomy, inguinal hernia repair.

Analgesia
- Postoperative analgesia for breast surgery, thoracic surgery, cholecystectomy, renal surgery, appendicectomy, inguinal hernia repair.
- Fractured ribs.
- Liver capsule pain, neuralgia, pancreatic pain.

Introduction

LA can be placed in the PVS anywhere along the vertebral column, resulting in a paravertebral block (PVB). The corresponding spinal nerves, rami communicantes, and sympathetic chain will be blocked on the injected side. LA spreads up and down the paravertebral space, into the intercostal space or along the spinal nerves, so that >1 dermatome can be blocked with a single injection. Intense somatic and autonomic neuronal blockade results, which can be sufficient for surgery without further supplementation. However, sedation or GA is usually administered as well. A catheter can be placed to prolong analgesia.

Prolonged analgesia can be provided that is equal or superior to epidural block, with less risk of bilateral sympathetic block or neurological damage.

PVB has been shown to reduce chronic pain after thoracic and breast surgery. This is possibly because of the intense blockade of both the sympathetic and somatic nerves, preventing sensitization of the CNS and NMDA receptor 'wind up'. Tumour recurrence may also be inhibited after breast surgery; however, this remains to be proven.

Anatomy

Paravertebral space
- The PVS is wedge shaped in all 3 planes, anteroposteriorly (axial), mediolaterally (coronal) and sagittally. It is widest medially (see Fig. 31.1):
  - The medial wall is formed by the body of the vertebra, the intervertebral discs and the intervertebral foramen
  - Posteriorly, the PVS is limited by the transverse process, the superior costotransverse ligament (CTL) and the head of the rib. The lower ribs lie slightly cranially and all the ribs are anterior to the transverse processes

- Anterolaterally, the space is bounded by the parietal pleura, the remnants of the innermost intercostal membrane, the subserous and endothoracic fascia.
- The PVS is continuous cranially and caudally. The space also communicates freely with:
  - The thoracic intercostal spaces
  - The epidural space, by the intervertebral foramen
  - The opposite PVS—under the anterior longitudinal ligament and endothoracic fascia.

  The CTL is continuous laterally with the posterior (internal) intercostal membrane (PIM).

- The PVS contains the endothoracic fascia, the subserous fascia, the intercostal nerves, rami communicantes and the sympathetic chain.
- The distance from the skin to the transverse process varies with body habitus, being most superficial in the mid thoracic region. At T4, the mean distance is 25mm (range 15–38mm) in females. The mean distance from the transverse process to the pleura (the PVS) was estimated to be 44mm (range 26–59mm), 35mm from the midline.

Specific contraindications

- Coagulopathy is a relative contra-indication.
- Due to the risk of pneumothorax, and the resulting paralysis of the intercostal muscles, careful consideration in patients with severe respiratory disease.

Side effects and complications

- Failure, ether partial or complete, is ~10% even in expert hands.
- Clinically significant pneumothorax occurs with a frequency of 1:100 (cranial approach) to 1:1000 (caudad approach).
- Haemothorax has been described.
- Hypotension. Although the sympathetic chain is reliably blocked on the affected side, the contralateral side is usually not affected, so that hypotension is rarely a problem and will usually respond rapidly to IV fluids and/or vasopressors.
- Epidural extension occurs in at least 10% if a single bolus is used.
- Total spinal and cardiovascular collapse are exceedingly rare.
- LAs are rapidly absorbed from the PVS and LA toxicity can result.
- No permanent neurological injuries have been reported with conventional local anaesthetics, but these are theoretically possible if the needle deviates medially into the neuraxis, the spinal nerve is penetrated, or if neurotoxic agents are used.
- Horner's syndrome occurs commonly after high thoracic PVB and is a good sign of an effective block.
- If the block is to be performed in a conscious patient, entry and injection into the PVS is often painful. PVBs are commonly performed under GA.
- No infectious complications have been reported.

Landmark techniques

Landmarks
- Spinous process of corresponding vertebrae.

Technique
- If performing the block awake or under conscious sedation, the patient should be seated with the neck and back flexed. A nurse should face the patient, to provide reassurance and stabilization.
- If GA is to be administered first, the patient is positioned in the lateral position, with the operative side uppermost.
- The tips of the appropriate spinous processes are marked in the midline.
- At the same level, a mark is made 25mm laterally from the midline. These marks should be equidistant, both from the midline and from each other. These are the injection points. See Fig. 31.2.
- Prepare the skin with 0.5% chlorhexidine in 70% alcohol. Wait until the skin is dry.
- If the block is being performed awake or under sedation, superficial and deep LA infiltration will be required. To limit the total dose of LA, 0.5% lidocaine plus 1:200,000 epinephrine is recommended. A volume of 3–4mL should be sufficient at each level.
- An 18–22G Tuohy epidural needle is used.
- The needle is connected to extension tubing with the chosen LA dose attached.
- Insertion is at the previously identified marks in a directly anteroposterior direction. The forefinger should be placed at the 35mm depth mark on the needle.
- Bone contact should be sought. If this is not achieved then the needle should be withdrawn to the skin and redirected in a slightly caudal and then cranial direction. If bone contact is still not realized, then the finger 'guard' should be replaced at 40mm, 45mm, and 50 mm, repeating the procedure at each depth until bone is contacted. Slight lateral angulation is also acceptable.
- Once bone has been contacted, the depth should be noted and the forefinger 'guard' moved 10mm posteriorly. The needle should then be withdrawn to the skin and re-inserted in a caudal and slightly lateral direction up to the forefinger guard mark.
- The CTL should be penetrated and the PVS will be encountered within 10–15mm. This is sometimes associated with a palpable click.
- Together with the described procedure, PVS penetration can be confirmed by the use of a syringe of air, saline, or 5% dextrose, noting the change in resistance to injection. This should *not* be a complete loss of resistance, which indicates *pleural puncture*.
- Further confirmation can be sought by the use of a nerve stimulator, set at 2Hz, 0.3msec, and 2mA. Intercostal or abdominal muscle contraction may be apparent.

- If it is not possible to move off bone, angle more laterally. If this is still impossible, re-insert the needle more caudally and repeat the process. Finally, attempt a cranial angulation with an insertion depth of 15mm greater than initial bone contact.
- Aspiration should be attempted to prevent subsequent intravascular injection.
- A test dose of LA should be administered, noting any increase in heart rate if epinephrine is used.
- Inject 5–7mL of LA for multiple blocks or 15–20mL as a single injection.
- Add 1:200,000 epinephrine and 1 microgram/kg of clonidine to 0.5% levobupivacaine or ropivacaine for maximum duration. 4–12 hours of intense analgesia can be anticipated, sufficient for awake surgery, or with sedation.
- A catheter can be inserted to a depth of 10–20mm to extend analgesia. Deeper insertion risks epidural location or anterior misplacement. If catheter insertion is very easy, it is likely that it is in the interpleural space. Pig-tail catheters aid insertion.
- Continuous infusion of 0.1mL/kg/hour of 0.1–0.2% levobupivacaine or ropivacaine will prolong analgesia.

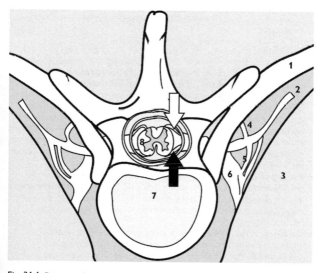

Fig. 31.1 Diagram of the cross-section of the paravertebral space. **1** rib; **2** ventral ramus; **3** lung; **4** dorsal ramus; **5** sympathetic rami communicantes; **6** sympathetic ganglion; **7** vertebra; **8** spinal cord; White arrow, dorsal root; Black arrow, ventral root.

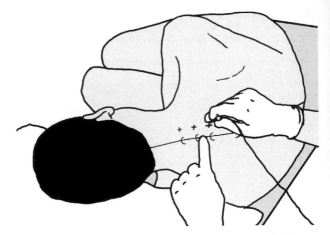

Fig. 31.2 Landmark technique for thoracic paravertebral block. The index finger of the left hand is palpating the spinous processes and the needle insertion is 25mm lateral to these.

Level of block

- If only 1–4 dermatomes need to be blocked, e.g. for lumpectomy or simple mastectomy, a single-level PVB might be chosen, at or below (cranial spread better than caudad) the mid dermatomal level.
- The level is established by palpating the spinous processes and counting down from C7 (the vertebra prominens), or up from L4 at the intercristal line. The spine of the scapula points to T3 and the lower border of the scapula is at the level of T8.
- In the thoracic region, due to the caudad angulation of the spinous processes, the injection into the PVS will be one level lower than that of the spinous process palpated if a caudal approach is used.
- If a spread >4 dermatomes is required, then multiple injections will block the whole area more reliably. For example, for mastectomy and axillary dissection, a block from at least T1–T6 will be required. It is suggested that for this procedure, blocks should be performed at T1, T3, and T5.
- For blocks in the lumbar region it is recommended that separate injections are performed at each level. For example, for inguinal herniorrhaphy, blocks should be performed at T12, L1, and L2.

Ultrasound technique

PVBs can be placed with the aid of US but is a developing technique. The US can be used to identify the anatomy and measure the depth to transverse process and PVS, to assist a landmark-based technique or used in real time to guide block placement. There are several different probe orientations and needle trajectories described but the 2 main approaches—out-of-plane, sagittal and in-plane, transverse—are described here.

Preliminary scan: parasagittal out-of-plane approach

- Place the probe in the parasagittal plane about 5cm from the midline.
- The rib, PIM, and pleura are then identified. See Fig. 30.2.
- The probe is then moved medially, to show the bony transition from rib to the more superficial (posterior) transverse process.
- The pleura will become less distinct at this point, so the probe is angled laterally to improve the view.
- The CTL and the PVS beyond are identified. See Fig. 31.3.

Ultrasound settings: parasagittal out-of-plane approach

- Probe: high-frequency linear L38 broadband probe
- Settings: MB—resolution/general
- Depth: 3–8cm
- Needle: 50mm
- US plane: parasagittal
- Needle approach: out-of-plane.

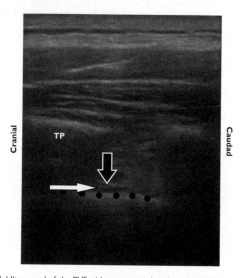

Fig. 31.3 Ultrasound of the PVS with a parasagittal probe orientation. TP, transverse process; Black arrow, costotransverse ligament; White arrow, paravertebral space; Black dots, pleura.

Technique: parasagittal out-of-plane approach

- The position of the transverse process can be marked and the distances from the skin to the transverse process and to the pleura can be measured (The actual needle-to-bone distance is usually slightly greater due to tissue compression by the probe.) This information can then be used to improve accuracy and safety of the technique described earlier.
- In the US-guided approach, the needle is inserted into the PVS alongside the probe in the out-of-plane approach. An in-plane approach is also possible.
- As LA is injected, the space between the pleura and CTL will be seen to expand, with the pleura being displaced anteriorly.
- This expansion can be followed cranially and caudally to assess the need for additional injections. A catheter can then be inserted and its position checked by injecting air.

Preliminary scan: transverse in-plane approach

- Place the probe in a slightly oblique transverse (axial) plane between 2 ribs.
- Identify the pleura laterally and the transverse process medially.
- The PIM can then be identified. See Fig. 31.4.
- The CTL and PVS are obscured by the acoustic shadow of the transverse process.

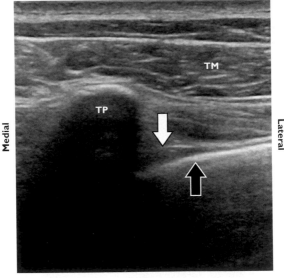

Fig. 31.4 Ultrasound from a transverse probe position to show the PIM, pleura, and TP of the vertebrae. The CTL and PVS are themselves obscured by the acoustic shadow of transverse process. TM, trapezius muscle; TP, transverse process; White arrow, PIM; Black arrow, pleura.

Ultrasound settings: transverse in-plane approach

- Probe: high-frequency linear L38 broadband probe
- Settings: MB—general
- Depth: 3–8cm
- Needle: 50–80mm
- US plane: transverse (axial)
- Needle approach: in-plane.

Technique: transverse in-plane approach

- The needle can be introduced in-plane into the space between the PIM and pleura, noting the expansion as the LA is injected.
- This is actually a very medial intercostal block, with medial spread into the PVS.
- During injection the pleura can be seen to be displaced anteriorly.

Ultrasound versus landmark techniques

- US requires expensive equipment and considerable expertise.
- Aseptic US techniques are time consuming compared with the landmark approaches.
- US views are hampered when the block is deep, so that the technique is less useful in larger patients and in the lumbar region. The extensive local bony anatomy makes good definition of anatomical structures and the needle difficult.
- US is particularly applicable in the paediatric population.
- US may improve the success rate of these blocks, reduce the number of injections required, and minimize the risk of complications, particularly pneumothorax.

Further reading

Cheema SP, Ilsley D, Richardson J, et al. (1995). A thermographic study of paravertebral analgesia. Anaesthesia, 50(2),118–21.

Eason MJ, Wyatt R. (1979). Paravertebral thoracic block-a reappraisal. Anaesthesia 34(7), 638–42.

Karmakar, M (2001). Thoracic paravertebral block. Anesthesiology, 95(3), 771–80.

Lonnqvist PA, MacKenzie J, Soni AK, et al. (1995). Paravertebral blockade: failure rate and complications. Anaesthesia, 50(9), 813–15.

Luyet C, Siegenthaler A, Szucs-Farkas Z, et al. (2012). The location of paravertebral catheters placed using the landmark technique. Anaesthesia, 67(12), 1321–6.

Pusch F, Wildling E, Klimscha W, et al. (2000). Sonographic measurement of needle insertion depth in paravertebral blocks in women. Br J Anaesth, 85(6), 841–3.

Shelley B, and Macfie A (2012). Where now for thoracic paravertebral blockade? Anaesthesia, 67(12), 1317–20.

Tighe SQ, Karmaker MK. (2013). Serratus plane block: do we need to learn another technique for thoracic wall blockade? Anaesthesia, 68(11), 1103–6.

Transversus abdominis plane block

Background

Landmark: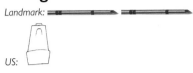

US:

Indications

Analgesia

- Unilateral transversus abdominis plane (TAP) block:
  - Appendicectomy
  - Inguinal herniorrhaphy
  - Femoral herniorrhaphy
  - Cholecystectomy.
- Bilateral TAP block:
  - Midline laparotomy
  - Laparoscopic abdominal/pelvic surgery
  - Caesarean section
  - Total abdominal hysterectomy.

Anatomy

- The anterior abdominal wall is innervated by the thoracolumbar segmental nerves T6–L1.
- These nerves course through the abdominal wall in the neurofascial plane between internal oblique and transversus abdominis (TAP—see Fig. 32.1) as far as the midaxillary line, where a cutaneous branch pierces the internal and external oblique muscles to supply the skin of the anterior abdominal wall.
- The rest of the nerve continues through the TAP until it pierces the posterior rectus sheath to supply the skin about the midline of the abdomen.
- At the level of the lumbar triangle of Petit the muscle of the external and internal oblique muscles become fascia prior to insertion into the perilumbar fascia.
- The lumbar triangle of Petit is an easily palpable landmark found posterior to the midaxillary line. The triangle is bounded posteriorly by the lateral edge of the latissimus dorsi muscle, anteriorly by the external oblique muscle, inferiorly by the iliac crest, with the external oblique aponeurosis as the floor.

Introduction

The TAP block is relatively easy and quick to perform with few associated risks. It has been associated with significant improvement in patients' perception of pain post abdominal surgery when used as a part of a multimodal analgesic regimen. The ↑ analgesia results in ↓ requirement of opioids in the postoperative period resulting in less opioid related side effects. The ability of a single-shot technique to provide significant analgesia for up to 48 hours postoperatively allows prolonged benefit of the decreased opioid consumption facilitating earlier mobilization.

The ability to perform the block in the anaesthetized patient means less stress and discomfort for the patient in the perioperative period. Added to this, the safety profile associated with the TAP block means that postoperatively there is no requirement for the supplemental observation necessary when central neuraxial blockade is utilized.

This technique can be performed without expensive imaging or stimulation equipment, providing an alternative to opioid medication in arenas where it may otherwise be difficult to provide adequate analgesia. Due to the neurological innervation of the abdominal wall the TAP block can be provided unilaterally when the intended surgery is to be limited to one side of the mid line.

The TAP block will only provide analgesia of the abdominal wall and therefore the lack of visceral analgesia does require some opiate administration perioperatively for intra-abdominal surgery, but it is usually modest and of limited duration.

Side effects and complications

Complications

- Vascular injection is possible—inject slowly with repeated aspiration.
- Peritoneal perforation if the needle is advanced through the transversus abdominis muscle.

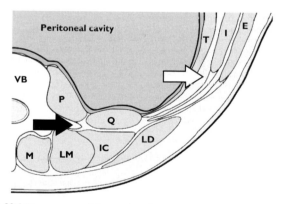

Fig. 32.1 The transversus abdominis plane. E, external oblique muscle; I, internal oblique muscle; T, transversus abdominis muscle; White arrow, transverus abdominis plane (TAP); P, psoas major muscle; Q, quadratus lumborum muscle; VB, vertebral body; Black arrow, transverse process; LD, latissimus dorsi muscle; IC, iliocostalis muscle; LM, longissimus muscle; M, multifidis muscle.

Landmark technique

Landmarks
- The lumbar triangle of Petit
- Iliac crest
- Lateral boarder of latissimus dorsi muscle
- Posterior border of the external oblique muscle.

Technique
- The patient is placed in the supine position, the lumbar triangle of Petit is identified by palpation of the lateral border of the latissimus dorsi muscle just superior to the iliac crest and the posterior boarder of the external oblique muscle and is marked using a skin marker. See Fig. 32.2.
- Prepare the skin with 0.5% chlorhexidine in 70% alcohol. Wait until the skin is dry.
- Anaesthetize the skin with LA for awake patients.
- Using a short-bevelled regional anaesthesia needle the skin is pierced ~1cm cephalad to the iliac crest. See Fig. 32.3.
- Gentle advancement of the needle in the coronal (horizontal) plane is then performed until resistance is encountered. This resistance indicates that the tip of the needle is at the external border of the external oblique fascia.
- Gentle advancement of the needle results in a 'pop' sensation as the needle enters the plane between the external and internal oblique muscles/fascia.
- Further gentle advancement of the needle results in a 2nd 'pop' being appreciated. This 2nd 'pop' indicates entry into the transversus abdominis fascial plane, having pierced the internal oblique fascia.
- After careful aspiration to exclude vascular puncture, 20–30mL of LA solution is then injected through the needle (care being taken not to exceed the maximal allowable dosage of the LA solution).
- The TAP block can then be performed on the opposite side using an identical technique if required.

Clinical notes
- The operator should stand on the contralateral side to the block side to maintain best control of the needle during the block.
- An assistant can be used to deliver the LA solution injection.
- This block can be performed safely in anaesthetized patients. In anaesthetized patients, lateral displacement of the lower limbs away from the side to be blocked aids identification of the triangle of Petit and performance of the block by 'stretching' of the fascial layers.
- The use of muscle relaxant decreases the perception of the passage of the needle through the fascial extensions of the external and internal oblique muscles and therefore the block should be performed prior to muscle relaxation to increase the safety profile and the success rate.
- As the needle starts to pass through the fascial extension of both external and internal oblique muscles the pressure applied to the needle should be lessened to avoid advancement of the needle into and through the next layer.

- This block can easily be performed in awake patients by providing local infiltration to the skin prior to performance of the block. In awake patients palpation of the triangle of Petit and block performance can be aided by asking the patient to raise their head from the bed, and by so doing ↑ tension can be exerted on the fascial extensions of the external and internal oblique muscles.
- In the obese patient the adipose layer is usually attenuated at the level of the iliac crest and displacement of the surplus skin and adipose tissue cranially by an assistant will aid the performance of the block.

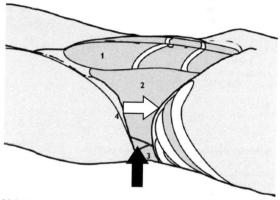

Fig. 32.2 Diagram to indicate the markings of the Lumbar triangle of Petit. **1** rectus abdominis muscle; **2** external oblique muscle; **3** latissimus dorsi muscle; **4** iliac crest; White arrow, inferior costal margin; Black arrow, lumbar triangle of Petit.

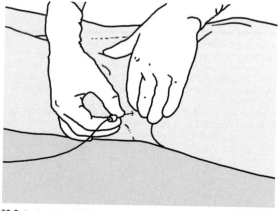

ig. 32.3 Performing a TAP block using the lumbar triangle of Petit approach.

Ultrasound technique

The use of US aids needle tip positioning within the TAP. There have been many different approaches described in the literature:

Preliminary scan
- The probe is placed in an axial orientation on the lateral aspect of the abdomen. Various exact positions have been described, as described in ➔ Technique, p. 368.
- Identify the 3 muscle layers; external oblique, internal oblique, and transversus abdominis. See Fig. 32.4.

US settings
- Probe: high-frequency (>10MHz) linear L38 broadband probe. Occasionally a curvilinear probe may be needed
- Settings: MB—general/penetration
- Depth: 3–8cm
- Orientation: axial/oblique
- Needle: 100mm short-bevel needle of choice.

Technique
- The patient is in the supine position.
- Prepare the skin with 0.5% chlorhexidine in 70% alcohol. Wait until the skin is dry.
- Anaesthetize the skin with LA for awake patients.
- An in-plane approach from the anterior end of the probe is recommended.
- Advance the needle in-plane until the tip is situated in the TAP. The needle can be introduced almost perpendicular to the US beam allowing good needle visibility, although this also results in a flat approach to the fascia, making it more difficult to pierce.
- After negative aspiration, 20mL of LA is injected in 5mL aliquots with repeated aspiration.
- The 2 muscles should separate cleanly if in the correct plane.
- Whilst gaining proficiency with the technique, injecting saline initially until the correct tissue plane is identified can help prevent placing significant amounts of the LA within the muscles.
- It can be useful to advance the needle tip fractionally through the plane and then inject slowly whilst gently withdrawing the needle until the correct tissue plane is found by the separation of the 2 muscles.
- Unpublished research suggests that volume is more important than concentration.
- The maximal allowable dose should never be exceeded and the dose should be divided in 2 for bilateral blockade. Alter the concentration to maintain a volume of 20mL for each side, without exceeding maximal doses.

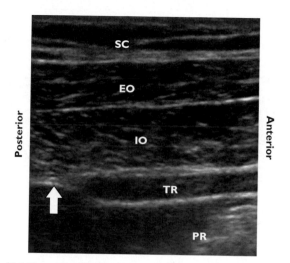

SC

EO

IO

TR

PR

Posterior

Anterior

Fig. 32.4 Ultrasound showing the 3 muscle of the abdominal wall. External oblique, internal oblique and transversus abdominis. SC, subcutaneous tissue; EO, external oblique muscle; IO, internal oblique muscle; TR, transversus abdominis muscle; White arrow, edge of transversus abdominis muscle becoming fascia.

Injection sites

The most common approach is to place the probe *over the midaxillary line* (see Fig. 32.5), at this point the 3 abdominal muscular layers are evident and a needle can be introduced under direct vision. The limitation of this approach is the extent of analgesia achieved with the block being limited to the infraumbilical region.

Another approach is to orientate the probe *subcostally* along the inferior aspect of the ribcage, again identifying the 3 abdominal muscles. The needle is then inserted in an in-plane manner under direct vision until the needle tip is seen within the TAP. Care has to be taken to avoid neuro-vascular trauma as the needle is generally orientated at right angles to the vessels in the plane. This block is generally used for supraumbilical surgery. A catheter may be placed with this approach as the effect is localized to within the TAP.

The last approach is to place the probe *posterior to the midaxillary line*, identify the posterior aspect of the abdominal wall muscles and the quadratus lumborum muscle further posteriorly/medially. The needle is advanced in-plane under direct vision to lie superficial to the transversalis fascia at the lateral border of the quadratus lumborum muscle. Prior to administering the LA solution care is taken to ensure that the needle tip is extravascular. With this approach LA solution has been shown to spread locally within the TAP, but more importantly superomedially to the thoracic paravertebral space. This paravertebral extension mimics the spread pattern associated with the landmark-based approach and helps explain the effective field and duration of analgesia, through probable involvement of the thoracic-lumbar sympathetic ganglia.

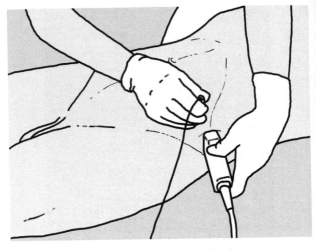

Fig. 32.5 An ultrasound-guided TAP block in the midaxillary line.

Further reading

Carney J, Finnerty O, Rauf J, et al. (2011). Studies on the spread of local anaesthetic solution in transversus abdominis plane blocks. *Anaesthesia*, **66**(11), 1023–30.

Carney J, McDonnell JG, Bhinder R, et al. (2007). Ultrasound guided continuous transversus abdominis plane block for post-operative pain relief in abdominal surgery. *Reg Anesth Pain Med*, **32**(Suppl 1), 24.

Hebbard P (2008). Subcostal transversus abdominis plane block under ultrasound guidance. *Anesth Analg*, **106**(2), 674–5.

McDonnell JG, Curley G, Carney J, et al. (2008). The analgesic efficacy of transversus abdominis plane block after cesarean delivery: a randomized controlled trial. *Anesth Analg*, **106**(1), 186–91.

Rozen WM, Tran TMN, Ashton MW, et al. (2008). Refining the course of the thoracolumbar nerves: a new understanding of the innervation of the anterior abdominal wall. *Clin Anat*, **21**(4), 325–33.

Ilioinguinal and iliohypogastric nerve blocks

Background

Landmark: ▬▬▬

US:

Indications

Anaesthesia
- Inguinal herniorrhaphy

Analgesia
- Postoperative: inguinal hernia repair, orchidopexy, varicocoele, hydrocoele repair
- Diagnostic block for groin pain or nerve entrapment following herniorrhaphy.

Introduction

- This block is safe and easy to perform and provides effective postoperative analgesia in both adults and children.
- Ilioinguinal/iliohypogastric nerve blocks are as effective as caudal blocks for postoperative analgesia following inguinal surgery in children.
- In adult patients undergoing hernia surgery, this block is associated with reduced postoperative analgesic requirements and improved mobility.
- Ultrasound guidance increases the success rate and safety of this block and reduces the amount of LA used.

Anatomy

- The iliohypogastric, ilioinguinal, and genitofemoral nerves are branches of the lumbar plexus.
- The iliohypogastric and ilioinguinal nerves arise from the ventral ramus of T12 and the upper division of the L1 nerve root. The genitofemoral nerve is formed by L2 and a contribution from the lower division of L1.
- The iliohypogastric and ilioinguinal nerves appear from the lateral border of the psoas major muscle and run anteriorly and obliquely across the quadratus lumborum muscle.
- At the lateral border, the nerves pierce the lumbar fascia to run anteriorly and medially between the transversus abdominis and internal oblique muscles.
- The iliohypogastric nerve then perforates the internal oblique muscle to lie deep to the external oblique muscle. This occurs variably but is described as being ~ 2cm medial to the anterior superior iliac spine (ASIS). It continues medially then pierces the external oblique aponeurosis ~ 3cm above the superficial inguinal ring, supplying the skin above the pubis and the medial half of the inguinal ligament.
- The ilioinguinal nerve perforates the internal oblique muscle inferior and medial to the iliohypogastric nerve and traverses the inguinal canal to emerge from the superficial inguinal ring and supply the skin over the root of the penis and scrotum as well as structures within the canal.

- The genitofemoral nerve perforates psoas major to appear on its anterior surface and runs distally until it divides into 2 terminal branches just above the inguinal ligament.
- See Fig. 33.1.

Side effects and complications

Complications
- Block of the femoral nerve
- Block of the lateral cutaneous nerve of thigh
- Bowel/viscus perforation
- Subcutaneous/pelvic haematoma
- Nerve injury
- Intravascular injection
- Local anaesthetic toxicity.

Clinical notes

- Care should be taken to deliver a safe total dose of LA.
- If using a landmark-guided technique, a blunt needle provides better appreciation of the 'click' as muscle layers are penetrated.
- An alternative insertion point is 5cm posterior and superior to the ASIS: at this point the muscle layers and nerves may be more easily visualized with US and the nerves are more likely to be lying in the same plane deep to internal oblique.

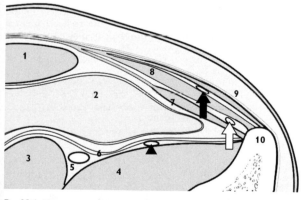

Fig. 33.1 Cross-section of the abdomen to show the positions of the iliohypogastric and ilioinguinal nerves. Black arrow, iliohypogastric nerve; White arrow, ilioinguinal nerve; 1 rectus abdominis muscle; 2 peritoneal cavity; 3 psoas major muscle; 4 iliacus muscle; 5 femoral nerve; 6 fascia iliaca; 7 transversalis muscle; 8 internal oblique muscle; 9 external oblique muscle; 10 iliac crest; Black triangle, lateral cutaneous nerve of the thigh.

Landmark technique

Landmarks
- ASIS
- Pubic tubercle (PT).

Technique
- This block is most commonly performed under GA with the patient in the supine position.
- Prepare the skin with 0.5% chlorhexidine in 70% alcohol. Wait until the skin is dry.
- Anaesthetize the skin with local anaesthetic for awake patients.
- At a point 1cm medial and 1cm inferior to the ASIS a 21G 35mm needle is advanced perpendicular to skin.
- As the external oblique muscle is pierced a characteristic 'click' or 'pop' is felt, 6–8mL of LA is injected here to block the iliohypogastric nerve.
- As the needle is advanced further a second 'click' is felt as the internal oblique muscle is pierced, a further 6–8mL of is injected at this point to block the ilioinguinal nerve.

Field block for herniorrhaphy
Hernia repair may be performed entirely under LA.

In addition to ilioinguinal and iliohypogastric nerve blocks, further injections are made to block the cutaneous branches of the subcostal nerve and the genital branch of the genitofemoral nerve. From a point just anterior to the ASIS, 3–5mL of LA is infiltrated subcutaneously in a fan-shaped manner superomedially and inferolaterally and a similar injection is made over the PT. Finally, the surgeon injects 5mL of LA into the fascial coverings of the spermatic cord, once it is exposed, to block the genitofemoral nerve and sympathetic fibres.

Ultrasound technique

Preliminary scan

- The US probe is placed immediately superior and medial to the ASIS, along a line joining the ASIS and the umbilicus and at right angles to the course of the nerves. See Fig. 33.2.
- Identify the 3 muscle layers (external oblique, internal oblique, and transversus abdominis) and the peritoneum.
- In this location, both the nerves may still be deep to the internal oblique muscle and are visualized as hypoechoic structures with hyperechoic rims lying between transversus abdominis and internal oblique. See Fig. 33.3.
- However, sometimes the iliohypogastric has pierced internal oblique to lie between internal and external oblique.
- Use the Doppler to identify any small blood vessels near the target area.

US settings

- Probe: high frequency (>10MHz) linear L38 broadband probe
- Settings: MB—general/resolution
- Depth: 3–6cm
- Orientation: sagittal oblique
- Needle: 50mm short-bevel needle of choice.

Technique

- The patient is in the supine position.
- Prepare the skin with 0.5% chlorhexidine in 70% alcohol. Wait until the skin is dry.
- Anaesthetize the skin with LA for awake patients.
- An in plane approach from the caudad end of the probe is recommended to maximize needle tip visibility, although an out-of-plane approach is also used.
- If a good image of the nerves is identified then adequate spread of LA around the nerves can be achieved with volumes of 0.075mL/kg (~5mL for adults), however if the nerves are not well seen volumes of 10–15mL may be more appropriate to ensure adequate spread in the tissue plane and successful block.

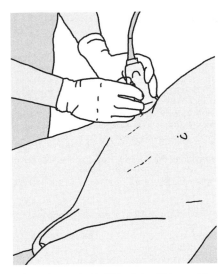

Fig. 33.2 Setup for an ultrasound-guided ilioinguinal and iliohypogastric nerve block.

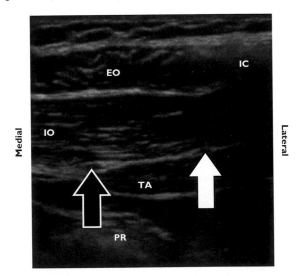

Fig. 33.3 Ultrasound image showing the ilioinguinal and iliohypogastric nerves between the internal oblique and transversus abdominis. IC, iliac crest; EO, external oblique muscle; IO, internal oblique muscle; TA, transversus abdominis muscle; White arrow, ilioinguinal nerve; Black arrow, iliohypogastric nerve; PR, bowel/peritoneal cavity.

Further reading

Eichenberger U, Greher M, Kirchmair L, et al. (2006). Ultrasound-guided blocks of the ilioinguinal and iliohypogastric nerve: accuracy of a selective new technique confirmed by anatomical dissection. Br J Anaesth, 97(2),238–43.

Hannallah RS, Broadman LM, Belman AB, et al. (1987). Comparison of caudal and ilioinguinal/iliohypogastric nerve blocks for control of post-orchiopexy pain in pediatric ambulatory surgery. Anesthesiology, 66(6), 832–4.

Nehra D, Gemmell L, Pye JK (1995). Pain relief after inguinal hernia repair: a randomized double-blind study. Br J Surg, 82(9), 1245–7.

Willschke H, Bosenberg A, Marhofer P, et al. (2006). Ultrasonographic-guided ilioinguinal/iliohypogastric nerve block in pediatric anaesthesia: what is the optimal volume? Anesth Analg, 102(6), 1680–4.

Willschke H, Marhofer P, Bosenberg A, et al. (2005). Ultrasonography for ilioinguinal/Iliohypo-gastric nerve blocks in children. Br J Anaesth, 95(2), 226–30.

Rectus sheath block

Background

Landmark:

US:

Indications

Anaesthesia
• Paraumbilical herniorrhaphy.

Analgesia
• Paraumbilical herniorrhaphy
• Radical retropubic prostatectomy
• Midline abdominal surgery.

Introduction
• The rectus sheath block was first described in 1899 for surgery performed about the umbilicus and has been extensively used in a paediatric population. However recent developments with US have led to a resurgence of the block among general anaesthetists for midline incisions of the anterior abdominal wall.
• US has made this block simple, safe, and effective to perform, even in the obese.
• The ability to perform the block in the anaesthetized patient means less stress and discomfort for the patient in the perioperative period.
• Avoiding the hypotensive side effects of central neuraxial techniques can reduce the requirement for the supplemental observations postoperatively.
• The lack of visceral analgesia does require some opiate administration perioperatively for intra-abdominal surgery, but it is usually modest and of limited duration.

Anatomy
• The aponeuroses of the lateral abdominal wall muscles fuse medially to form the rectus sheath about the recti muscles.
• The internal oblique cleaves in 2 in order to envelope the recti muscles. It fuses anteriorly with the external oblique aponeurosis and posteriorly with the transversalis aponeurosis before fusing in the midline, with the corresponding aponeurosi from the contralateral side, to form the linea alba.
• The anterior rectus sheath fuses with the recti muscles to form up to 6 tendinous intersections.
• Below the level of the arcuate line the posterior wall of the rectus sheath is deficient with only the thin transversalis fascia deep to the muscle belly, before the peritoneum is encountered.
• The anterior abdominal wall is innervated by the thoracolumbar nerves T6–L1.

- These segmental nerves course in the abdomen through the neurofascial plane between internal oblique and transversus abdominis as far as the midaxillary line, where a cutaneous branch pierces the internal and external oblique muscles to supply skin of the abdominal wall.
- The rest of the nerve continues medially until they pierce the posterior rectus sheath to supply the skin about the midline of the abdomen.

Side effects and complications

- Vascular injection. The courses of the superior and inferior epigastic vessels are variable.
- Systemic absorptions especially if large doses are injected into the rectus muscles.
- Peritoneal perforation especially below the arcuate line.

Landmark technique

Landmarks
- Lateral border of the rectus sheath
- Umbilicus
- Pubic crest
- Arcuate line
- Linea alba
- Costal margin.

Technique
- Patient in the supine position. Usually performed in anaesthetized patients, but can be done awake with LA infiltration.
- The lateral border of the rectus sheath (linea semilunaris) is identified and marked. It is unimportant at which level the block is performed above the arcuate line.
- Prepare the skin with 0.5% chlorhexidine in 70% alcohol. Wait until the skin is dry.
- Anaesthetize the skin with LA for awake patients.
- A 50mm, 24G short-bevelled needle is inserted above or below the umbilicus roughly 0.5cm medial to the linea semilunaris in a vertical plane. See Fig. 34.1.
- The needle is advanced until the anterior rectus sheath is encountered whereby a loss of resistance is felt as the needle passes through the fascial layer, the needle is advanced through the belly of the rectus muscle until resistance is encountered at the posterior rectus sheath.
- The rectus sheath is described as being rough when the needle is moved along the surface.
- After careful aspiration LA solution is injected with repeated aspirations.
- The volume injected is 0.15–0.2mL/kg of bupivacaine 0.25%, on each side.
- A single site of injection on each side should be sufficient as the LA should spread freely all along the posterior rectus sheath.
- Resistance to injection may mean that the needle tip is still situated within the muscle body.

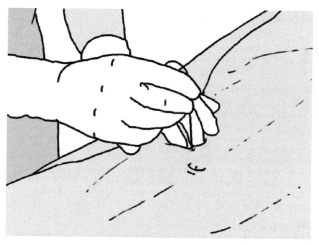

Fig. 34.1 Landmark technique for rectus sheath block.

Ultrasound technique

The advent of US has revolutionized this technique and enabled the technique to be offered to a wider population. The ability to visualize the passage of the needle allows for ↑ safety and precision in LA solution deposition (Fig. 34.2).

Preliminary scan

- Place the probe transversely (axial) anywhere in the midline of the abdomen above the arcuate line.
- Identify the linea alba and the 2 recti muscles either side.
- Slide the probe laterally observing the rectus muscle and posterior to this the 'tram lines' of the posterior rectus sheath.
- Bowel can often be seen deep to this.
- Continue laterally to the lateral border of the rectus muscle identifying external oblique, internal oblique, and transversalis.
- Use the Doppler to check for branches of the superior and inferior epigastric arteries.

US settings

- Probe: medium/high-frequency (>8MHz) linear L38 broadband probe
- Settings: MB—general
- Depth: 3–6cm
- Orientation: transverse (axial) or parasagittal
- Needle: 50–80mm of choice.

Technique

- Supine position of the patient. Stand by the patient's side with the US machine on the opposite side.
- Prepare the skin with 0.5% chlorhexidine in 70% alcohol. Wait until the skin is dry.
- Anaesthetize the skin with LA for awake patients.
- The needle should be introduced in an in-plane approach, although the orientation of the probe and the injection site is less important.
- The needle is then directed until it lies posterior to the rectus muscle.
- After careful aspiration LA is injected in 5mL aliquots, up to 20mL per side.
- The LA should be seen to 'peel' the rectus muscle off the posterior rectus sheath.
- Scanning proximally and distally after the injection should confirm the spread of the LA along the posterior rectus sheath.
- Repeat on the opposite side.

Clinical notes

- Where possible US should be used to increase the safety and efficacy of the block.
- This block has to be performed on both sides for surgery involving the midline.
- This block can be performed safely in anaesthetized patients.
- These techniques will only provide analgesia of the abdominal wall, so control of any visceral pain will also needs attention.
- Avoid injecting below the arcuate line due to the absence of the posterior rectus sheath.
- Unpublished research suggests that volume is more important than concentration. Adjust the concentration to ensure the maximum dose is not exceeded, whilst using 20mL for each side.
- Catheters are easily placed once the rectus muscle is 'hydrodiseccted' off the posterior rectus sheath. They can often then be visualized with the US. Inserting them in the upper abdomen and then tunnelling them superiolaterally over the costal margin removes them from the surgical field. Full aseptic precautions should be used for catheter techniques.
- Intermittent bolus techniques are perhaps more effective than continuous infusion regimens with catheters.

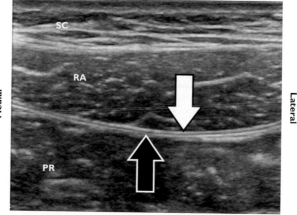

Fig. 34.2 Ultrasound image of the rectus muscle showing the posterior rectus sheath. SC, subcutaneous tissue; RA, rectus abdominis muscle; PR, peritoneal cavity; White arrow, posterior rectus sheath; Black arrow, peritoneum.

Further reading

Dolan J, Lucie P, Geary T, *et al.* (2009). The rectus sheath block: accuracy of local anesthetic placement by trainee anesthesiologists using loss of resistance or ultrasound guidance. *Reg Anesth Pain Med*, **34**(3), 247–50.

Willschke H, Bösenberg A, Marhofer P, *et al.* (2006). Ultrasonography-guided rectus sheath block in paediatric anaesthesia – a new approach to an old technique. *Br J Anaesth*, **97**(2), 244–9.

Yentis SM, Hills-Wright P, Potparic O (1999). Development and evaluation of combined rectus sheath and ilioinguinal blocks for abdominal gynaecological surgery. *Anaesthesia*, **54**(5), 475–9.

Penile block

Background

Landmark: ▰▰▰▰▰▰▰✎

Indications
- Reduction of paraphymosis
- Analgesia following circumcision, meatotomy, or dorsal slit.

Introduction
- This block is simple to perform and is very safe provided the correct technique is employed.
- The block can be safely performed under GA reducing patient discomfort.
- In children undergoing circumcision, dorsal penile block provides more effective postoperative analgesia than systemic opiates, NSAIDs, or paracetamol and it is associated with longer-lasting postoperative analgesia than application of EMLA® cream.
- This technique avoids the motor block and urinary retention associated with caudal block, which can delay patient discharge from day surgery units.

Anatomy
- The somatic innervation of the penis is from the sacral plexus.
- The dorsal nerve of the penis is a terminal branch of the pudendal nerve formed by the ventral rami of S2–S4.
- The dorsal nerve arises in the pudendal canal and passes along the ramus of the ischium. It then runs anteriorly along the margin of the inferior ramus of the pubis to pierce the suspensory ligament to enter the subpubic space.
- The subpubic space is enclosed anteriorly by (the deep) Buck's fascia and also contains the dorsal arteries and deep dorsal vein of the penis running medially.
- It enters Buck's fascia (the fibrous tissue investing the corpus cavernosum) and supplies the skin and the glans of the penis.
- The base of the penis receives additional innervation from cutaneous branches of the genital branch of the genitofemoral nerve.
- The autonomic innervation is from the inferior hypogastric plexus with fibres running in the pudendal nerves or accompanying blood vessels.

Side effects and complications
- Bleeding/haematoma/oedema at injection site.
- Intravascular injection of LA.
- Ischaemia/gangrene of the penis is associated with poor technique or vasoconstrictors.

Landmark technique

Landmarks

- The pubic symphysis.

Technique

- This block is most commonly performed under GA with the patient in the supine position.
- The pubic symphysis is identified and a finger placed underneath in the midline.
- Prepare the skin with 0.5% chlorhexidine in 70% alcohol. Wait until the skin is dry.
- A 23G 2.5–5cm needle is inserted in the midline, perpendicular to skin and then angled 20° laterally (to avoid the blood vessels).
- The needle is advanced under the pubis until Buck's fascia is traversed (a 'pop' is often felt at this point) and then needle enters the subpubic space.
- After careful aspiration 5mL of 0.25–0.5% plain bupivacaine is injected.
- The needle is then withdrawn into the subcutaneous tissue and redirected to the other side.
- For complete anaesthesia, another 5–10mL of solution is injected around the base of the penis in a loose subcutaneous 'ring'.

Clinical notes

- No resistance should be felt on injection; forced injection of large volumes of LA within Buck's fascia may compromise the arterial supply and cause penile gangrene.
- Beware of only passing through the superficial fascia.
- An alternative technique is to aim to contact the inferior edge of the pubis and 'walk off' inferiorly.
- Epinephrine-containing and other vasoconstrictor solutions should be avoided because of the potential to cause ischaemia.
- This is a very vascular area and frequent aspiration is necessary to avoid intravascular injection.
- Subcutaneous ring block alone does not provide optimal analgesia post-circumcision.

Further reading

Choi WY, Irwin MG, Hui TW, *et al.* (2003) EMLA cream versus dorsal penile nerve block for postcir-
    cumcision analgesia in children. *Anesth Analg,* **96**(2), 396–9.
Holder KJ, Peutrell JM, Weir PM (1997). Regional anaesthesia for circumcision. Subcutaneous ring
    block of the penis and subpubic penile block compared. *Eur J Anesth,* **14**(5), 495–8.
Sara CA, Lowry CJ (1985). A complication of circumcision and dorsal nerve block of the penis.
    Anaesth Intensive Care, **13**(1), 79–82.
Serour F, Mori J, Barr J (1994). Optimal regional anesthesia for circumcision. *Anesth Analg,* **79**(1),
    129–31.

Posterior lumbar plexus (psoas compartment, lumbar plexus) block

Background

PNS: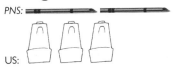

US:

Indications

Anaesthesia
- All lower limb surgery in combination with a sciatic nerve block.
- Surgery on anterior thigh (e.g. muscle biposy).

Analgesia
- Hip and femoral fracture surgery, knee surgery (± sciatic nerve block).

Anatomy

- The lumbar plexus is formed by the anterior 1° rami of the spinal nerves of T12–L3 within the body of the psoas major muscle.
- The spinal nerves coalesce into the lumbar plexus within the posterior 1/3 of the muscle forming the major branches:
  - femoral
  - obturator
  - lumbar component to the lumbosacral trunk.
- Other branches include the iliohypogastric, ilioinguinal, genitofemoral, and lateral cutaneous nerve of the thigh and these leave the lateral border of the psoas muscle (except for the genitofemoral which pierces the anterior surface) passing around the pelvis to supply the skin of the lower anterior abdominal wall, anterior perineum, and anterolateral surface of the thigh.

Side effects and complications

- The lumbar plexus block (LPB) has the highest incidence of major complication as compared to any other lower limb block, including intravascular injection/rapid LA absorption (LA toxicity) and epidural spread.
- LA toxicity. This is in part due to the fact that this is, in essence, just an intramuscular injection (the psoas muscle is very vascular) and the consequent blood levels associated with this block can be high. Added to this, volumes in excess of 50mL have been commonly employed in the past. Volumes in excess of 25mL are to be avoided and a very slow incremental injection should be employed.

- Epidural spread/injections. Published reports put the incidence of epidural spread variably between 3–27% with about 7% as a realistic overall figure. The effects can be unilateral or bilateral, and it is the loss of sympathetic tone that results in the major consequences. Most patients will tolerate a unilateral sympathectomy, but it may cause haemodynamic instability. Cardiovascular collapse can result from a profound, bilateral epidural block from misplaced LA. Medial placement of the needle encourages spread into the epidural space.
- Intrathecal injections have been reported and the resultant high volume total spinal produces profound cardiovascular collapse.
- Retroperitoneal haematomas and abscesses have been reported.
- Renal capsule haematomas have also occurred (needle too cranial).

Peripheral stimulator technique: posterior approach

- The posterior approach to the lumbar plexus is preferred to the anterior approach, i.e. high-volume femoral nerve block (3 in 1 block is an obsolete term) because of the more reliable blockade of all 3 major nerves, femoral, obturator, and lateral cutaneous nerve of thigh.
- First described by Winnie and initially termed 'psoas compartment block', the initial description was confusing as it indicated the needle placement was posterior to psoas and anterior to quadratus lumborum terming this space as the 'psoas compartment'. Although the anatomical description of the compartment may not have survived close scrutiny, the superficial landmarks used have borne the test of time.
- Further approaches have been described: Chayen in 1976 and Dekrey in 1989, but will not be discussed here.
- More recently Capdevila (in 2002) produced a modification of Winnie's approach.
- A comparative study between the approaches of Winnie and Capdevila showed no difference in success rates for femoral (90% vs 93%), lateral cutaneous nerve of the thigh (93% vs 97%) or obturator (80% vs 90%) blockade while the incidence of bilateral spread (10% vs 12%) was the same.

Landmarks

- Posterior superior iliac spine (PSIS)
- Lumbar spinous processes (SP)
- Iliac crest and Tuffier's line.

Technique

- Position the patient in the lateral recumbent position with the hips flexed to 90° with the operative side up.
- Palpate the lumbar spine marking the L4 spinous process. This can be achieved by drawing a line vertically down from the highest point of the iliac crest to cross the vertebral column (Tuffier's line). This should pass through the L4–L5 interspace and the first SP cranial to this line should be L4.
- Palpate and mark the PSIS (feels like a sugared almond).

Winnie's approach

- Needle insertion is at a point where Tuffier's line is crossed by a line drawn parallel to the spine passing through the PSIS. See Fig. 36.1.
- Prepare the skin with 0.5% chlorhexidine in 70% alcohol. Wait until the skin is dry.
- Anaesthetize the skin with a subcutaneous injection of 1% lidocaine at the needle insertion point.
- Insert a 100mm, 21G, insulated short-bevelled stimulating needle attached to a nerve stimulator set to 1.5 mA, 0.1msec, 2Hz pulses.

- Winnie's original description suggests a slight medial inclination, but many opt for a perpendicular trajectory to reduce the risk of neuraxial spread or injection. However, a perpendicular approach risks being too lateral and missing the plexus.
- The needle should pass between L4 and L5 transverse processes and the plexus should be within 70–100mm from the skin.
- If the transverse process is encountered, redirect the needle caudad to 'walk off' the bone. Advance the needle a maximum of 2cm beyond the transverse process until an elicited motor response is seen in the quadriceps muscle (patella dance).
- By small movements of the needle, maximize the motor response and reduce the current to maintain contractions between 0.3mA and 0.5mA.
- After gentle aspiration, inject 1–2mL of LA. The motor response should disappear. Disconnect the syringe to exclude passive reflux of blood (i.e. intravascular needle placement), reconnect and inject 20–25mL slowly in 5mL aliquots, aspirating regularly to detect intravascular injection.

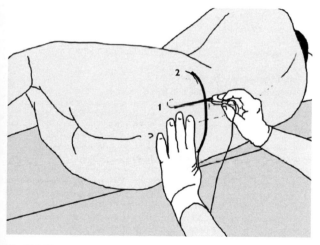

Fig. 36.1 The intersection of the lines from the posterior superior iliac spine (**1**) (parallel to the spinous processes) and Tuffier's line (from the iliac crest (**2**)) is the needle insertion point for Winnie's posterior approach to the lumbar plexus.

Capdevila's approach

- Mark up the back as for Winnie's approach.
- The needle insertion point is at the junction of the lateral 1/3rd and medial 2/3rd of a line between the SP of L4 and a line parallel to the spinal column passing through the PSIS. The SP of L4 is estimated to be 1cm cephalic to Tuffier's line.
- Prepare the skin with 0.5% chlorhexidine in 70% alcohol. Wait until the skin is dry.
- Anaesthetize the skin with a subcutaneous injection of 1% lidocaine at the needle insertion point.
- Insert a 100mm, 21G, insulated short-bevelled stimulating needle attached to a nerve stimulator set to 1.5 mA, 0.1msec, 2Hz pulses perpendicular to the skin.
- Contact with the transverse process should be encountered at between 4cm and 8cm depending on the patient's body habitus.
- Redirect the needle to pass caudally and advance the needle by a maximum of 2cm until an elicited motor response is seen in the quadriceps muscle (patella dance). (Table 36.1.)
- By small movements of the needle, maximize the motor response and reduce the current to maintain contractions between 0.3mA and 0.5mA.
- After gentle aspiration, inject 1–2mL of LA. The motor response should disappear. Disconnect the syringe to exclude passive reflux of blood (i.e. intravascular needle placement), reconnect and inject 20–25mL slowly in 5mL aliquots, aspirating regularly to detect intravascular injection.

Clinical notes

- The commonest use of the LPB is in hip & knee arthroplasty and fractured neck of femur surgery. Analgesia obtained by LPBs, in most cases, is short lived, 4–8 hours. To improve the length of analgesia, continuous lumbar plexus catheters can be used.
- In clinical practice within the UK, LPBs are commonly used where spinal anaesthesia is unsuccessful, contraindicated, and/or in patients in whom a femoral nerve block is deemed insufficient.
- This technique relies on the patient being truly lateral. Care should be taken when the patient either rotates forwards or backwards as this will encourage either medial or lateral needle placement. If the patient has a marked kyphoscoliosis, true lateral is impossible (unless you use US). Avoid the LPB and consider performing a femoral approach instead.
- The need for 150mm needles is small, do not use routinely and only in experienced hands.
- Lumbar plexus catheter—see Chapter 14.
- An optional check to minimize the risk of paravertebral placement of the needle and consequent epidural spread can be performed:
  - Advance the needle further until the motor response is lost. There should be *no contact with bone* if the needle is safely within the psoas muscle. Withdraw the needle slowly reconfirming the motor response
  - If bone is contacted this indicates the needle is too medial and in contact with the vertebral body (i.e. paravertebral and close to the intervertebral foramen)—withdraw the needle and redirect more laterally.

Table 36.1 Possible responses to nerve stimulation and how to adjust

Response	Stimulation	Needle position	Action
Quadriceps contractions	L3–L4 root	PERFECT	Stabilize the needle reduce current threshold 0.3–05mA and inject
Hamstrings contaction	L4 component to lumbosacral plexus	Too caudad and may be too medial	Withdraw needle and insert more cephelad
Hip flexion	Direct psoas muscle stimulation	Too deep	Withdraw needle
Abdominal wall contraction	Direct muscle stimulation of muscles of the abdominal wall	Too far laterally	Check landmarks, withdraw needle and insert more medially
No response	Not close to lumbar plexus	Probably too lateral/too cephelad	Check landmarks—find transverse process and redirect

Ultrasound techniques

- The lumbar plexus is difficult to visualize in adults due to its depth (less resolution) from the surface (7–10cm) and its location within the psoas muscle (more attenuation). The added problem of a limited US window created by the transverse processes (TP) of the lumbar vertebrae all adds to its difficulty.
- It is necessary to use a low-frequency probe (2–5MHz) in most cases, but this limits the visibility due to the low resolution.
- Because of the poor visibility, the combined use of a peripheral nerve stimulator is often employed to confirm the position of the plexus.

Preliminary scan

- Place the probe longitudinal in the paramedian sagittal plane at the level of the TP of the lumbar vertebrae.
- Identify the TP; these will be seen as dark fingers with the hyperechoic periosteum of the TP superficial and resultant acoustic 'drop out' shadow beneath.
- The psoas muscle can be seen between the TP. This picture is often referred to as the 'Trident sign'. See Fig. 36.2.
- Anterior (deep) to the psoas muscle, peristalsis movement of abdominal viscera may be seen, distinguishing the anterior boarder of the psoas muscle.
- More superficial to the psoas the erector spinae muscle can be seen.
- By moving the probe caudad, identify the sacrum (flat hyperechoic line), then moving the probe cephalad, identify and count the transverse processes of the lumbar vertebrae L5, L4, and L3. The L5 lumbar TP is short and thicker than the subsequent transverse processes, with the L4 TP being the longest (widest).
- Continue moving cephalad; note how the psoas muscle becomes thinner and at L1–L2 the lower pole of the kidney can be seen anterior to the psoas muscle.
- Move the probe caudad, identifying the TP of L3 and L4; mark the skin.
- Turn the probe through 90° to obtain a transverse picture of the lumbar spine at the level of the L3 TP. The bony reflection of the TP obscures any deeper structures and the psoas muscle cannot be identified.
- Move the probe caudad between the L3 and L4 TP until the hyperechoic shadow of the TP disappears and the deeper structures are seen.
- The psoas muscle will now appear as a rounded structure, the hyperechoic nerve roots may be seen as lines spreading laterally in the posterior third of the muscle. Medial to the psoas muscle the entrance of the intervertebral foramina may be seen. See Fig. 36.3.

Ultrasound settings

- Probe: adults, low-frequency (<5MHz) curvilinear. Children, high-frequency (8–18MHz) linear.
- Settings: MB—abdomen, general /penetration.
- Depth: 8–12cm.
- Needle: 100mm of choice.

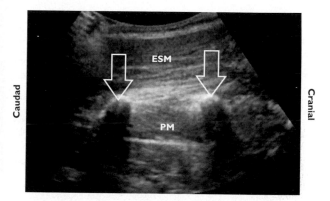

Fig. 36.2 Ultrasound in the paramedian sagittal plane, showing the transverse processes and the psoas muscle deep to them. ESM, erector spinae muscle; Arrows, transverse processes; PM, psoas major muscle.

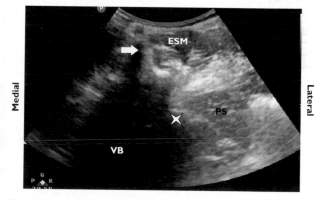

Fig. 36.3 Ultrasound scan in the transverse (axial) plane showing the erector spinae muscle and the psoas muscle. The vertebral body can be seen on the medial side of the image. ESM, erector spinae muscle; White arrow, spinous process; White star, position of intervertebral foramina; PS, psoas major muscle; VB, vertebral body.

Technique
- Prepare the skin with 0.5% chlorhexidine in 70% alcohol. Wait until the skin is dry.
- Anaesthetize the skin with a subcutaneous injection of 1% lidocaine.
- Use an in-plane (lateral to medial) needle approach.
- The plexus is often not seen as a distinct entity but more as a hyperechoic band within the psoas muscle (transverse scan), seen through the intratransverse process window in the posterior 1/3 of the psoas muscle.
- Where the plexus is not visualized the needle can be directed onto the transverse process and then guided by US 2cm deep to the TP and then either motor response is sought or the injection performed under real-time US guidance, observing the spread of LA.

Clinical notes
- Combine the nerve stimulator with US for this approach ('dual technique'). Ideally a good needle position in the posterior 1/3 of the psoas muscle on US and an appropriate motor response is obtained, but it is important to use ONLY one or other as an endpoint.
- In cases of difficult visibility use the US just to identify the level, position and depth of the TP and use this to aid PNS.

Further reading

Capdevila X, Marcaire P, Dadurec D, et al. (2002). Continuous psoas compartment block for post-operative analgesia after total hip arthroplasty: new landmarks, technical guidelines and clinical evaluation. Anesth Analg, 94(6), 1606–13.

Karmakar MK, Ho NH, Li X, et al. (2008). Ultrasound guided lumbar plexus block through the acoustic window of the lumbar ultrasound trident. Br J Anaesth, 100(4), 533–7.

Kirchmair L, Entner T, Wissel J (2001). A study of the paravertebral anatomy for ultrasound-guided posterior lumbar plexus block. Anesth Analg, 93(2), 477–81.

Mannion S , O'Callaghan S, Walsh M, et al. (2005). In with the new, out with the old? Comparison of two approaches for psoas compartment block. Anaesth Analg, 101(1), 259–64.

Touray ST, De Leeuw MA, Zuurmond WWA, et al. (2008). Psoas compartment block for lower extremity surgery: a meta-analysis. Br J Anaesth, 101(6), 750–60.

Femoral nerve block

Background

PNS:

US:

Indications

Anaesthesia

- Sole technique for surgery on anterior thigh (skin graft/muscle biopsy).
- In combination with sciatic popliteal block for foot and ankle surgery.
- In combination with proximal obturator and sciatic nerve blocks for all surgery on the leg (excluding hip surgery).

Analgesia

- Fracture of femur (neck and shaft).
- Total hip replacement.
- Knee surgery (anterior cruciate reconstruction and total knee replacement).
- The use of continuous catheters for extending the block in the postoperative period is common in total knee replacements.

Anatomy

- The femoral nerve is formed from the anterior 1° rami of L2–L4, within the body of the psoas muscle.
- Emerging from the lateral border of the psoas muscle the nerve travels in the gutter formed by the psoas and iliacus muscles (the nerve gives branches to iliacus in the pelvis).
- Passing beneath the midpoint of the inguinal ligament the nerve enters the femoral triangle into the anterior thigh, lateral to the femoral sheath (femoral artery, veins, and lymphatics).
- In the thigh the nerve lies deep to the fascia iliacus (on the iliacus muscle), with the thickened medial border of the fascia iliacus (iliopectineal band) separating the nerve from the femoral sheath. See Fig. 37.1 and Fig. 37.2.
- As soon as the nerve enters the anterior thigh, it divides into superficial and deep components.
- The superficial branches include:
  • the musculocutaneous branch which both innervates sartorius and continues as the intermediate cutaneous nerve, which divides into the lateral and medial branches—supplying sensory innervation to the skin on the medial and lateral aspects of anterior thigh
  • the medial anterior cutaneous nerve supplying skin over the medial thigh
  • the nerve to pectineus (passing deep to the femoral sheath)—also supplying anterior part of hip joint
  • the nerve to rectus femoris—also supplying anterior part of the hip joint.
- The deep branches include:
  • the nerve to vastus lateralis (branch to the capsule of the knee joint)
  • nerve to vastus intermedius (branch to the capsule of the knee joint)
  • nerve to vastus medialis—passing with the common femoral artery into the adductor canal (branch to the capsule of the knee joint)

- saphenous nerve—passing with the common femoral artery into the adductor canal—supplying sensory innervation to the knee (infrapatellar branch) and the medial aspect of the lower leg to the base of the 1st metatarsal.
- The closer to the inguinal ligament, the more superficial the femoral nerve is and the more compact its components are. The lateral circumflex femoral *artery* may pass between the superficial branches of the femoral nerve at this level.

Side effects and complications

- Vascular puncture and injection. This is easy with PNS technique as the edges of the artery can be difficult to locate.
- Nerve damage. This may be less likely as the nerve will often separate out into its branches.

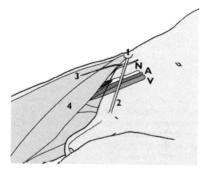

Fig. 37.1 Illustration of the anatomy of the femoral nerve as it passes under the inguinal ligament, lateral to the femoral vessels. **1** anterior superior iliac spine; **2** inguinal ligament; **3** lateral cutaneous nerve of the thigh; **4** sartorius muscle; N, femoral nerve; A, femoral artery; V, femoral vein.

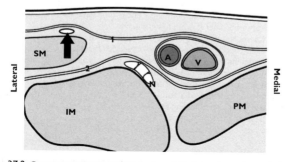

Fig. 37.2 Cross-sectional anatomical illustration of the femoral nerve beneath the fascia iliaca. **1** fascia lata; **2** fascia iliaca; Black arrow, lateral cutaneous nerve of the thigh; N, femoral nerve; A, femoral artery; V, femoral vein; IM, iliacus muscle; PM, pectineus muscle; SM, sartorius muscle.

Peripheral nerve stimulator technique

Prior to the introduction of the PNS, blockade of the femoral nerve was achieved by direct injection using a combination of loss of resistance, blind infiltration, and/or paraesthesia.

In 1973 Winnie coined the term '3-in-1 block', which used a high-volume technique via an anterior femoral perivascular approach to achieve blockade of the lumbar plexus (femoral, obturator, and lateral cutaneous nerve of thigh). The evidence for predictable proximal spread of LA to the lumbar plexus is inconclusive, especially for reliable blockade of the obturator nerve (4–30% by this approach). The term 3:1 block is now considered a misnomer and its use is not encouraged.

The blockade of the lateral cutaneous nerve of thigh is commonly (>60%) achieved during a femoral nerve block and can be ↑ by using a more lateral landmark technique (see Chapter 38).

Landmarks

- ASIS
- PT
- Inguinal ligament
- Femoral artery.

Technique

- Palpate the ASIS and PT, mark a line joining these 2 points, this is the surface marking of the inguinal ligament.
- Palpate the femoral artery (midpoint of inguinal ligament) and mark a point 1–2cm distal to the inguinal ligament and 1cm lateral to the femoral artery. See Fig. 37.3.
- Prepare the skin with 0.5% chlorhexidine in 70% alcohol. Wait until the skin is dry.
- Anaesthetize the skin with a subcutaneous injection of 1% lidocaine at the point of needle insertion.
- Insert a 50mm short-bevelled needle through the skin at an angle of 30–45° in a cephalad direction.
- 2 distinct losses of resistance or 'pops' should be felt as the needle is advanced: 1st fascia lata, 2nd fascia iliacus. The nerve is usually located at a depth of 12mm ± 4mm from the skin.
- Look for stimulation of the quadriceps muscles from the posterior division of the femoral nerve 'patella twitch' (Table 37.1).
- Manipulate the needle until stimulating current is between 0.3 and 0.5mA. Disconnect syringe before injection to exclude passive reflux of blood and inject 5mL aliquots of LA, aspirating regularly to exclude intravascular injection.
- 20–30mL of LA is sufficient.

Clinical notes

- Sartorius twitch may indicate either stimulation of the motor branch to sartorius (part of the superficial division of the femoral nerve) or direct muscle stimulation, but the spread of LA to the posterior division cannot be guaranteed with injection at this point.
- Note that the nerve can be up to 3cm lateral to the artery.
- Commonest cause of failure is to be too far distal from the inguinal crease, the nerve is now a collection of branches.
- If you obtain contraction of the medial bulk of the quadriceps redirect the needle more laterally, vice versa if contraction of the lateral bulk of quadriceps.

Table 37.1 Possible responses to nerve stimulation and how to adjust

Response	Stimulation	Needle position	Action
Patella twitch	Posterior division branches to the quadriceps	PERFECT	Stabilize the needle reduce current threshold 0.3–0.5mA and inject
Sartorius twitch	Nerve to sartorius	Too superficial and maybe too lateral (or medial)	Reposition more medial (or lateral) and insert needle deeper
Local twitch	Iliacus muscle	Too deep	Withdraw needle
No response	In subcutaneous tissues	Too medially or more likely too lateral	Often found in obese patients. Withdraw needle, repalpate and start nearer the femoral artery
Vascular puncture	Femoral artery	Too medially	Withdraw and insert more laterally

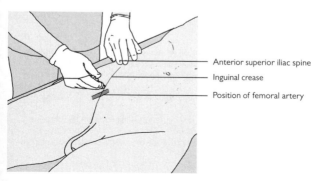

Anterior superior iliac spine

Inguinal crease

Position of femoral artery

Fig. 37.3 PNS technique for femoral nerve block.

Ultrasound technique

The femoral nerve is a large, superficial nerve with clearly identifiable landmarks (the femoral artery) and is therefore suitable for a US-guided block. However, achieving a good image of the nerve is not always easy and requires good control and manipulation of the probe and needle. The use of US has been shown to decrease the volume of LA needed and reduce the latency of onset of the block.

Preliminary scan
- Place the probe on the patient in a transverse/oblique position, i.e. longitudinally along the inguinal crease.
- Identify the femoral artery (pulsatile, anechoic) and the femoral vein (compressive distensible anechoic).
- Scan caudad and cephalad identifying the division of the common femoral artery into the superficial femoral and profunda femoris arteries and ensure you are above this level, close to the inguinal ligament.
- Scanning laterally identify the iliacus and sartorius muscles.
- From superficial to deep identify 2 hyperechoic fascia layers, the superficial fascia lata (this fascia continues medially, superficial to the femoral sheath) and the deeper fascia iliacus (enclosing the iliacus muscle, passing posterior to the femoral sheath). See Fig. 37.4.
- The femoral nerve can be identified *beneath* the iliacus fascia on the medial border of iliacus, lateral and deep to the femoral artery. The nerve appears as a hyperechoic structure in this triangle between the femoral artery, iliacus, and subcutaneous tissues. It may appear crescent shaped or flattened, often seen as a collection of nerves rather than a distinct nerve entity. Angulation of the probe may help with identification.

Ultrasound settings
- Probe: high-frequency (>10MHz) linear L38 broadband probe
- Settings: MB—resolution
- Depth: 3–4cm
- Needle: 50–80mm
- Orientation: transverse (slightly oblique).

Technique
- Either an in-plane or an out-of-plane technique can be used. In-plane (from lateral to medial) is preferable to achieve good spread of LA around the nerve, but an out-of-plane technique is better for catheter insertions.
- Prepare the skin with 0.5% chlorhexidine in 70% alcohol. Wait until the skin is dry.
- Anaesthetize the skin with a subcutaneous injection of 1% lidocaine at the point of needle insertion.
- For either technique, aim to introduce the needle just lateral to nerve just underneath the fascia iliaca.

- After aspiration, inject 1mL of LA to confirm position deep to fascia iliaca (hydrolocation).
- Aim to 'peel' the nerve off the fascia above and the muscle below (hydrodissection) with fractionated injections of LA and careful needle repositioning.
- Aim for circumferential spread around the nerve.
- 15–20mL of LA should be sufficient.

Clinical notes

- The femoral nerve can be difficult to visualize, and the use of a dual technique using US and PNS is often helpful, but does not improve success.
- Always approach the lateral aspect of the femoral nerve using US as the medial edge of the femoral nerve may be obscured by lateral shadowing from the femoral artery.
- To achieve good spread of LA it is best to place the needle beneath the femoral nerve using the in-plane technique. The femoral nerve will often then be seen to float up into the LA, becoming brighter and also splitting into its component branches.
- Always scan distally and proximally confirming circumferential spread around the nerve.

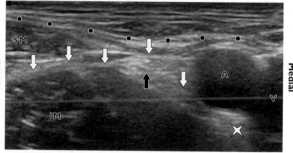

Fig. 37.4 Ultrasound of the femoral nerve. Black dots, fascia lata; SM, sartorius muscle; White arrows, fascia iliaca; Black arrow, femoral nerve; A, femoral artery; V, femoral vein; IM, iliacus muscle; White star, post cystic enhancement (not nerve).

Further reading

Anns JP, Chen EW, Nirkavan N, *et al.* (2011). A comparison of sartorius versus quadriceps stimulation for femoral nerve block: a prospective randomized doudouble blind controlled trial. *Anest Analg*, **112**(3), 725–31.

Casati A, Baciarello M, Di Cianni S, *et al.* (2007). Effects of ultrasound guidance on the minimum effective anaesthetic volume required to block the femoral nerve. *Br J Anaesth*, **98**(6), 823–7.

Paul JE, Arya A, Hurlbert L, *et al.* (2010). Femoral nerve block improves analgesia outcomes after total knee arthroplasty: a meta-analysis of randomized controlled trials. *Anesthesiology*, **113**(5), 1144–62.

Soong J, Scafhalter-Zoppoth I, Gray T (2005). The importance of transducer angle to ultrasound visibility of the femoral nerve, *Reg Anesth Pain Med*, **30**(5), 505.

Winnie A, Ramamurthy S, Durrani ZI (1973). The inguinal paravascular technique of lumbar plexus anesthesia: the '3-in-1 block'. *Anesth Analg*, **52**(6), 989–96.

Fascia iliaca block

Background

Landmarks:

US:

Indications

Anaesthesia
• Sole technique for surgery on anterior thigh (skin graft/muscle biopsy).

Analgesia
• Hip and shaft of femur fractures and surgery to the knee.

Introduction

This technique was initially developed as an alternative to the femoral 'perivascular 3:1 block' in children. The advantage of this block is that it reliably blocks the femoral nerve with minimal risk of inadvertent femoral artery, vein, or nerve puncture, thereby increasing the safety and simplicity of technique.

It also has a higher associated blockade of the lateral cutaneous nerve of the thigh (LCNTH) than the perivascular approach, but will not reliable block the obturator nerve.

Its popularity has ↑ significantly with its use for early pain control in patients with a femoral neck or shaft fractures. In these cases the 1° benefit is from paralysis and loss of spasm of the quadriceps muscle rather than direct analgesia of the femur.

Such is its safety and simplicity that it is regularly performed by non-physicians (e.g. paramedics, nurses, or physicians' assistants) in the pre-hospital, emergency room, or ward environment. This technique does not use a PNS or need an US as it safety relies on the injection site being well lateral to the femoral artery.

Anatomy

• This is a fascial plane block, which takes the advantage of the anatomical relationship of the femoral nerve to the fascia iliaca.
• This fascia is adherent to and covers the internal surface of the iliacus muscle.
• At its cephalad attachment it fuses with the posterior lumbar fascia at its origin from the iliac crest. Laterally it fuses with the origin of iliacus and medially with the psoas fascia, which is tightly adherent to the muscle within the pelvis and covered anteriorly by the parietal peritoneum. Inferiorly it covers the iliacus as it passes behind the inguinal ligament and then fuses with the fascia of the muscles of the thigh, thickening medially into the iliopectineal ligament.
• Because of its defined borders, injection of LA in this subfascial space (compartment) gives a predictable and reliable pattern of spread.
• Spreading medially and cephalad it will surround the femoral nerve and spreading cephalad and laterally (beneath the inguinal ligament) it will surround the LCNTH.

Side effects and complications

- As this is not a perineural injection and is away from major vessels complications should be low.
- Bleeding and bruising is possible.
- LA toxicity.
- Deep (retroperitoneal) abscesses with catheters.

Landmark technique

Landmarks
- ASIS
- PT
- Inguinal ligament
- Femoral artery.

Technique
- With the patient supine and the leg in a neutral position, palpate the ASIS and the PT and draw a line between the 2; this is the surface marking of the inguinal ligament.
- Divide this line into 3; at the junction of the middle and lateral 1/3 mark a point 1–2cm inferiorly. This is the needle insertion point. See Fig. 38.1.
- Prepare the skin with 0.5% chlorhexidine in 70% alcohol. Wait until the skin is dry.
- Anaesthetize the skin with a subcutaneous injection of 1% lidocaine at the point of needle insertion.
- Insert a 25–50mm short-bevelled needle perpendicular through the skin (or at 30° cephalad if intending to place a catheter).
- This technique relies on 2 fascial pops, clicks, or a loss of resistance. As the needle is gently inserted a click or pop will be felt as the needle initially passes through the fascia lata, the second is when the needle passes through the fascia iliaca.
- This is *not* a perineural injection so a PNS is not needed or useful.
- Stabilize the needle, aspirate, and inject 20–25mL of LA.

Clinical notes
- The injection point should always be 2–3 finger breadths lateral to the artery.
- When injecting, if the subcutaneous tissues swell, this indicates that the needle placement is too superficial above the fascia iliaca—withdraw the needle and reposition.
- If it is difficult to inject, then the needle is probably too deep, within the muscle of iliacus—withdraw the needle and reposition.
- Using short-bevelled needles may aid in the detection of the pops when passing through the fascial planes.

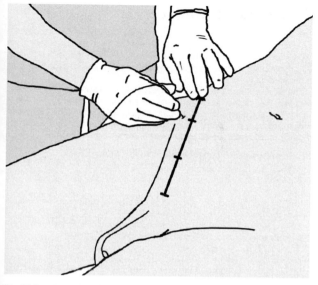

Fig. 38.1 Landmarks for a fascia iliaca block. Needle insertion 1–2cm inferior to junction of middle 1/3 and lateral 1/3 of the inguinal ligament (between the ASIS and pubic tubercle).

Ultrasound technique

Although this block can be carried out with US, the benefit of this technique is its non-reliance on technology, e.g. PNS or US. With the assistance of an US it may be better to perform an US-guided femoral nerve block—see ⊃ Ultrasound technique, p. 410. However, the technique is described later in this section.

The block can be carried out in a similar fashion to a femoral nerve block, although the injection is more lateral (away from the nerve), or there is a more recent description of a suprainguinal fascia iliaca block (described later in this section). With this injection being more proximal, there is less reliance on proximal spread to achieve blockade of the LCNTH.

Preliminary scan: suprainguinal fascia iliaca block

- Position the patient supine.
- Place the probe on the patient in a sagittal plane over the inguinal ligament, close to the ASIS.
- Identify the hyperechoic reflection of the internal surface of the Ilium, with the Iliacus muscle superficial to it.
- The hyperechoic fascia iliaca covers the iliacus muscle. Tilting the more laterally may enhance the visibility of the fascia.
- The iliacus muscle angles deep in the pelvis superiorly and is then covered by the abdominal wall muscle. The peritoneum may sit between these, but the pressure of the probe should exclude abdominal contents from here.
- Scan inferiomedially along the inguinal ligament, until the femoral artery is seen.
- Scan back superior-laterally looking for the anterior *inferior* iliac spine as a small peak on the surface of the ilium. This will be lateral to the femoral nerve and marks the needle insertion point.
- Use the colour Doppler to try to identify the deep circumflex iliac artery superficial to the fascia iliaca.
- See Fig. 38.2.

Ultrasound settings: suprainguinal fascia Iliaca block

- Probe: high-frequency (>10MHz) linear L38 broadband probe (occasially a lower frequency curvilinear probe in obese patients).
- Settings: MB/general/penetration.
- Depth: 4–6cm.
- Needle: 80–100mm.
- Orientation: parasagittal.

Technique: suprainguinal fascia Iliaca block

- Prepare the skin with 0.5% chlorhexidine in 70% alcohol. Wait until the skin is dry.
- Anaesthetize the skin with a subcutaneous injection of 1% lidocaine at the point of needle insertion.
- An in-plane technique is used, inserting the needle at the inferior end of the probe, *inferior* to the inguinal ligament.

- The needle should pierce the fascia iliaca approximately at the level of the inguinal ligament.
- After aspiration, inject 1mL of LA. This should form a small bleb, or 'lens' deep to fascia iliaca.
- Gently advance the needle into this bleb and further LA is injected.
- The LA should inject easily and pass freely over the top of the iliacus muscle.
- Inject 20mL of LA.
- Turn the probe through 90° to image the spread of LA medially to the femoral nerve.

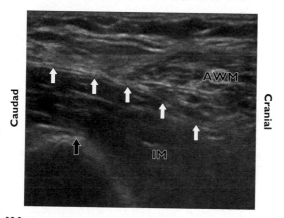

Fig. 38.2 Ultrasound scan of the iliac fossa for a fascia iliaca block. AWM, abdominal wall muscles; IM, iliacus muscle; White arrows, fascia iliaca; Black arrow, anterior inferior iliac spine.

Further reading

Capdavila X, Biboulet P, Bouregba M, *et al.* (1998). Comparison of the three in one and fascia iliaca compartment block in adults: clinical and radiological analysis. *Anesth Analg*, **86**(5), 1039–44.

Dolan J, Williams A, Murney E, *et al.* (2008). Ultrasound guided fascia iliacus block: A comparison with loss of resistance technique. *Reg Anesth Pain Med*, **33**(6), 526–31.

Foss NB, Kristensen BB, Bundgaard M, *et al.* (2007). Fascia iliaca compartment block for acute pain control in hip fracture patients: a randomised, placebo controlled trial. *Anesthesiology*, **106**(4), 773–8.

Hebbard P, Ivanusic J, Sha S. (2011). Ultrasound guided supra-inguinal fascia iliaca block: a cadaveric evaluation of a novel approach. *Anaesthesia*, **66**(4), 300–5.

Wathen JE, Gao D , Merritt G, *et al.* (2007). A randomised controlled trial of fascia iliaca compartment nerve block to traditional systemic analgesia for femur fractures in a paediatric emergency department. *Ann Emerg Med*, **50**(2), 162–71.

Lateral cutaneous nerve of the thigh block

Background

PNS/landmarks: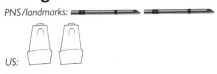

US:

Indications

Anaesthesia
- Diagnostic and treatment for meralgia paraesthetica.

Analgesia
- For surgery and/or incisions on the lateral aspect of the thigh including skin graft harvesting.

Anatomy
- The LCNTH, or lateral femoral cutaneous nerve, is formed in the body of the psoas muscle from the posterior rami of L2–L3.
- Emerging form the lateral boarder of psoas it passes obliquely across the iliacus muscle beneath iliacus fascia towards the ASIS.
- Here it supplies the parietal peritoneum of the iliac fossa and is crossed superficially by the deep circumflex iliac artery.
- The nerve passes either behind or through the inguinal ligament at a variable distance medial (commonly 1cm) or inferiorly to the anterior superior iliac spine.
- It then passes inferolaterally either through or anterior to sartorius, dividing into its anterior and posterior branches. See Fig. 39.1.
- The anterior branch pierces fascia lata more distal than the posterior branch (8.0cm distal to inguinal crease) and supplies the skin on the anterior thigh, connecting more distally with the infrapatella branch of the saphenous nerve and anterior cutaneous femoral nerves to form the patella plexus.
- The posterior branch supplies the skin over the lateral surface of the thigh from the greater trochanter to mid-thigh.

Side effects and complications
- Femoral nerve block
- Bleeding and bruising.

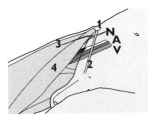

Fig. 39.1 Anatomy of the LCNTH. **1** anterior superior iliac spine; **2** inguinal ligament; **3** lateral cutaneous nerve of the thigh; **4** sartorius muscle; **N**, femoral nerve; **A**, femoral artery; **V**, femoral vein.

Landmark technique

The lateral cutaneous nerve of the thigh is a wholly sensory nerve and as such blockade is commonly performed by subcutaneous infiltration above and below the fascia lata in the anterior thigh. The use of PNS, can improve the success rate but is not commonly employed, as eliciting paraesthesia can be difficult.

Landmarks
- ASIS.

Technique
- Mark a point 2cm medial and 2cm inferior to the ASIS.
- Prepare the skin with 0.5% chlorhexidine in 70% alcohol. Wait until the skin is dry.
- Anaesthetize the skin with a subcutaneous injection of 1% lidocaine for awake patients.
- Insert a 25mm short-bevelled needle perpendicular to the skin.
- Elicit a loss of resistance as the needle passes through the fascia lata.
- Inject up to 10mL of LA in a fan-wise fashion below and above the fascia lata.

Clinical notes
- Femoral nerve blockade is common and will increase as the volume is increased—mobilize with assistance especially if done as a day case.

Ultrasound technique

The LCNTH is a small nerve with a high level of anatomical variability. This makes the nerve difficult to locate and visualize with US. It is therefore very important to use a high-frequency probe >12Mhz and to have a structured examination of the area.

Preliminary scan

- Place the probe transversely on the anterior thigh, medial to the ASIS above the inguinal ligament.
- Scanning distally identify the origin, and the developing body, of the sartorius muscle and the fascia lata coving it.
- More distally, lateral to the sartorius, identify the tensor fascia lata muscle and posteriorly is the developing rectus femoris muscle.
- Scanning distally over the sartorius from its origin, look for a small hyperechoic structure (or structures) often composed of bubbles (individual fascicle and branches—up to 3–4 branches) passing from medial to lateral over the surface of the muscle, deep to fascia lata—this is the LCNTH. See Fig. 39.2.
- Once identified, follow the nerve cephalad to where it disappears under the inguinal ligament. At this point the nerve makes a sharp angle as it goes into the abdomen (often difficult to visualize without acutely angling the probe).
- Within the abdomen the LCNTH can often be visualized in thin individuals and children as it sweeps round the pelvis beneath the fascia iliaca on the iliacus muscle, as it is crossed by the circumflex iliac vessels (use colour flow Doppler to identify). At this point in some individuals the femoral nerve can also be visualized medial to the LCNTH.
- Blockade of the nerve is best achieved as close to the inguinal ligament as possible.
- If the nerve is not easily identified over sartorius (the nerve may pass through sartorius), start scanning more distally; identify the (fat-filled) triangle between sartorius and tensor fascia lata, the nerve may be seen here, or identified when scanning more proximally.

Ultrasound settings

- Probe: high-frequency (>10MHz) linear L38 broadband probe
- Settings: MB—resolution
- Depth: 1–3cm
- Orientation: transverse
- Needle: 25–50mm of choice.

Technique

- Prepare the skin with 0.5% chlorhexidine in 70% alcohol. Wait until the skin is dry.
- Anaesthetize the skin with a subcutaneous injection of 1% lidocaine for awake patients.
- Either an in-plane or out-of-plane approach can be used.
- Inject 3–4mL of LA around nerve.
- If you cannot see the nerve, infiltrate in the triangle between the sartorius and tensor fascia lata muscles with up to 10mL of LA.

Clinical notes

• Use the highest frequency probe possible.

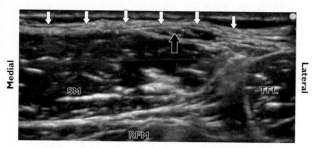

Fig. 39.2 Ultrasound of the LCNTH. White arrows, fascia lata; Black arrow, lateral cutaneous nerve of the thigh; SM, sartorius muscle; TFL, tensor fascia lata muscle; RFM, rectus femoris muscle.

Further reading

Hebbard P, Ivanusic J, Sha S (2011). Ultrasound-guided supra-inguinal fascia iliaca block: a cadaveric evaluation of a novel approach. *Anaesthesia*, **66**(4), 300–5.

Hopkins PM, Ellis FR, Halsall PJ (1991). Evaulation of local anaesthetic blockade of the lateral cutaneous nerve. *Anaesthesia*, **46**(2), 95–6.

Shannon J, Lang SA, Yip RW, et al. (1995). Lateral cutaneous nerve block revisited. A nerve stimulator technique. *Reg Anesth*, **20**(2), 100–4.

Tumber PS, Bhatia A, Chan VW (2008). Ultrasound-guided lateral femoral cutaneous nerve block for meralgia paresthetica. *Anesth Analg*, **106**(3), 1021–2.

Saphenous nerve block

Background

Landmarks:

US:

Indications

Anaesthesia
- In combination with popliteal sciatic nerve block for all surgery on the foot and lower leg.

Analgesia
- For all surgery involving the medial aspect of the leg and foot.

Anatomy
- The saphenous nerve is the largest cutaneous branch of the femoral nerve.
- The branch originates form the posterior division (deep part) of the femoral nerve and follows the femoral artery into the adductor canal covered anteriorly by the sartorius muscle.
- Initially it lies lateral to the artery then crosses it anteriorly to lie medial to the artery at the distal end of the canal. Here it leaves the artery piercing the overlying fascia of the canal, accompanied by the saphenous branch of the descending genicular artery.
- It then passes vertically down beneath sartorius on the medial aspect of the knee exiting between the tendons of sartorius and gracilis into subcutaneous tissues. See Fig. 40.1.
- In the mid-thigh region the saphenous nerve gives off a branch to the subsartorial plexus and as it leaves the canal its infrapatella branch, which pierces sartorius and fascia lata to supply the prepatella skin, connects with the other femoral cutaneous branches and forms the patella plexus.
- In the lower leg the nerve accompanies the long saphenous vein to the ankle along the posterior border of the tibia.
- Dividing into 2 branches, it supplies the skin over the medial border of the tibia and passing anterior to the medial malleolus, supplies the skin on the medial side of the foot. Its cutaneous distribution is highly variable as it connects with the superficial peroneal nerve but may extend distally to the 1st metatarsophalangeal junction.

Side effects and complications
- Bleeding and bruising
- Paraesthesia and nerve dysfunction
- LA toxicity and intravascular injection.

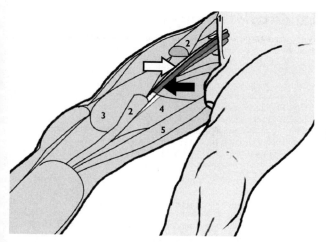

Fig. 40.1 Diagram to show the saphenous nerve running with the femoral artery in the adductor canal deep to sartorius (cut away). **1** inguinal ligament; **2** sartorius muscle (cut); **3** quadriceps muscles; **4** adductor muscles; **5** gracilus muscle; White arrow, saphenous nerve; Black arrow, femoral artery.

Landmark technique

The saphenous nerve is wholly sensory and so classically, blockade of this nerve has been performed by subcutaneous infiltration, either at the level of the tibial condyle or at the medial malleolus.

Alternative techniques have been devised to improve the success rates:
- Trans-sartorial approach with a loss of resistance.
- Paravenous approach.
- High PNS technique.
- Low PNS technique.
- Using PNS, either a surrogate motor response from a motor nerve such as the nerve to vastus medialis is used, (as it is from the same component of the femoral nerve and is in close proximity to the saphenous nerve) or paraesthesia in the distribution of the saphenous nerve.

A recent comparative study of 5 techniques (perifemoral-PNS, trans-sartorial-PNS, block at the medial femoral condyle, below-knee field block, and medial malleoli blocks) showed varying success rates. The best success rates were obtained from the trans-sartorial (100%) and perifemoral blocks (70%), with the below-knee field block 70% and medial malleolus block (60%) being more successful than the medial femoral condyle infiltration (10%). As expected, the perifemoral block (low femoral nerve block) had a high incidence of hip flexor and leg extensor weakness >60%.

The common innervation of the medial aspect of the foot by the medial dorsal cutaneous branch of the peroneal nerve makes it difficult in many cases to get complete anaesthesia of the medial aspect of the foot with the saphenous nerve block alone.

Landmarks
- Inguinal ligament
- Femoral artery
- Sartorius muscle and its insertion
- Patella
- Tibial condyle and tibial tuberosity
- Long saphenous vein
- Medial malleolus.

Techniques

Infiltration at the tibial condyle
- Palpate medial tibial condyle.
- Prepare the skin with 0.5% chlorhexidine in 70% alcohol. Wait until the skin is dry.
- At the level of the tibial tuberosity insert a needle in an anterior to posterior direction, infiltrate 5–10mL of LA subcutaneously medially over the medial tibial condyle to the dorsomedial aspect of the calf.
- The use of a thigh tourniquet may help identify the long saphenous vein and paravenous infiltration may be used in addition.

Infiltration at the medial malleolus
- Palpate the medial malleolus.
- Prepare the skin with 0.5% chlorhexidine in 70% alcohol. Wait until the skin is dry.

- 1–2 finger breadths above the medial malleoli infiltrate 5mL of LA subcutaneously from the posterior border of the medial malleoli to the anterior border of the tibia.

Trans-sartorial

- With the leg extended and slightly raised identify the belly of the sartorius muscle on the medial side of the knee. At point 1–2 finger breadths above the patella, drop a perpendicular line to cross the sartorius muscle.
- Prepare the skin with 0.5% chlorhexidine in 70% alcohol. Wait until the skin is dry.
- Anaesthetize the skin with a subcutaneous injection of 1% lidocaine.
- Insert a needle in a slightly caudad and dorsal direction. As the needle passes through the belly of sartorius a loss of resistance will be elicited as the needle passes into the subsartorial space. See Fig. 40.2.
- After careful aspiration, inject 10mL of LA.

Perifemoral

- Identify the inguinal ligament and the femoral artery.
- Prepare the skin with 0.5% chlorhexidine in 70% alcohol. Wait until the skin is dry.
- Anaesthetize the skin with a subcutaneous injection of 1% lidocaine.
- At a distance 4–6cm distal to the inguinal ligament, insert a 50mm needle 1cm lateral to the femoral artery.
- A motor response from the medial part of the femoral nerve is elicited, e.g. ideally contraction of vastus medialis, but rectus femoris or patella twitch is acceptable.
- After careful aspiration 10mL (low volume femoral block) of LA is injected.

Clinical notes

- To minimize the motor weakness, perform the block as distally as possible but if motor weakness is not a problem—then a more proximal technique can be used.
- A femoral nerve block is still the most reliable technique to block the saphenous nerve.

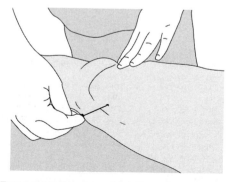

Fig. 40.2 Trans-sartorial saphenous nerve block. The needle insertion point is in line with 2 finger breadths above the superior end of the patella.

Ultrasound technique

The saphenous nerve is small (3–6mm) and potentially deep at its most consistent site, subsartorially, and as such can be difficult to visualize accurately in all cases.

Preliminary scan

- Position the patient supine, with the leg slightly abducted and knee slightly flexed.
- Place the probe transversely on the medial aspect of the thigh 2 finger breadths above the patella; identify the sartorius muscle. The muscle has a distinct fattened triangular appearance (and if followed cephalad will cross the anterior thigh to its origin at the anterior superior Iliac spine). See Fig. 40.3.
- With the body of the muscle in the middle of the image, scan cephalad, identifying the common femoral artery and vein beneath sartorius in the subsartorial canal.
- The saphenous nerve enters the canal lateral to the artery with the nerve to vastus medialis, then crosses the artery superiorly to lie superomedial to the artery in the lower part of the canal.
- The saphenous nerve may be identified lateral to the artery high in the canal as a hyperechoic structure, but often it is not clearly seen. See Fig. 40.4.
- Scanning caudally, follow the artery till it starts to pass posteriorly into the adductor canal. At this point the artery will give off a major branch 'the descending genicular artery' and the saphenous nerve will leave the canal at this level accompanied by the saphenous branch of this artery.
- The nerve can be followed inferiorly as it passes beneath sartorius, then between sartorius and gracilis into the subcutaneous tissues of the medial thigh. A small hyperechoic branch 'infrapatellar' can often be identified beneath sartorius before the nerve becomes superficial.

US settings

- Probe: high-frequency (>10MHz) linear L38 broadband probe
- Settings: MB—resolution
- Depth: 2–4cm
- Orientation: transverse (axial)
- Needle: 50–80mm of choice.

Technique

- Identify the sartorius muscle with the femoral artery and vein beneath it.
- If the saphenous nerve can clearly be seen within the canal, blockade of the nerve can be performed at any level.
- Prepare the skin with 0.5% chlorhexidine in 70% alcohol. Wait until the skin is dry.
- Anaesthetize the skin with a subcutaneous injection of 1% lidocaine.
- Alternatively, if the nerve is not clearly identified, inject in the tissue plane deep to sartorius and superficial to the femoral artery.
- An in-plane technique is used and the needle can be directed to pass between sartorius and vastus medialis.
- 5mL of LA is sufficient if the nerve is clearly seen; if not a volume of 10mL is injected.

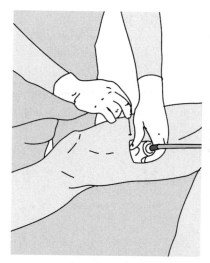

Fig. 40.3 Set up for an ultrasound-guided subsartorial saphenous nerve block.

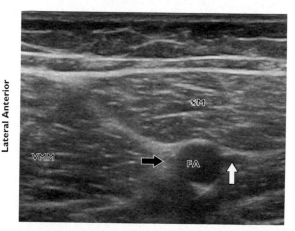

Fig. 40.4 Ultrasound of the subsartorial canal showing the femoral artery, the descending genicular artery, and the saphenous nerve. SM, sartorius muscle; VMM, vastus medialis muscle; FA, femoral artery; Black arrow, saphenous nerve; White arrow, descending genicular artery.

Further reading

Benzon HT, Sharma S, Calimaran A (2005). Comparison of the different approaches to the saphenous nerve. *Anesthesiology*, **102**, 633–8.

Horn JI, Pitsch T, Salinas F, Benninger B (2009). Anatomic basis to the ultrasound-guided approach for saphenous nerve blockade. *Reg Anesth Pain Med*, **34**(5), 486–9.

Manickam B, Perlas A, Duggan E, *et al*. (2009). Feasibility and efficacy of ultrasound-guided block of the saphenous nerve in the adductor canal. *Reg Anesth Pain Med*, **34**(6), 578–80.

Van der Wal M, Lang S, Yip R (1993). Transsartorial approach for saphenous nerve block. *Can J Anesth*, **40**, 542–6.

Obturator nerve block

Background

PNS:

US:

Indications

Anaesthesia

- Used in combination with proximal sciatic and femoral nerve block for 'completeness' in knee surgery.
- Can be used as sole technique to paralyse the adductor muscles in cases of spasm (spasticity, transurethral bladder resections).

Analgesia

- For operations on and painful conditions of the hip and knee. Note: the cutaneous innervation of this nerve is so variable and unpredictable that for incisions on the medial aspect of the thigh and knee it is not recommended. Even for total knee replacements, routine blockade of the obturator nerve is not routinely done (see ➋ Clinical notes, p. 431).

Anatomy

- The obturator nerve arises from the anterior primary rami of L2–L4, with its major component from L3.
- Forming within the body of the psoas muscle it pierces the medial border of psoas at the level of the pelvic brim, behind the common iliac artery and lateral to the internal iliac vessels.
- Passing down on obturatus internus, close to the wall of the bladder and anterosuperior to the obturator vessels, it passes through the upper part of the obturator foramen into the thigh giving off a branch to the hip joint.
- In the thigh the nerve divides into its anterior and posterior branches, separated initially by fibres of the obturator externus then by the adductor brevis.
- The anterior branch descends in the thigh behind pectineus and adductor longus, anterior to adductor brevis.
- At the lower border of adductor brevis the nerve communicates with the medial cutaneous nerve of the thigh and saphenous nerve to form the subsartorial plexus (which supplies the skin on the medial side of the thigh).
- The terminal branches of the anterior obturator nerve terminate on the femoral artery (which it supplies). It also supplies adductor longus, gracilis, usually adductor brevis, and occasionally pectineus. If there is an accessory obturator nerve it usually connects with the anterior branch.
- The anterior obturator nerve has a highly variable connection with the cutaneous nerves of the femoral nerve. This is reflected in the highly variable cutaneous innervation of the obturator nerve and in some cases there is none.

- The posterior branch descends through the thigh between adductor brevis and adductor magnus which it supplies.
- It gives an articular branch which either pierces adductor magnus or passes with the femoral artery into the popliteal fossa where it pierces the oblique posterior ligament to supply the articular capsule. Its terminal branches also supply the popliteal artery.
- An accessory obturator nerve can be present (seen in 69/800 dissections). This small nerve arises from the ventral rami of L3–L4 descending on the medial border of psoas passing into the thigh in front of the superior pubic rami (*not* through the obturator foramen) and onto the posterior surface of pectineus. Here it can divide into up to 3 branches: 1 that supplies pectineus, 1 that innervates the hip joint, and 1 that communicates with the anterior branch of the obturator nerve.

Side effects and complications

- Vascular puncture—intravascular injection, bleeding, and bruising
- Nerve damage.

Peripheral nerve stimulation technique

To guarantee complete blockade of both the anterior and posterior branches of the obturator nerve (complete cutaneous and articular sensory block and motor blockade of the adductor muscles) the main nerve trunk of the obturator nerve needs to be identified above its bifurcation, as close to its exit from the obturator canal as possible (stimulation of just the posterior division will only reliably give adductor magnus contraction—not easy to differentiate). There are 2 approaches described.

Landmarks
- PT
- Adductor longus tendon
- Femoral artery
- Inguinal crease.

Technique

Classical
- With the patient supine and the leg to be blocked abducted 30°, identify and mark the PT.
- Mark a point 1cm lateral and 1cm caudad to the PT.
- Prepare the skin with 0.5% chlorhexidine in 70% alcohol. Wait until the skin is dry.
- Anaesthetize the skin with a subcutaneous injection of 1% lidocaine.
- Insert a 50–80mm short-bevelled needle perpendicular to the skin.
- Advance until contact with the inferior boarder of the superior pubic ramus is achieved (2–4cm).
- Withdraw the needle slightly and redirect 45° laterally and slightly posteriorly to pass under the superior pubic ramus into the obturator foramen—advance the needle until contraction of the adductor muscles is visible.
- Carefully manipulate the needle until stimulating current is between 0.3mA and 0.5mA. After careful aspiration, 10–15mL of LA is injected slowly in 5mL aliquots.

Inter-adductor approach
- With the patient supine and the hip adducted and the knee flexed identify the tendon of adductor longus, medial to the femoral artery.
- Prepare the skin with 0.5% chlorhexidine in 70% alcohol. Wait until the skin is dry.
- Anaesthetize the skin with a subcutaneous injection of 1% lidocaine.
- At the level of the inguinal crease insert a 50–80mm needle posterior to the adductor longus tendon, directed laterally and cranially aiming in the direction of the ASIS but with a slight posterior inclination. See Fig. 41.1.
- Advance the needle into the obturator foramen until contraction of the adductor muscles is visible.
- Carefully manipulate the needle until stimulating current is between 0.3mA and 0.5mA. After careful aspiration, 10–15mL of LA is injected slowly in 5mL aliquots.

Clinical notes

- Place hand on the adductor muscle to distinguish direct muscle stimulation from a true adductor motor response.

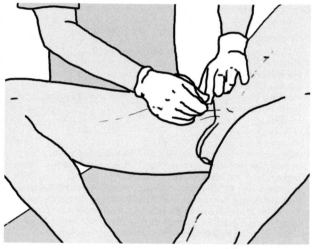

Fig. 41.1 Inter-adductor approach to the obturator nerve.

Ultrasound technique

Individual localization of the 2 branches of the obturator nerve is difficult using PNS and US has the potential to improve the accuracy and success. Visualization of the individual nerves can be difficult as they are small flattened nerves lying in fascial planes between muscles. There are few accompanying structures that run with the nerves to aid identification, but the fascial planes are easily identified.

Preliminary scan

- Position the patient supine and the leg abducted 30°.
- Place the probe parallel to the inguinal ligament in the inguinal crease. Identify the femoral artery, femoral vein, and pectineus muscle (deep and medial).
- Move the probe medially identifying the adductor muscles, from superficial to deep:
  - longus
  - brevis
  - magnus.
- After passing beneath the medial part of pectineus the anterior branch of the obturator nerve lies in the fascial plane between adductor longus (superficially) and adductor brevis (posteriorly).
- Scan proximally and distally, looking for a hyperechoic structure passing within this fascial plane that moves more medially as you scan more distally.
- The anterior branch is often accompanied by an artery (use colour Doppler to help confirm its presence).
- Once identified, follow the anterior obturator nerve proximally. In a number of cases it is possible to follow this nerve to the bifurcation of the obturator nerve and visualize the obturator trunk (this is often facilitated by turning the probe through 90° to scan the nerve longitudinally).
- The posterior branch is deeper, in the fascial plane between adductor brevis and adductor magnus, and is often not clearly seen.
- See Fig. 41.2.

Ultrasound settings

- Probe: linear L38 or curvilinear broadband probe
- Settings: MB—general or penetration
- Depth: 4–8 cm
- Orientation: transverse
- Needle: 80–100 mm of choice.

Technique

- Prepare the skin with 0.5% chlorhexidine in 70% alcohol. Wait until the skin is dry.
- Having identified the adductor muscle and ideally the nerve, anaesthetize the skin with a subcutaneous injection of 1% lidocaine.
- An in-plane technique from the anterior side of the probe is recommended, although ensure this trajectory does not involve the femoral vessels. An out-of-plane approach is acceptable.

- If the nerves are not clearly visualized, inject within the fascial planes between abductor longus/brevis and adductor brevis/magnus.
- After careful aspiration, inject 5mL around each nerve or within the fascial planes.

Clinical notes
- A high-volume saphenous nerve block in the lower part of the adductor canal may block the articular branches of the posterior obturator nerve.
- Interfascial plane blocks are probably easier, and just as effective as trying to isolate the individual nerves.
- If the main trunk of the obturator is easily visible, this is probably the best place to block the nerve.

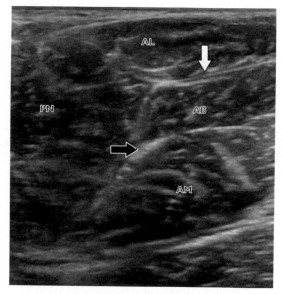

Fig. 41.2 Ultrasound showing the adductor longus, brevis and magnus muscle, with the anterior and posterior divisions of the obturator nerve in the fascial planes between them. AL, adductor longus muscle; AB, adductor brevis muscle; AM, adductor magnus muscle; PN, pectineus; White arrow, anterior obturator nerve; Black arrow, posterior obturator nerve.

Further reading

Bouaziz H, Vial F, Jochum D, *et al.* (2002). An evaluation of the cutaneous distribution of the obturator nerve block. *Anesth Analg*, **94**(2), 445–9.

Parks CR, Kennedy WF (1967). Obturator nerve block: a simplified approach. *Anesthiology*, **28**(4), 775–8.

Sinha SK, Abrams JH, Houle TT, *et al.* (2009). Ultrasound-guided obtutator nerve block: an interfascial injection approach without nerve stimulation. *Reg Anesth Pain Med*, **34**(3), 261–4.

Soong J, Schafhalter-Zoopoth I, Gray AT (2007). Sonographic imaging of the obturator nerve for regional block. *Reg Anest Pain Med*, **32**(2), 146–51.

Wassef M (1993). Interadductor approach to obturator nerve blockade in spastic conditions of adductor thigh muscles. *Reg Anesth*, **18**(1), 13–17.

Parasacral approach to sacral plexus block

Background

PNS: ▰▰▰▰▰   ▰▰▰▰▰   ▰▰▰▰▰

US: N/A

Indications

Anaesthesia
- All lower limb surgery (but invariably needs to be combined with blockade of components of the lumbar plexus for complete anaesthesia).
- Foot and ankle surgery may be possible under sacral plexus block alone, although the medial side of ankle (and foot) is innervated by the saphenous branch of femoral nerve.

Analgesia
- Lower limb amputations, foot surgery, knee surgery, hip surgery (innervation to posterior capsule via nerve to quadratus femoris and superior gluteal nerve).

Introduction
- Reliable, easy to learn lower limb block with a success rate of 94% and a mean onset time of 13 minutes.
- First described by Mansour in 1993.

Anatomy
The sacral plexus is formed by the lumbosacral trunk (L4, L5, and S1–S4). It lies anterior to the sacrum and to piriformis muscle but deep to the pelvic fascia. It forms the sciatic and pudendal nerves giving off pelvic branches which are released before the sciatic component leaves through the greater sciatic foramen. These pelvic branches include the posterior cutaneous nerve of the thigh and the nerve to quadratus femoris and superior and inferior gluteal nerves.

Side effects and complications
- Obturator nerve (L2–L4) may occasionally be blocked causing anaesthesia in its dermatomal distribution and weakness of the leg adductors.
- Sacral parasympathetics blockade, perineal and pudendal nerves may be blocked leading to urinary retention/incontinence.
- Intravascular injection (beware internal iliac vessels).
- Perforated pelvic viscera.

Peripheral nerve stimulator technique

Landmarks
- PSIS
- Ischial tuberosity (IT)
- See Fig. 42.1.

Technique
- Position the patient in the lateral recumbent position and draw a line joining the PSIS and the IT.
- Mark a point 6cm distal to the PSIS. See Fig. 42.2.
- Prepare the skin with 0.5% chlorhexidine in 70% alcohol. Wait until the skin is dry.
- Anaesthetize the skin with a subcutaneous injection of 1% lidocaine.
- Insert a 100mm, 21G, insulated short-bevelled stimulating needle attached to a nerve stimulator set to 1.5mA, 0.1msec, 2Hz pulses, perpendicular to the skin.
- Advance until either a motor response is elicited or bone is contacted. If bone is reached (margin of the greater sciatic notch (GSN)), reinsert needle caudally and walk off into the greater sciatic foramen.
- Do not advance needle further than 2cm past the depth of the GSN.
- Usual depth is 60–80mm.
- Accept plantar flexion of the foot (tibial nerve). If dorsiflexion/ eversion of the foot is seen (peroneal nerve) redirect needle medially. (Significantly higher success rate of complete block achieved with tibial nerve stimulation).
- Manipulate the needle until stimulating current is between 0.3 and 0.5mA. Inject 5mL aliquots of LA to 20–30mL total aspirating regularly to exclude intravascular injection. Disconnect syringe before injection of first aliquot to exclude passive reflux of blood.

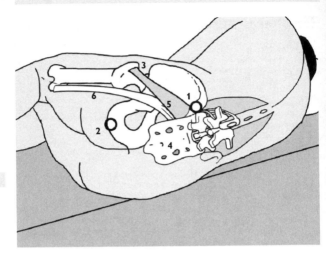

Fig. 42.1 Diagram showing the sciatic nerve passing anterior to piriformis and exiting the pelvis through the greater sciatic notch. The landmarks of the PSIS and IT are marked. **1** posterior superior iliac spine (PSIS); **2** ischial tuberosity (IT); **3** greater trochanter of femur; **4** sacrum; **5** piriformis muscle; **6** sciatic nerve.

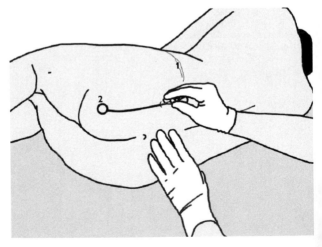

Fig. 42.2 Landmarks for a parasacral approach to a sacral plexus block. The needle insertion is 6cm distal to the PSIS on the line between the PSIS and the IT. **1** iliac crest; **2** ischial tuberosity (IT).

Further reading

Gaertner E, Lascurain P, Venet C, et al. (2004). Continuous parasacral sciatic block: a radiographic study. *Anesth Analg*, **98**(3), 831–4.

Hagon BS, Itani O, Bidgoli JH, et al. (2007). Parasacral sciatic nerve block: does the elicited motor response predict the success rate? *Anesth Analg*, **105**(1), 263–6.

Helayel PE, Ceccon MS, Knaesel JA, et al. (2006). Urinary incontinence after bilateral parasacral sciatic-nerve block: report of two cases. *Reg Anesth Pain Med*, **31**(4), 368–71.

Mansour NY (1993). Reevaluating the sciaitc nerve block: another landmark for consideration. *Reg Anesth*, **18**(5), 322–3.

Ripart J, Cuvillon P, Nouvellon E, et al. (2005). Parasacral approach to block the sciatic nerve: a 400-case survey. *Reg Anesth Pain Med*, **30**(2), 193–7.

Proximal sciatic nerve block

Background

PNS:

US:

Indications

Anaesthesia

- All lower limb surgery (but invariably needs to be combined with blockade of components of the lumbar plexus for complete anaesthesia).
- Foot and ankle surgery may be possible under sciatic nerve block alone, although the medial side of ankle (and foot) is innervated by the saphenous branch of femoral nerve.

Analgesia

- Lower limb amputations, foot surgery, ankle surgery, knee surgery, hip surgery.

Anatomy

- The sciatic nerve (L4, L5, S1–3) is formed from the sacral plexus and is the largest nerve in the body (may be as wide as 1–2cm). In reality it is made up of the common peroneal nerve laterally and the tibial nerve medially which are held within a common fibrous sheath.
- They usually divide at the apex of the popliteal fossa, however anatomical studies demonstrate that the sciatic nerve divides in 27% of subjects at 20cm distal to the greater trochanter (GT) and in 90% at 30cm. Indeed 10% separate as high up as the sacral plexus and in such circumstances, the peroneal component often pierces through the piriformis muscle.
- As, or before, it leaves the pelvis through the greater sciatic foramen it releases cutaneous collateral branches including the posterior cutaneous nerve of the thigh and muscular collateral branches including the nerve to quadratus femoris, the superior and inferior gluteal nerves. Branches to semitendinosus, semimembranosus, the ischial head of adductor magnus, and the short and long heads of biceps femoris arise outside the pelvis. Of these only the short head of biceps femoris is supplied by the lateral (peroneal) side of the sciatic nerve. This, in part, may explain why nerve stimulation and deposition of LA around the tibial component (plantar flexion) of the sciatic nerve produces a more reliable nerve block than the peroneal component. Innervation to the posterior part of the hip capsule is via the sacral plexus (see ➔ Background, p. 444) via superior gluteal nerves and nerve to quadratus femoris. A branch of the inferior gluteal artery runs within the substance of the sciatic nerve to the lower part of the thigh.
- On exiting the pelvis through the greater sciatic foramen, below the piriformis muscle, the sciatic nerve is deep to the gluteus maximus

muscle on the posterior surface of the ischium. It runs over obturator internus and gemelli muscle and lies between the quadratus femoris muscle anteriorly and gluteus maximus superficially and is roughly midway between the ischial tuberosity and the GT. The posterior cutaneous nerve of the thigh runs just medial to the sciatic nerve in this subgluteal space.

- At the infragluteal level the sciatic nerve sits on adductor magnus anteriorly and biceps femoris crosses it superficially from the medial side.
- The sciatic nerve descends down the midline of the back of the leg until it separates into its 2 components. See Fig. 43.1.

Advantages of ultrasound over stimulation

- US visualization of the proximal sciatic nerve can be difficult due to the depth of the nerve from the skin.
- There is little evidence that US improves the procedural time or block quality except in lateral mid-femoral approaches.
- US offers advantages when muscle group contraction is undesirable through nerve stimulation such as in trauma patients.
- US has a place in cases of peripheral vascular disease, diabetes, neuropathy or ischemia where the response to nerve stimulators can be unreliable.

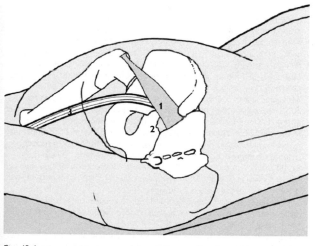

Fig. 43.1 Diagram of the course of the sciatic nerve. 1 piriformis muscle; 2 greater sciatic notch; 3 sciatic nerve.

Peripheral nerve stimulator technique: posterior approach (Labat)

- Credited to Gaston Labat in 1923, but similarly described by Victor Pauchet in 1920.
- More reliably blocks the posterior cutaneous nerve of the thigh (tourniquet analgesia) and has a faster onset and higher success rate with less LA requirements than other approaches. Turning patient on the side and requiring leg flexion may limit its use in some patients.

Landmarks

- PSIS
- GT
- Sacral hiatus (SH)
- See Fig. 43.2.

Technique

- Position the patient in lateral recumbent position (block side up) with the top knee flexed at 90° and the hip flexed so that the long axis of the femur forms a continuous line from the PSIS to the GT. (Otherwise known as the Sim's position although this strictly speaking describes a left-side up position facilitating rectal suppository administration!)
- Draw a line connecting the PSIS and the GT. Mark the midway point and drop a perpendicular 5cm below this. The tip of this line should meet a line drawn from the GT to the SH. This intersection is the needle insertion point. See Fig. 43.3.
- Prepare the skin with 0.5% chlorhexidine in 70% alcohol. Wait until the skin is dry.
- Anaesthetize the skin with a subcutaneous injection of 1% lidocaine.
- Insert a 100–150mm, 21G, insulated short-bevelled stimulating needle attached to a nerve stimulator set to 1.5mA, 0.1msec, 2Hz pulses perpendicular to the skin.
- Advance until either a motor response is elicited or bone is contacted.
- At 50–100mm, plantar flexion of the foot/toes (tibial nerve lies medially in the sciatic bundle) or dorsiflexion/eversion of the foot (peroneal nerve lies laterally in the sciatic bundle) will be elicited. Higher success rates are seen with tibial nerve stimulation.
- Double injection techniques identifying both sciatic components improve success rates at 45 minutes (75–100% vs 55–80%) and provide a quicker onset. Performance time is ↑ however.
- Direct gluteal muscle stimulation will be seen superficially. Ignore hamstring stimulation. If bone is contacted, redirect caudally as the GSN has probably been encountered.
- If no stimulus is elicited, redirect needle in 5° increments along the perpendicular line.
- Manipulate the needle until stimulating current is between 0.3 and 0.5mA. Disconnect syringe before injection to exclude passive reflux of blood. Inject 5mL aliquots of LA to 20–30mL total aspirating regularly to exclude intravascular injection (ED95 = 17mL).

Complications

- LA toxicity (note: aspiration check through 100mm insulated needle yields a high number of false negatives). This is a very vascular area with the inferior gluteal artery/vein and pudendal artery/vein nearby. This block is commonly used in combination with a lumbar plexus or femoral nerve block; care must be exercised to avoid exceeding the maximum recommended LA dose.
- Nerve injury. It may be appropriate to avoid epinephrine-containing solutions as the sciatic nerve has a poor intrinsic blood supply and use may increase the risk of neuronal ischaemia. The risk should be balanced at all times with the benefits of detecting intravascular injection.

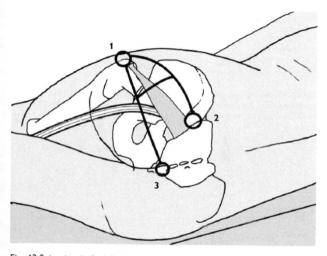

Fig. 43.2 Landmarks for Labat's approach to sciatic nerve block. 1 greater trochanter of femur; 2 posterior superior iliac spine (PSIS); 3 sacral hiatus.

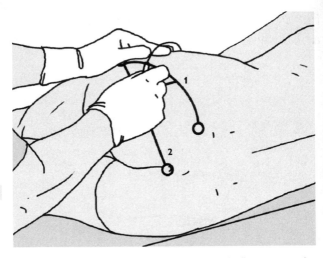

Fig. 43.3 Labat's posterior approach to the sciatic nerve. Needle insertion is at the intersection of: **1** The perpendicular from the midpoint of the line from the PSIS to the GT; **2** The line from the GT to the sacral hiatus.

Peripheral nerve stimulator technique: anterior approach (Beck)

- First described by Beck in 1963.
- Patient can be kept in supine position; particularly useful for patients with poor mobility or painful fractures.
- Stimulating needle passes through significant muscle bulk potentially making this block uncomfortable to perform.
- With the knee in a neutral position, the sciatic nerve is not accessible below the lesser trochanter in 40% of cases. (Improved with internal rotation of the thigh.)
- It is likely that if the insertion point is adjusted more distally to that described by Beck, the lesser trochanteric obstruction can be avoided.
- Less reliably blocks the posterior cutaneous nerve of the thigh than Labat's approach.

Landmarks

- ASIS
- GT
- PT.

Technique

- Position the patient in the supine position.
- Draw a line connecting the ASIS to the pubic tubercle. Draw a further, parallel, line from the greater trochanter and drop a perpendicular from the 1st line at the junction of the middle 1/3 and medial 1/3, marking where it crosses the 2nd line. This intersection is the needle insertion point. See Fig. 43.4.
- Chelly described an alternative method of defining the same entry point. Draw a line between the inferior border of the ASIS and the superior angle of the pubic symphysis tubercle. At its midpoint, a perpendicular line is dropped 8cm distally.
- Prepare the skin with 0.5% chlorhexidine in 70% alcohol. Wait until the skin is dry.
- Anaesthetize the skin with a subcutaneous injection of 1% lidocaine at the needle insertion point.
- Insert a 100–150mm, 21G, insulated short-bevelled stimulating needle attached to a nerve stimulator set to 1.5 mA, 0.1msec, 2Hz pulses perpendicular to the skin.
- The needle passes lateral to sartorius and medial to rectus femoris while the sciatic nerve at this level sits immediately below the lesser trochanter and posterior to adductor magnus.
- Advance with slight lateral intent until either a motor response is elicited or bone is contacted (femur). If bone is contacted, redirect medially and advance a further 2–5cm. (Put non-dominant hand under the buttocks with a finger on the ischial tuberosity. Aim the stimulating needle 1–2cm lateral to this finger.)
- At 80–100mm, plantar flexion of the foot/toes (tibial nerve lies medially in the sciatic bundle) or dorsiflexion/eversion of the foot (peroneal

nerve lies laterally in the sciatic bundle) will be elicited. Higher success rates are seen with tibial nerve stimulation.
• Manipulate the needle until stimulating current is between 0.3 and 0.5mA. Disconnect syringe before injection to exclude passive reflux of blood. Inject 5mL aliquots of LA to 20–30mL total aspirating regularly to exclude intravascular injection (ED95 = 17mL).

Complications
• LA toxicity (note: aspiration check through 100mm insulated needle yields a high number of false negatives.) This block is commonly used in combination with a lumbar plexus or femoral nerve block; care must be exercised to avoid exceeding the maximum recommended LA dose.
• Vessel puncture. The femoral artery lies just medial to the needle trajectory.
• Nerve injury. It may be appropriate to avoid epinephrine-containing solutions as the sciatic nerve has a poor intrinsic blood supply and use may increase the risk of neuronal ischaemia. The risk should be balanced at all times with the benefits of detecting intravascular injection. The femoral nerve is also just medial to the needle trajectory, although at this level it is usually divided into its terminal braches that should easily move out of the way of a short-bevelled needle without damaging them.

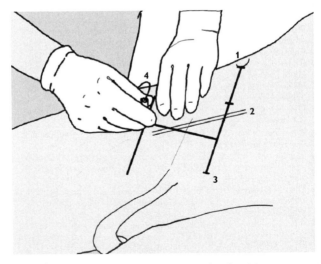

Fig. 43.4 Landmarks for the anterior (Beck's) approach to the sciatic nerve.
1 anterior superior iliac spine (ASIS); 2 femoral artery; 3 pubic tubercle; 4 greater trochanter of femur.

Peripheral nerve stimulator technique: lateral approach

- Patient can be kept in supine position.
- Faster onset time than lateral popliteal block and lower risk of vascular puncture (vascular bundle medial and anterior to nerve).
- No posterior cutaneous nerve of the thigh block; tourniquet pain.
- Sciatic nerve can be blocked at any point along the length of the thigh.

Landmarks
- GT.

Technique
- Draw a line from the posterior border of the GT along the length of the femur distally.
- Prepare the skin with 0.5% chlorhexidine in 70% alcohol. Wait until the skin is dry.
- Anaesthetize the skin with a subcutaneous injection of 1% lidocaine.
- High approach = at level of ischial tuberosity.
- Mid-thigh approach = half way along thigh. See Fig. 43.5.
- Insert a 50–100mm, 21G insulated short-bevelled stimulating needle attached to a nerve stimulator set to 1.5 mA, 0.1msec, 2Hz pulses perpendicular to the skin.
- Advance with slight anterior intent until either a motor response is elicited or bone is contacted (femur). If bone is contacted, redirect posteriorly and advance a further 2–5cm.
- At 30–80mm (up to 100mm with high approach), plantar flexion of the foot/toes (tibial nerve lies medially in the sciatic bundle) or dorsiflexion/eversion of the foot (peroneal nerve lies laterally in the sciatic bundle) will be elicited. Higher success rates are seen with tibial nerve stimulation. Often peroneal component stimulated first; rotating thigh internally helps identify tibial component.
- Manipulate the needle until stimulating current is between 0.3 and 0.5mA. Disconnect syringe before injection to exclude passive reflux of blood. Inject 5mL aliquots of LA to 10–20mL total aspirating regularly to exclude intravascular injection. (ED95 = 17mL).

Complications
- LA toxicity (note: aspiration check through 100mm insulated needle yields a high number of false negatives). This block is commonly used in combination with a lumbar plexus or femoral nerve block; care must be exercised to avoid exceeding the maximum recommended LA dose.
- Nerve injury. It may be appropriate to avoid epinephrine-containing solutions as the sciatic nerve has a poor intrinsic blood supply and use may increase the risk of neuronal ischaemia. The risk should be balanced at all times with the benefits of detecting intravascular injection.

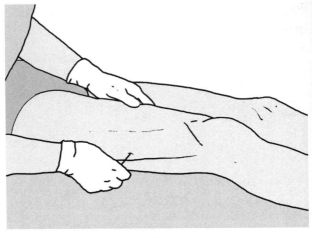

Fig. 43.5 Mid-thigh lateral approach to sciatic nerve.

Peripheral nerve stimulator technique: posterior subgluteus approach (Di Benedetto)

- Less painful than Labat's technique.
- Less reliably blocks the posterior cutaneous nerve of the thigh than Labat's.
- More accurately described as the infragluteal approach as it is at, or below, the caudad margin of this muscle.

Landmarks

- GT
- IT.

Technique

- Position the patient in the lateral recumbent position with the top knee flexed at 90° and the hip flexed so that the long axis of the femur forms a continuous line from the PSIS to the GT.
- Draw a line connecting the GT to the IT and mark 4cm distal to its midpoint (this often corresponds to a palpable, or visible, longitudinal groove formed by the lateral edge of the long head of biceps femoris).
- Prepare the skin with 0.5% chlorhexidine in 70% alcohol. Wait until the skin is dry.
- Anaesthetize the skin with a subcutaneous injection of 1% lidocaine.
- Insert a 50–100mm, 21G, insulated short-bevelled stimulating needle attached to a nerve stimulator set to 1.5mA, 0.1msec, 2Hz pulses perpendicular to the skin.
- At 30–60mm, plantar flexion of the foot/toes (tibial nerve lies medially in the sciatic bundle) or dorsiflexion/eversion of the foot (peroneal nerve lies laterally in the sciatic bundle) will be elicited. Higher success rates are seen with tibial nerve stimulation.
- Manipulate the needle until stimulating current is between 0.3 and 0.5mA. Disconnect syringe before injection to exclude passive reflux of blood. Inject 5mL aliquots of LA to 20–30mL total aspirating regularly to exclude intravascular injection (ED95 = 17mL).

Complications

- LA toxicity (note: aspiration check through 100mm insulated needle yields a high number of false negatives). This block is commonly used in combination with a lumbar plexus or femoral nerve block; care must be exercised to avoid exceeding the maximum recommended LA dose.
- Nerve injury. It may be appropriate to avoid epinephrine-containing solutions as the sciatic nerve has a poor intrinsic blood supply and use may increase the risk of neuronal ischaemia. The risk should be balanced at all times with the benefits of detecting intravascular injection.

Peripheral nerve stimulator technique: inferior approach (Raj)

- First described in 1975.
- Patient can be kept in supine position.
- Sciatic nerve more superficial, making block easier to perform/learn.
- Less reliably blocks the posterior cutaneous nerve of the thigh than Labat's.
- An assistant will be required to support the leg.

Landmarks
- GT
- IT.

Technique
- Position the patient in the supine position and flex the hip and knee to 90°. (Unilateral lithotomy position.)
- Draw a line connecting the GT to the IT and mark its midpoint (this often corresponds to a palpable, or visible, longitudinal groove formed by the lateral edge of the long head of biceps femoris). See Fig. 43.6.
- Prepare the skin with 0.5% chlorhexidine in 70% alcohol. Wait until the skin is dry.
- Anaesthetize the skin with a subcutaneous injection of 1% lidocaine.
- Insert a 50–100mm, 21G, insulated short-bevelled stimulating needle attached to a nerve stimulator set to 1.5mA, 0.1msec, 2Hz pulses perpendicular to the skin with slight medial intent.
- The needle passes through the gluteal muscles causing direct muscle stimulation.
- At 40–80mm, plantar flexion of the foot/toes (tibial nerve lies medially in the sciatic bundle) or dorsiflexion/eversion of the foot (peroneal nerve lies laterally in the sciatic bundle) will be elicited. Higher success rates are seen with tibial nerve stimulation.
- Manipulate the needle until stimulating current is between 0.3 and 0.5mA. Disconnect syringe before injection to exclude passive reflux of blood. Inject 5mL aliquots of LA to 20–30mL total aspirating regularly to exclude intravascular injection (ED95 = 17mL).

Complications
- LA toxicity (note: aspiration check through 100mm insulated needle yields a high number of false negatives). This block is commonly used in combination with a lumbar plexus or femoral nerve block; care must be exercised to avoid exceeding the maximum recommended LA dose.
- Nerve injury. It may be appropriate to avoid epinephrine-containing solutions as the sciatic nerve has a poor intrinsic blood supply and use may increase the risk of neuronal ischaemia. The risk should be balanced at all times with the benefits of detecting intravascular injection.

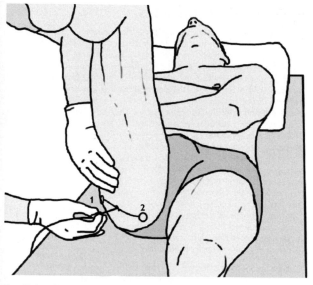

Fig. 43.6 Set up and landmarks for inferior (Raj) approach to sciatic nerve.
1 greater trochanter; 2 ischial tuberosity.

Ultrasound techniques

- The sciatic nerve has the largest cross-sectional diameter of a nerve within the human body, but the proximal sciatic nerve block is still considered as one of the more difficult US-guided nerve blocks to perform. Although not always easy, the nerve can be visualized throughout its length from its subgluteal location through to its bifurcation above, or within the popliteal fossa. The best images are reported to be between 7cm and 11cm distal to the gluteal crease.
- *Subgluteal* and *infragluteal* approaches are often confused. The subgluteal space represents the area between the anterior surface of the gluteus maximus muscle and the posterior surfaces of the quadratus femoris, gemellius, or obturator internus muscles (depending in level). Both the sciatic nerve and the posterior cutaneous nerve of the thigh lie in this space and can be simultaneously blocked in 70% of cases. True infragluteal approaches are caudad to the inferior border of the gluteus maximus muscle and often the posterior cutaneous nerve of the thigh has moved out of close proximity with the sciatic nerve.
- Theoretically, the sciatic nerve can be blocked at any point it can be visualized. Lateral and anterior approaches to nerve visualization have been described although no clear advantage has been demonstrated other than supine patient positioning.

Preliminary scan: subgluteal approach

- Position the patient in the lateral 'Sim's' position, operative side up.
- Place the probe in a transverse position across the buttock midway between the IT medially and the GT laterally.
- A curvilinear probe helps probe orientation as both the IT and GT can be visualized in the same US window. See Fig. 43.7.
- Adjust the depth of field to suit the patient and then identify the gluteus maximus muscle superficially and quadratus femoris muscle deep to this.
- The sciatic nerve will appear as a bright hyperechoic oval or flattened structure sandwiched between these two muscles. See Fig. 43.8.
- Often the inferior gluteal vessels can be visualized medially.
- Because of its depth from the skin, anisotropic nature of the nerve and the large muscle mass overlying, the sciatic nerve can often be difficult to locate. Adjust angulation, rotation, and tilt to obtain the best image of what is normally a bright hyperechoic round or triangular structure.
- To help confirm nerve identity it may be useful to scan in the longitudinal plane, identifying the nerve in its long-axis view (the sciatic nerve is the only tubular structure present in the buttock and posterior thigh). See Fig. 43.9.

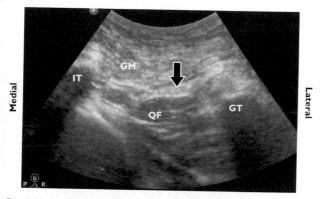

Fig. 43.7 Ultrasound of the sciatic nerve in the subgluteal space with a curvilinear probe showing both the GT and IT. GM, gluteus maximus muscle; QF, quadratus femoris muscle; IT, ischial tuberosity; GT, greater trochanter; Black arrow, sciatic nerve.

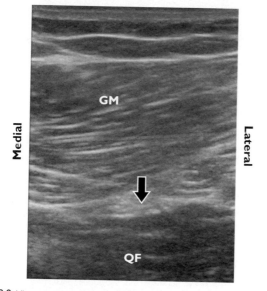

Fig. 43.8 Ultrasound image of subgluteal sciatic nerve. GM, gluteus maximus muscle; QF, quadratus femoris muscle; Black arrow, sciatic nerve.

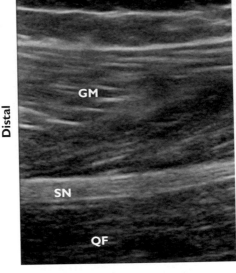

Fig. 43.9 Long-axis view of the sciatic nerve in the subgluteal space. GM, gluteus maximus muscle; SN, sciatic nerve; QF, quadratus femoris muscle.

Ultrasound settings: subgluteal approach
- Probe: low-frequency (<5MHz) curvilinear C60 (linear L38 broadband probe may be used in thin individuals).
- Settings: MB—abdomen, general /penetration.
- Depth: 4–8cm.
- Needle: 100mm of choice.

Technique: subgluteal approach
- Prepare the skin with 0.5% chlorhexidine in 70% alcohol. Wait until the skin is dry.
- Anaesthetize the skin with a subcutaneous injection of 1% lidocaine.
- An in-plane (lateral to medial) approach is recommended, but an out-of-plane approach is also described. See Fig. 43.10.
- A nerve stimulator may be used to help identify the nerve in case of difficult anatomy.
- Aim to inject 10–20mL of LA.
- Since the sciatic nerve sits within this 'subgluteal space', injection of LA away from the nerve often leads to 'filling' of the space and convenient circumferential spread of LA.
- Care must be taken to avoid the infragluteal vessels.

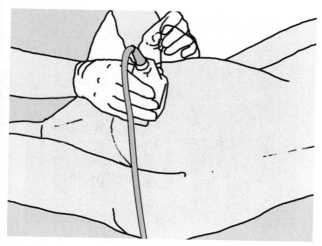

Fig. 43.10 Set up for an ultrasound-guided subgluteal approach to the sciatic nerve.

Preliminary scan: infragluteal approach

- Position the patient in the prone position.
- Lack of bony landmarks can make the initial identification of the sciatic nerve difficult at this level, however it is at its most superficial about 5cm distal to the gluteal crease and is most easily visualized by US between 7cm and 11cm.
- Place the probe in a transverse orientation across the proximal thigh.
- Identify the lateral border of the biceps femoris muscle (characteristically half oval in shape) just lateral to the midline. This muscle covers the sciatic nerve as it passes from the lateral side of the leg to insert medially on the IT.
- More medially are the semitendinosus and semimembranosus muscles.
- Proximally these 3 muscles form tendons that insert into the IT. They appear similar to the sciatic nerve on US, but the nerve always lies deep and laterally. At this point they are covered by the inferior margin of the gluteus maximus.
- Distally the sciatic nerve is seen under the belly of the long head of biceps femoris (see Fig. 43.11), which further down the leg will sit on the lateral side of the nerve.

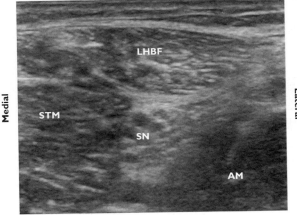

Fig. 43.11 Ultrasound image of infragluteal sciatic nerve. LHBF, long head of biceps femoris muscle; STM, semitendinosus muscle; SN, sciatic nerve; AM, adductor magnus muscle.

Ultrasound settings: infragluteal approach

• Probe: linear L38 broadband probe (low-frequency (<5MHz) curvilinear C60 in obese individuals may be necessary.
• Settings: MB—general/penetration.
• Depth: 3–6cm.
• Needle: 50–100 mm of choice.
• US plane: transverse.

Technique: infragluteal approach

• Prepare the skin with 0.5% chlorhexidine in 70% alcohol. Wait until the skin is dry.
• Anaesthetize the skin with a subcutaneous injection of 1% lidocaine.
• Use an in-plane (lateral to medial) needle approach, although an out-of-plane approach is also acceptable. See Fig. 43.12.
• A nerve stimulator may be used to help identify the nerve in case of difficult anatomy.
• After careful aspiration, inject 10–20mL of LA.

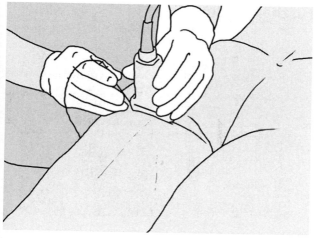

Fig. 43.12 Set up for an ultrasound-guided infragluteal sciatic nerve block.

Further reading

Partridge BL (1991). The effects of local anesthetics and epinephrine on rat sciatic nerve blood flow. *Anesthesiology*, **75**(2), 243–50

Taboada M, Rodríguez J, ALvarez J, et al. (2004). Sciatic nerve block via posterior Labat approach is more efficient than lateral popliteal approach using a double-injection technique: a prospective, randomised comparison. *Anesthesiology*, **101**(1), 138–42

Taboada M, Alvarez J, Cortés J, et al. (2004). The effects of three different approaches on the onset time of sciatic nerve blocks with 0.75% ropivicaine. *Anesth Analg*, **98**(1), 242–7

Taboada M, Rodríguez J, Valiño C, et al. (2006). What is the minimum effective volume of local anaesthetic required for sciatic nerve blockade? A prospective, randomised comparison between a popliteal and a subgluteal approach. *Anesth Analg*, **102**(2), 593–7

Taboada M, Atanassoff PG, Rodriguez J, et al. (2005). Plantar flexion seems more reliable than dorsiflexion with Labat's sciatic nerve block: a prospective, randomized comparison. *Anesth Anag*, **100**, 250–4.

44444444

4444444444444444444

Chapter 44

469

Popliteal fossa sciatic nerve block

Background

PNS:

US:

Indications

Anaesthesia
- Below knee amputations, hind and forefoot surgery (in combination with a saphenous, or femoral nerve block).

Analgesia
- Below knee amputations, hind and forefoot surgery (in combination with a saphenous, or femoral nerve block).

Anatomy
- The boundaries of the popliteal fossa are formed superior medially by the semitendinosus muscle, superior laterally by the biceps femoris muscle, inferior medially by the medial head of the gastrocnemius muscle, and inferior laterally by the lateral head of the gastrocnemius muscle.
- It contains the popliteal artery and vein and either an intact or bifurcated sciatic nerve forming the common peroneal and tibial nerves respectively.
- Superiorly in the popliteal fossa, the sciatic nerve is immediately superficial to adductor magnus; however, lower down in the popliteal fossa it sits superficial to the femur. See Fig. 44.1.
- By virtue of the fact that the sciatic nerve may bifurcate at any point from its origin, a popliteal fossa block may represent a sciatic nerve block or an individual common peroneal or tibial nerve block.

Side effects and complications
- Vascular puncture and LA toxicity
- Neuropraxia.

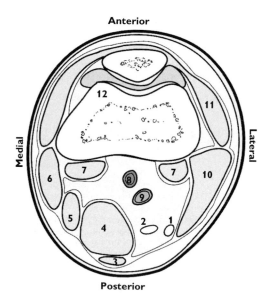

Fig. 44.1 Cross-sectional anatomy in the popliteal fossa. **1** common peroneal nerve; **2** tibial nerve; **3** semitendinosus muscle; **4** semimembranosus muscle; **5** gracilis muscle; **6** sartorius muscle; **7** heads of gastrocnemius muscle; **8** popliteal artery; **9** popliteal vein; **10** biceps femoris muscle; **11** vastus lateralis muscle; **12** femur.

Peripheral nerve stimulator technique: lateral approach

- This approach has the advantage that it is carried out with the patient in the supine position although it may take longer to perform than a posterior approach.
- Block onset time 20–30 min for surgical anaesthesia.

Landmarks
- The lateral groove between vastas lateralis above and the long head of biceps femoris below.
- The patella.

Technique
- Position the patient supine with the leg slightly flexed to help identify the lateral groove. Sometimes actively tensioning the ventral and dorsal thigh muscles against resistance can help to delineate this groove. Alternatively, with the leg straight, the groove is in line with a line extended from the lateral margin of the fibula. See Fig. 44.2.
- Mark the point of intersection between the groove and a line droped from the superior border of the patella.
- Prepare the skin with 0.5% chlorhexidine in 70% alcohol. Wait until the skin is dry.
- Anaesthetize the skin with a subcutaneous injection of 1% lidocaine at the point of intersection.
- Insert a 50mm, 21G, insulated short-bevelled stimulating needle attached to a nerve stimulatand set to 1.5mA, 0.1msec, 2Hz pulse.
- Direct 30° posteriorly and 5–10° caudally and advance until either a motor response is elicited or the needle has been inserted more than the radius of the leg.
- The peroneal nerve, often stimulated first, is found more superficially and usually within 10–20mm of the skin. The tibial nerve is usually found within 30–50mm of the skin.
- If no stimulus is elicited, redirect needle in 5° increments along an anterior posterior line. Note: more anterior angulation increases the chance of popliteal vascular injection. Also, if direct muscle stimulation is elicited check needle puncture site is situated *between* vastas lateralis and biceps femoris.
- One common error is made by searching for the nerve too deeply. (The nerve's position is usualy more superficial than one thinks.)
- Double injection techniques identifying both peroneal and tibial nerve have an improved success rate (88% vs 54%). If single injection techniques are used, ↑ success rates are found with plantar flexion (tibial nerve) as the endpoint.
- Manipulate the needle until stimulating current is between 0.3 and 0.5mA. Disconnect syringe before injection to exclude passive reflux of blood and inject 5mL aliquots of LA to 10–15mL for each component, aspirating regularly to exclude intravascular injection. Volume rather than concentration of LA is a better predictor of block duration.
- Expect your block to last about 16 hours with 0.5% bupivacaine.
- Clonidine added to the LA significantly prolongs the length of analgesia.

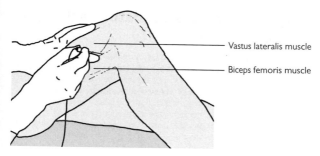

Fig. 44.2 Lateral approach to popliteal sciatic nerve block.

Peripheral nerve stimulator technique: posterior approach

- This is the traditional and first described popliteal block.
- It can either be carried out with the patient in the prone, lateral, or supine position. If supine, the leg needs to be held with the hip and knee flexed to 90° by an assistant; in the case of a heavy leg, this can be difficult.
- Generally a more proximal approach than the lateral approach, so more likely to block the sciatic nerve before it has bifurcated.
- Block onset time 20–30 min for surgical anaesthesia.

Landmarks
- Semimembranosus
- Biceps femoris
- The popliteal crease.

Technique
- Position the patient prone, lateral or supine (with knee and hip flexed to 90°) and draw out the isosceles triangle formed by the landmarks. The popliteal crease represents the base of the triangle and the superior emergence of the biceps femoris, and semimembranosus muscles form the apex. See Fig. 44.3.
- Flexion of the knee against resistance may accentuate these landmarks.
- Draw a line from the apex to the middle of the popliteal crease.
- The puncture site is located 5–8cm cranial from the base of this triangle and about 1cm lateral to the mid line. This should also be ~ 1cm lateral to the palpable pulse of the popliteal artery.
- Prepare the skin with 0.5% chlorhexidine in 70% alcohol. Wait until the skin is dry.
- Anaesthetize the skin with a subcutaneous injection of 1% lidocaine at your insertion point.
- Insert a 50mm, 21G, insulated short-bevelled stimulating needle attached to a nerve stimulator and set to 1.5mA, 0.1msec, 2Hz pulse.
- Direct at 45–60° to the skin in a cranial direction. (The more proximal you are, the more likely you are to find an unbifurcated sciatic nerve.)
- Advance until a motor response is elicited, usually within 3–8cm. If no twitch is elicited or if bone is contacted, withdraw and redirect sequentially in 5° angles laterally and then medially. The peroneal component will usually be found just lateral to the tibial component.
- Double injection techniques do not improve the success rates especially if the 2 nerves are close together or within the same sheath. Tibial nerve stimulation with a single injection technique will result in a more reliable block if a single injection technique is employed.
- Manipulate the needle until stimulating current is between 0.3 and 0.5mA. Disconnect syringe before injection to exclude passive reflux of blood and inject 5mL aliquots of LA to 10–15mL for each component, aspirating regularly to exclude intravascular injection. Volume rather than concentration of LA is a better predictor of block duration. Expect your block to last about 16 hours with 0.5% bupivacaine.
- Clonidine added to the LA significantly prolongs the length of analgesia.

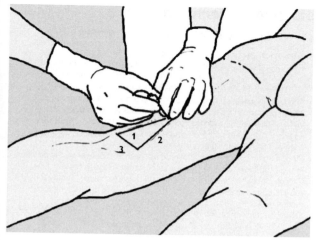

Fig. 44.3 Posterior approach to the popliteal sciatic nerve. **1** border of biceps femoris muscle; **2** border of semimembranosus muscle; **3** popliteal crease.

Ultrasound technique

- The sciatic nerve can be visualized throughout its length from its subgluteal location through to its bifurcation above, or within the popliteal fossa. The best images are reported to be between 7cm and 11cm distal to the gluteal crease.

Preliminary scan

- This block can be carried out with the patient in the prone, supine, or lateral position. The supine position is possible with the knee flexed at 90° and the heel supported by an assistant on the bed or raised up on a pillow. Adequate space around the posterior aspect of the thigh is required to allow for placement of the probe.
- Place a linear probe in a transverse position at the level of the popliteal crease and firstly identify the popliteal artery and vein (colour flow Doppler may be useful). To further aid nerve location, identify the muscle bellies of semimembranosus medially and the long head of biceps femoris laterally. The nerves sit between these muscles.
- Often the nerves can be difficult to visualize as they are generally of similar echogenicity to the surrounding muscle. The rotational movement of the nerves as induced by dorsiflexion and plantar flexion of the foot (seesaw sign) can often enhance their visibility.
- The nerves here are also anisotropic, and tilting of the probe is often required to see the nerves more clearly. Usually the probe needs to be angled distally (as the nerve is becoming more superficial).
- The larger tibial nerve can be seen as a hyperechoic oval structure superficial and medial to the artery while the smaller hyperechoic oval common peroneal nerve can be seen superficial and lateral. See Fig. 44.4. At this level the sural communicating nerve can also be seen to 'peel off' from the peroneal nerve as it descends toward the head of the fibula.
- Scan proximally while observing the tibial nerve move to the lateral side of the artery and gradually converge with the common peroneal nerve to form the sciatic nerve. See Fig. 44.5.
- The sciatic nerve can either be blocked as a single injection technique or separately as a double injection technique after its bifurcation (but beware of missing the sural communicating nerve).

Ultrasound settings

- Probe: high-frequency linear L38 broadband probe
- Settings: MB—resolution/general
- Depth: 3–6cm
- Needle: 50–100 mm of choice.

Technique

- Prepare the skin with 0.5% chlorhexidine in 70% alcohol. Wait until the skin is dry.
- Anaesthetize the skin with a subcutaneous injection of 1% lidocaine.
- Either an in-plane (lateral), or out-of-plane approach can be used. See Fig. 44.6a and Fig. 44.6b.
- A nerve stimulator may be used to help identify the nerve in case of difficult anatomy. Aim to inject 10–20mL of LA with a single injection or 10mL to each component for a double-injection technique.

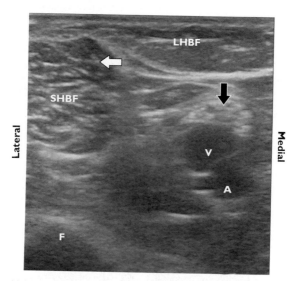

Fig. 44.4 Ultrasound of the popliteal fossa showing popliteal artery, vein, tibial nerve, and common peroneal nerve. LHBF, long head of biceps femoris muscle; SHBF, short head of biceps femoris muscle; White arrow, common peroneal nerve; Black arrow, tibial nerve; V, popliteal vein; A, popliteal artery; F, femur.

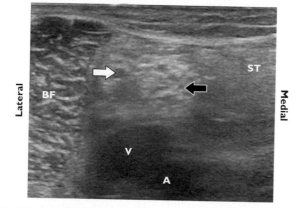

Fig. 44.5 Ultrasound scan showing the convergence of the tibial and common peroneal nerves. BF, biceps femoris muscle; ST, semimembranosus muscle; White arrow, common peroneal nerve; Black arrow, tibial nerve; V, popliteal vein; A, popliteal artery.

Advantages of ultrasound over stimulation

- Even in expert hands nerve stimulator popliteal blocks can be time consuming and may require multiple needle passes. Adding to the complexity of the procedure is the biological variability in location of the division of the sciatic nerve into its common peroneal and tibial components within the popliteal fossa. US visualization minimizes the impact of this variability and reduces block performance time while improving patient comfort.
- US guidance enhances the quality of popliteal sciatic nerve block compared with single-injection, nerve stimulator-guided block using either tibial or peroneal endpoints. It results in higher success rate, faster onset, without increasing complications.
- When muscle group contraction is undesirable through nerve stimulation, such as in trauma patients, US can be used.
- US can also be useful in diabetics and those with peripheral vascular disease who may have an impaired response to nerve stimulators.

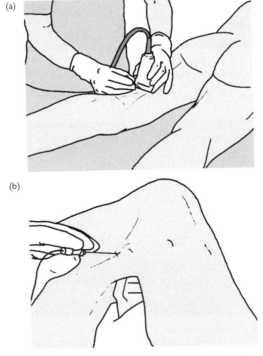

(a)

(b)

Fig. 44.6 Diagrams to show the (a) out-of-plane in a prone position and (b) in-plane (lateral) in a supine position US guided popliteal sciatic blocks

Further reading

Hadzic A, Vloka JD (1998). A comparison of the posterior versus lateral approaches to the block of the sciatic nerve in the popliteal fossa. *Anesthesiology*, **88**(6), 1480–6.

Perlas A, Brull R, Chan VW, *et al.* (2008). Ultrasound guidance improves the success of sciatic nerve block at the popliteal fossa. *Reg Anesth Pain Med*, **33**(3), 259–65.

Schafhalter-Zoppoth I, Younger SJ, Collins AB, *et al.* (2004). The 'seesaw' sign: improved sonographic identification of the sciatic nerve. *Anesthesiology*, **101**(3), 808–9.

van Geffen GJ, van den Broek E, Braak GJ, *et al.* (2009). A prospective randomised controlled trial of ultrasound guided versus nerve stimulation guided distal sciatic nerve block at the popliteal fossa. *Anaesth Intensive Care*, **37**(1), 32–7.

Vloka JD, Hadzic A, April E, *et al.* (2001). The division of the sciatic nerve in the popliteal fossa: Anatomical implications for popliteal nerve blockade. *Anesth Analg*, **92**(1), 215–17.

Ankle block

Background

PNS/landmark: ▬▬▬▬▬➤

US: ⌂

Indications

- Anaesthesia and/or analgesia for forefoot and toe surgery (calcaneal and ankle surgery will need a more proximal block).

Anatomy

The foot is innervated by the sciatic and femoral nerve via the following 5 branches. If complete anaesthesia of the foot is required, all nerves must be blocked:

- *Tibial nerve* (L4–S3, anterior divisions): this is the largest and most medial branch of the sciatic nerve which enters the calf deep to soleus after leaving the popliteal fossa. It then passes medially to the tendo-achilles where it lies behind the posterior tibial artery and between the tendons of flexor digitorum longus and flexor hallucis longus. See Fig. 45.1. The medial calcaneal nerve is released proximal to the flexor retinaculum to supply the medial side of the heel. Posterior to the medial malleolus and deep to the flexor retinaculum, the tibial nerve finally divides into its terminal branches, the medial and lateral plantar nerves which supply the medial and lateral sole of the foot as well as the bony structures of the mid and forefoot. They supply flexor hallucis brevis and flexor digitorum brevis and terminate as plantar digital nerves.
- *Sural nerve* (S1): this is a branch of the tibial nerve arising in the popliteal fossa descending on the posterior surface of the gastrocnemius and communicating with a branch from the common peroneal nerve. It descends alongside the small saphenous vein behind the lateral malleolus and along the lateral border of the foot. It has usually divided into several subcutaneous branches by this stage and it supplies the skin on the lateral side of the heel, foot, and 5th toe.
- *Common peroneal nerve* (L4–S2): descends on the lateral margin of the popliteal fossa and passing superficial to the lateral head of gastrocnemius, and then posterior to the head of the fibula, where it divides into its 2 principal braches.
- *Superficial peroneal nerve:* this nerve sits deep to peroneus longus and runs along the anterior intermuscular septum in the lateral compartment of the lower leg. It emerges superficially between peroneus longus (posteriorly) and extensor digitorum longus, then peroneus brevis (anteriorly) but deep to the fascia. It perforates through the crural fascia, before running more anteriorly superficial to the extensor retinaculum, terminating in subcutaneous branches which supply the dorsum of the foot and end as digital nerves.
- *Deep peroneal nerve:* after bifurcating from the common peroneal nerve, this nerve descends in the anterior compartment of the leg alongside and lateral to the anterior tibial artery. At the ankle, it passes deep to the extensor retinaculum between the 2 malleoli and usually lies lateral

to the dorsalis pedis artery, with the tendon of extensor hallucis longus medial and superficial to the nerve. The nerve then crosses to artery to lie medial and divides into medial and lateral terminal branches which supply the ankle joint and the skin of the 1st interdigit cleft.

- *Saphenous nerve:* this is the sensory terminal branch on the femoral nerve having become subcutaneous at the medial edge of the knee joint. It follows the great saphenous vein to the medial malleolus and supplies the skin over the medial side of the knee, leg, and foot.

Side effects and complications

- Vascular puncture
- Nerve damage.

Clinical notes

- Ankle blocks can be painful, due to the tight tissue planes and high volumes of LA. This may be due to the relative high volumes needed to overcome the lack of precision and reliability of the landmark-based techniques. Sedation is therefore advisable and often these blocks are performed in patients under GA. However, avoid the obvious pitfall of use of neuromuscular blockade and a nerve stimulator!
- Ankle (lower limb) tourniquets are often well tolerated allowing for awake surgery (± sedation).
- Block duration 10 hours with long-acting LAs but may be extended to 15 hours with clonidine.

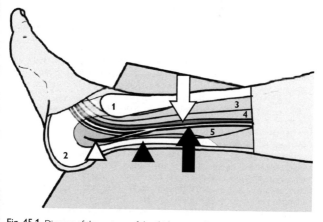

Fig. 45.1 Diagram of the anatomy of the tibial nerve at the ankle showing its relationship to the posterior tibial artery, flexor digitorum longus, and flexor hallux longus. **1** tibia; **2** calcaneum; **3** tibialis posterior muscle; **4** flexor digitorum longus muscle; **5** flexor hallucis longus muscle; White arrow, posterior tibial artery; Black arrow, tibial nerve; White triangle, medial calcaneal nerve; Black triangle, tendo achillis.

Landmark technique

Landmarks: tibial nerve

- *Retrotibial approach:*
  - draw a line joining the medial malleolus to the posterior border of the calcaneum
  - injection is just posterior to the posterior tibial pulse (~ half way). See Fig. 45.2.
- *Sustentaculum tali approach:*
  - palpate the inferior border of the sustentaculum tali (horizontal ridge of bone felt 1cm distal to the medial malleolus)
  - the tibial nerve consistently runs just inferior to this bony landmark
  - this technique is particularly useful in patients with peripheral vascular disease who may not exhibit a posterior tibial pulse
  - success rates approach 100% and may be more reliable than with the retrotibial approach.

Technique: tibial nerve

- This block can be performed with the patient supine with the knee flexed and leg externally rotated.
- Non-stimulating techniques are frequently described but carry a higher failure rate and slower onset.
- Prepare the skin with 0.5% chlorhexidine in 70% alcohol. Wait until the skin is dry.
- Anaesthetize the skin with a subcutaneous injection of 1% lidocaine.
- Insert a 25–50mm, insulated short-bevelled needle attached to a nerve stimulator set to 1.5mA, 0.1msec, 2Hz pulses perpendicular to the skin.
- Advance until plantar flexion of the toes is observed and manipulate needle until stimulation is lost at 0.3–0.5 mA.
- After negative aspiration, inject 5–8mL of LA.

Landmarks: deep peroneal (fibular) nerve

- Intermalleolar line: between the tendons of tibialis anterior and extensor hallucis longus.
- Midtarsal level: dorsalis pedis artery (tendon of extensor hallucis longus lies medially and extensor digitorum longus laterally to the artery).

Technique: deep peroneal (fibular) nerve

- Prepare skin with 0.5% chlorhexidine in 70% alcohol. Wait until the skin is dry.
- Insert a 23–25G needle at 90° to the skin until bone is contacted. Withdraw 1–2mm and inject LA.
- Intermalleolar line: inject 5–10mL in a fan-like manner through the same insertion point.
- Midtarsal level: inject 2–3mL medial and lateral to the artery.

Landmarks: superficial peroneal (fibular) nerve

- Ankle level: anterior border of the tibia and the lateral malleolus.
- Midtarsal level: insertion point as for deep peroneal nerve block to dorsum/plantar junction medially.

Technique: superficial peroneal (fibular) nerve

- Prepare skin with 0.5% chlorhexidine in 70% alcohol. Wait until the skin is dry.
- Infiltrate a subcutaneous wheel between the 2 landmarks with 5–10mL of LA.

Landmarks: sural nerve

- Lateral malleolus and lateral border of Achilles tendon.

Technique: sural nerve

- Prepare skin with 0.5% chlorhexidine in 70% alcohol. Wait until the skin is dry.
- Infiltrate a subcutaneous wheel between the 2 landmarks with 5mL of LA.

Landmarks: saphenous nerve (distal block)

- 1cm proximal and 1cm anterior to the medial malleolus.
- The long saphenous vein may be visible at this point especially if a tourniquet is applied.

Technique: saphenous nerve (distal block)

- Prepare the skin with 0.5% chlorhexidine in 70% alcohol. Wait until the skin is dry.
- Inject 5mL of LA with a 23–25G needle subcutaneously around the long saphenous vein.
- Avoid direct injection into the vein. Careful negative aspiration is essential.

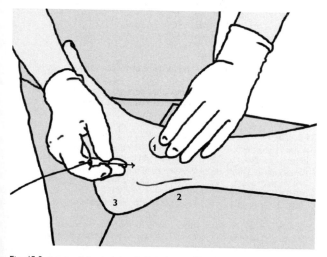

Fig. 45.2 Approach for the retrotibial tibial nerve block. **1** medial malleolus; **2** tendo achillis; **3** calcaneum.

Ultrasound technique

Preliminary scan: tibial nerve

- Position the patient supine with the knee flexed and abducted to reveal the medial aspect of the ankle.
- At a level posterior and superior to the medial malleolus, the transducer is placed transversely and a systematic scan is made to identify the important structures.
- The medial malleolus is identified by its hyperechoic periosteum and a dark underlying shadow.
- Move the transducer slightly posteriorly to identify the tibialis posterior and flexor digitorum longus tendons. Both tendons are found beneath the flexor retinaculum of the ankle. They display a sliding movement with ankle flexion and are usually hyperechoic, resembling the appearance of nerves.
- Scanning proximally helps to distinguish between nerve and tendon, as the tendons will develop into their respective muscles.
- The round hypoechoic pulsatile tibial artery (colour flow Doppler may be used to assist) is then located and the predominantly hyperechoic (may appear honeycombed, round or oval) tibial nerve is visualized posterior to this in transverse section. See Fig. 45.3.
- The tendon of flexor hallucis longus can be seen to lie deep/posterior to the nerve.
- Beware of the vein(s) adjacent to the artery and nerve.

Ultrasound settings: tibial nerve

- Probe: high-frequency (10MHz) linear probe
- Settings: MB resolution
- Depth: 1–2cm
- Needle: 50mm short-bevel needle.

Technique: tibial nerve

- Prepare the skin with 0.5% chlorhexidine in 70% alcohol. Wait until the skin is dry.
- An in-plane or out-of-plane approach can be used. See Fig. 45.4. The in-plane approach can be ergonomically awkward if entering from the posterior aspect and coming from the anterior aspect the medial malleolus can often be in the way. Moving a few centimetres proximally can help.
- A nerve stimulator may be used to help identify the nerve in case of difficult anatomy.
- Aim to inject 3–5mL of LA circumferentially around the nerve.

Preliminary scan: deep peroneal nerve

- Place the transducer transversely above the intermalleolar line on the anterior aspect of the leg.
- Identify the dorsalis pedis artery (use of colour flow Doppler can be helpful and beware of too much pressure with the transducer as the artery is easily compressible).
- The nerve can be visualized in its short-axis plane as a hyperechoic circle, (usually) lateral to and very close to the artery. See Fig. 45.5.

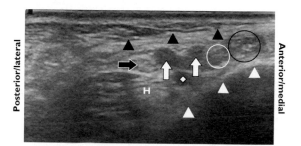

Fig. 45.3 Ultrasound of the tibial nerve and surrounding structures, just proximal to the medial malleolus. Black arrow, tibial nerve; Black triangles, flexor retinaculum; Black circle/outline, tibialis posterior tendon; White circle/outline, flexor digitorum longus tendon; White arrows, veins; White diamond, posterior tibial artery; H, flexor hallucis longus tendon; White triangles, tibia.

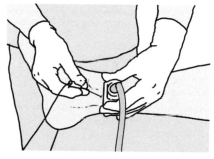

Fig. 45.4 Set up for an out-of-plane ultrasound-guided approach to the tibial nerve.

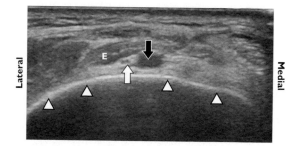

Fig. 45.5 Ultrasound of the deep peroneal nerve adjacent to the dorsalis pedis artery on the anterior if the ankle. E, extensor hallucis longus tendon; Black arrow, dorsalis paedis artery; White arrow, deep peroneal nerve; White triangles, anterior surface of tibia.

Ultrasound settings: deep peroneal nerve

- Probe: high-frequency (10MHz) linear probe
- Settings: MB resolution
- Depth: 1–2cm
- Needle: 50mm short-bevel needle.

Technique: deep peroneal nerve

- Prepare the skin with 0.5% chlorhexidine in 70% alcohol. Wait until the skin is dry.
- An in-plane or out-of-plane approach can be used.
- Inject 2–3mL of LA around the nerve.
- If the nerve cannot be easily visualized, inject 2–3mL either side of the artery.

Preliminary scan: superficial peroneal nerve

- Position the patient supine. Place the transducer transversely on the lateral aspect of the proximal lower leg.
- The superficial peroneal nerve can be seen as the large lateral branch of the common peroneal nerve as it crosses the fibula neck. Follow it as it enters the peroneal compartment under peroneus longus and then emerges superficially between peroneus longus and extensor digitorum longus.
- Identify the relationship of the nerve to the crural fascia (i.e. deep or superficial). This is important to ensure the LA is injected in the correct plane. See Fig. 45.6.
- The terminal branches of the superficial peroneal nerve are inconsistently visualized at the level of the ankle.

Ultrasound settings: superficial peroneal nerve

- Probe: high-frequency (10MHz) linear probe
- Settings: MB—resolution
- Depth: 1–2cm
- Needle: 50mm short-bevel needle.

Technique: superficial peroneal nerve

- Prepare the skin with 0.5% chlorhexidine in 70% alcohol. Wait until the skin is dry.
- An in-plane or out-of-plane approach can be used.
- Aim to inject 3–5mL of LA circumferentially around the nerve.
- It is important to ensure that LA is injected on the correct side of the crural fascia (the nerve pieces the crural fascia at some point in the distal lower leg).

Preliminary scan: sural nerve

- Place the patient supine.
- The medial contribution of the sural nerve can be imaged between the medial and lateral heads of the gastrocnemius muscles where it emerges piercing the fascia lata and joining the lateral branch, descending with the lesser saphenous vein within the subcutaneous tissue of the lateral aspect of the lower leg (being subcutaneous avoids confusion with tendons).
- The sural nerve is a hyperechoic circle seen immediately adjacent to the vein. See Fig. 45.7.

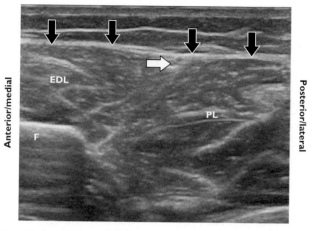

Anterior/medial

Posterior/lateral

Fig. 45.6 Superficial peroneal nerve, seen between peroneus longus and extensor digitorum longus, deep to the crural fascia. Black arrows, crural fascia; White arrow, superficial peroneal nerve; EDL, extensor digitorum longus muscle; PL, peroneus longus muscle; F, fibula.

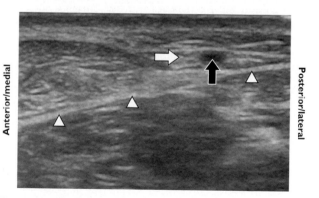

Anterior/medial

Posterior/lateral

Fig. 45.7 Ultrasound image of the sural nerve and the adjacent lesser saphenous vein within the subcutaneous tissue of the lateral aspect of the distal lower leg. Black arrow, lesser saphenous vein; White arrow, sural nerve; White triangles, fascia.

Ultrasound settings: sural nerve
- Probe: high-frequency (10MHz) linear probe
- Settings: MB—resolution
- Depth: 1–2cm
- Needle: 50mm short-bevel needle.

Technique: sural nerve
- Place the probe in a transverse plane at a midcalf level on the lateral aspect of the lower leg and identify the lesser saphenous vein and the adjacent sural nerve.
- Identifying the lesser saphenous vein can be enhanced with the use of a leg tourniquet.
- Prepare the skin with 0.5% chlorhexidine in 70% alcohol. Wait until the skin is dry.
- An in-plane or out-of-plane approach can be used.
- Aim to inject 3–5mL of LA circumferentially around the nerve.

Preliminary scan: saphenous nerve
- Position the patient supine with the knee flexed and abducted to reveal the medial aspect of the ankle.
- After emerging from between sartorious and gracilis, the saphenous nerve runs down the medial edge of the tibia immediately posterior to the great saphenous vein. It moves, with the vein, anterior to the medial malleolus.
- At a level proximal and anterior to the medial malleolus, the transducer is placed transversely to identify the great saphenous vein (a proximal tourniquet may be of help) in the subcutaneous tissue; the nerve itself can be difficult to identify.

Ultrasound settings: saphenous nerve
- Probe: high-frequency (10MHz) linear probe
- Settings: MB—resolution
- Depth: 1–2cm
- Needle: 50mm short-bevel needle.

Technique: saphenous nerve
- Prepare the skin with 0.5% chlorhexidine in 70% alcohol. Wait until the skin is dry.
- An in-plane or out-of-plane approach can be used.
- Aim to inject 3–5mL of LA circumferentially around the nerve.
- At this level, the saphenous nerve may not be visualized in which case a perivascular injection can be made around the great saphenous vein.
- The saphenous nerve may also be reliably blocked in the thigh. See Chapter 40.

Advantages of ultrasound over stimulation

- Intravascular injection, convulsions, and temporary paraesthesia have all been described with blind techniques for tibial nerve block. US may offer safety advantages.
- US has been shown to improve the success of surgical anaesthesia for ankle blocks compared to landmark techniques (84% vs 66%) as well as reduce supplemental opiates, supplemental LA and conversion to GA.
- A small study demonstrated that US improved the success rate of tibial nerve blocks at the ankle (72% vs 22%).
- Another similar small study found an improvement in onset but not success of deep peroneal nerve blocks at the ankle.
- US guidance using the lesser saphenous vein as a reference point results in a more complete and longer lasting sural nerve block than does a traditional approach using surface landmarks (94% vs 56%).
- US may be useful if vascular landmarks are not easily palpable (e.g. peripheral vascular disease) for tibial and deep peroneal nerve blocks.

Further reading

Chin KJ, Wong NW, Macfarlane AJ, et al. (2011). Ultrasound-guided versus anatomic landmark-guided ankle blocks: a 6-year retrospective review. *Reg Anesth Pain Med*, **36**(6), 611–18.

Doty RJ, Sukhani R, Kendall MC, et al. (2006). Evaluation of a proximal block site and the use of a nerve-stimulator-guided needle placement for posterior tibial nerve block. *Anesth Analg*, **103**(5), 1300–5.

Meyerson M, Ruland C, Allon S (1992). Regional anesthesia for foot and ankle surgery. *Foot Ankle*, **13**(5), 282–8.

Rudkin GE, Rudkin HK, Dracopoulos GC (2005). Ankle block success rate: a prospective analysis of 1000 patients. *Can J Anaesth*, **52**(2), 209–10.

Wassef MR (1991). Posterior tibial nerve block. A new approach using the boney landmark of the sustentaculum tali. *Anaesthesia*, **46**(10), 841–4.

Foot blocks

Background

PNS: ━━━━━▶
US: N/A

Indications

- Anaesthesia and/or analgesia for minor surgery of the forefoot and toe.

Anatomy

The tibial nerve divides into its terminal branches the medial and lateral plantar nerves which run along the dorsal side of the plantar fascia deep to flexor digitorum brevis. They supply the medial and lateral sole of the foot as well as the bony structures of the mid and forefoot. These then form and terminate as the digital nerves, which run down both sides of each toe along the plantar aspect.

Landmark technique

Landmarks: mid tarsal block
- 2cm proximal to the metatarsophalangeal joint (MTPJ) of the required toe.

Technique: mid tarsal block
- Prepare skin with 0.5% chlorhexidine in 70% alcohol. Wait until skin is dry.
- Insert a 21–23G needle vertically down the side of the metatarsal until it sits on the plantar fascia.
- Inject 2–3mL of LA and then withdraw needle, injecting a further 2–3mL.
- Repeat on the other side of the metatarsal.
- A further injection of 2–3mL subcutaneously will anaesthetize any ventrocutaneous innervation of the toe.

Landmarks: webspace block
- MTPJ of required toe.

Technique: webspace block
- Prepare skin with 0.5% chlorhexidine in 70% alcohol. Wait until skin is dry.
- Insert a 21–23G needle horizontally within the webspace towards the MTPJ.
- Inject 3–5mL of LA.
- Repeat on the other side of the required toe.

Landmarks: digital nerve block
- Base of the proximal phalanx of the required toe.

Technique: digital nerve block
- Prepare skin with 0.5% chlorhexidine in 70% alcohol. Wait until skin is dry.
- Insert a 21–23G needle vertically down the side of the phalanx until it sits on the plantar fascia.
- Inject 2–3mL of LA and then withdraw needle, injecting a further 2–3mL.
- Repeat on the other side of the phalanx.
- A further injection of 2–3mL subcutaneously will anaesthetize any ventrocutaneous innervation of the toe.

Complications
- Haematoma.

Clinical notes
Avoiding epinephrine for extremity blocks is weakly supported by limited numbers of case reports involving unknown concentrations of epinephrine and other confounding variables (e.g. infection). No case reports of digital gangrene exist following the use of commercial preparations of lidocaine with epinephrine and there are case series and randomized controlled trials to support its routine use. As always, a balance of risk should be struck between the risks of epinephrine in LAs and the potential advantages it may bring (the avoidance of mechanical tourniquets and prolonged analgesia).

Further reading

Denker K. (2001). A comprehensive review of epinephrine in the finger: to do or not to do. *Plast Reconstr Surg*, **108**(1), 114–24.

Thomson CJ, Lalonde DH. (2006). Randomised double-blind comparison of duration of anaesthesia among three commonly used agents in digital nerve block. *Plast Reconstr Surg*, **118**(2), 429–32.

Part 6

Neuraxial

General considerations for central neuraxial blocks

Anatomy

- Spinal cord delivers 31 pairs of spinal nerves.
- Cord ends at L1/2 (90%), L2/3 (10%) in adults.
- Vertebral column has normal curvatures—kyphosis in thoracic and sacral region, lordosis in cervical and lumbar regions. See Fig. 47.1.
- Transverse processes (TPs) are bifid in cervical region, caudal angulated and short in thoracic region, and broad and horizontal in lumbar region.
- Largest TP is L5.
- Spinous processes (SPs) are bifid in cervical region, caudal angulated ++ and cluttered in thoracic region, and tall and horizontal in lumbar region.
- The nerve supply of the spine is variable. Periosteum is innervated by branches from the sympathetic chain and rami communicantes. The ligaments have a sparse nerve supply either the same as the periosteum, or from the medial branches of the posterior 1° rami bilaterally.

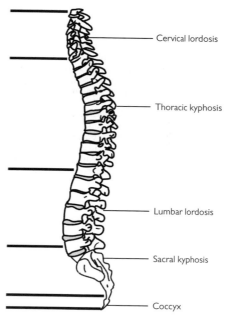

Cervical lordosis

Thoracic kyphosis

Lumbar lordosis

Sacral kyphosis

Coccyx

Fig. 47.1 Lateral view of spine showing usual kyphosis and lordosis.

Basic approach

The midline approach is the standard technique for central neuraxial blockade (CNB). Full asepsis is required; surgical scrub, gown, mask, gloves, hat, and a sterile field. Equipment should be prepared in advance and in a sterile manner.

- Position the patient. Sitting or lateral positions are standard depending on your patient and/or preference. Flexion of the spine usually improves access.
- Palpate SPs. Infiltrate subcutaneously with lidocaine just caudal to your chosen SP.
- Deeper infiltration either side of the ligaments may be needed for techniques using Tuohy needles; this may reduce discomfort from ligament distortion and diminish periosteal pain.
- The spinal or epidural needle should be directed with a slight cranial angulation. If an introducer needle is used, the tip of this should be passed into the 1st (supraspinous) ligament layer.
- The midline approach passes the needle through 3 ligamentous structures, the supraspinous and interspinous ligaments and the ligamentum flavum. When applying a loss of resistance technique, a characteristic medium–low–high resistance is felt as the needle is advancing.
- When passing through ligamentum flavum, solid resistance is usually felt. This suddenly 'gives' as the needle tip enters the epidural space.
- If advancing intrathecally, a further gentle 'click' or 'give' may be felt. The patient may also feel this. CSF should now be apparent.

Clinical notes

- Exact identification of a specific vertebra is difficult without image guidance. As a guide: the tip of the scapula sits at T8, the lowest ribs attach to T12, and the intercristine line/Tuffier's line (joining the 2 iliac crests) passes through L4. See Fig. 47.2.
- When you think you are at L3/4, stop. You are probably at L2/3 with a 10% chance of hitting spinal cord.
- Alterations to normal curvature—difficult technique and unknown needle direction (see ➔ Scoliosis, p. 504).
- The L5/S1 space is big and safe. However, it is too low for most epidurals, and spinal needles may need caudal angulation.
- Common approaches are midline or paramedian. Whichever approach is used for any reason, know the anatomy of the TP and SPs to avoid surprises.
- Spinals should not be performed above L2/3.
- Inserting the entire introducer needle may cause a dural puncture.
- Mid-thoracic epidurals may mandate a paramedian approach.
- The cervical epidural is in the remit of the expert and should not be attempted without expert supervision and extensive training.

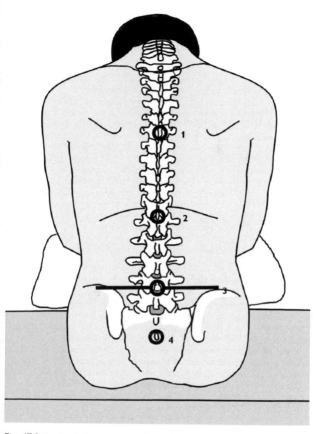

Fig. 47.2 Landmarks for estimation of vertebral level. **1** tip of scapula = T8; **2** costal margin = T12; **3** intercristine/Tuffier's line (between iliac crests) = L4; **4** sacral hiatus (apex of equilateral triangle with PSIS) = S5.

Central neuraxial blocks in special circumstances

Scoliosis

Scoliosis is a side-to-side curvature of the spine. This may include rotation as well as angulation. When using palpable landmarks to guide neuraxial blockade, scoliosis creates technical difficulty and increases the risk of complications. CNB may still be necessary. Explain to the patient that there is a higher risk of CNB failure. To improve success, try to imagine the spinal curvature of the back in front of you; review the patient's notes for relevant X-rays. The thoracic spine is attached to the rib cage; the sacrum is attached to the pelvis. The points of transition at the T12/L1 and L5/S1 intervertebral spaces may represent areas less likely to be rotated and angulated. A sitting patient may more clearly delineate spinal curvature. Pay attention to depth of bony landmarks as your needle is advancing; try to establish between SP/TP etc. Paraesthesiae may indicate nerve root proximation; withdraw and redirect away from the side of the paraesthesia. Use of a loss of resistance technique with a Tuohy needle may give a 'feel' for ligaments to aid advancement. Do not try relentlessly; this is more likely to result in dural puncture and ↑ patient discomfort. US may help to identify the SP and guide needle direction.

Spinal stenosis/disc herniation

The spinal canal is a cylindrical space with its contents bordered by the vertebral bodies anteriorly and the vertebral arch posterolaterally. It extends from foramen magnum to the sacrum and contains the spinal cord, all 31 pairs of nerve roots, CSF, meninges, spinal arteries and veins, and the epidural space. Any narrowing of this canal or encroachment of structures onto nerve roots decreases the available space for fluid to pass into; giving a bolus of injectate will increase pressure onto these structures. The risk of prolonged altered neurology in particular areas may therefore be ↑; there is also the possibility of a higher block for any given volume of injectate.

Previous spinal surgery

This may make CNB unwise, difficult, or unreliable. Decompression surgery may scar the epidural space, reducing LA spread. Laminectomy results in loss of bone and ligamentous tissue; therefore loss of resistance techniques cannot be used. Harrington, or other rod fixations reduce vertebral flexion; CNB will be technically more challenging. Kyphoscoliosis correction may make thoracic epidural techniques unwise or dangerous. Carefully consider the indications and benefits of the technique with the potential complications and difficulties you may encounter.

Cardiovascular disease

Severe cardiovascular disease requires careful consideration of any anaesthetic technique. Patients may be impossible to position lying down for CNB, or for the duration of intended surgery. Rapid swings in heart rate or blood pressure (BP) may cause acute decompensation of severe valvular disease; moderate drops in BP may impair coronary perfusion in ischaemic heart disease. Regurgitant valvular disease may improve with the reduction in systemic vascular resistance (SVR) associated with CNB; however, this SVR drop will return to normal, so caution must be exercised not to use excessive IV fluid perioperatively. The earliest physiological change with spinal anaesthesia is of venous dilatation leading to reduced venous return, and hypotension. This may mandate ↑ fluid administration and/or vasopressor treatment; both of which may be problematic with severe cardiovascular disease.

Respiratory disease

CNB represents a good option in severe respiratory disease; well-conducted CNB should barely interfere with respiratory mechanics as opposed to GA. CNB encroaching on thoracic levels will reduce FEV_1 and FVC; in patients with critical respiratory disease, this may cause decompensation. Use of continuous spinal anaesthesia enables a slow and incremental block to develop, which can prevent this.

Impaired coagulation

This increases the risk of neuraxial haematoma formation, which may compress the spinal cord and nerve roots resulting in permanent neurological deficit.

CNB should be avoided in frank coagulopathy.

Patients on warfarin should have their risk of thrombus formation estimated. If this is low, warfarin should be stopped 3 days prior to elective surgery, and INR checked on morning of surgery. An INR of <1.5 is acceptable. If risk is high, warfarin will be replaced by a heparin infusion or LMWH at therapeutic dose; this is likely to render CNB unachievable.

Patients on IV unfractionated heparin should have this stopped for >4 hours prior to CNB. This should not be restarted until at least 1 hour post-CNB. This also includes patients requiring intraoperative heparin.

Patients on prophylactic LMWH should have received their last dose >12 hours prior to CNB. Once CNB has been performed, administration of LMWH should be at least >4 hours after any manipulation of the spinal canal; i.e. removal of epidural catheter or spinal catheter; performance of any central block.

Patients on therapeutic dose LMWH should have received their last dose >24 hours prior to CNB.

Patients on aspirin may have received their morning dose. This represents an acceptable risk.

Patients on clopidogrel should have remained off this for >7 days prior to CNB. If this is not the case, elective surgery should be postponed. Certain patients represent a high-risk category that is required to continue their antiplatelet agents. These include patients with unstable coronary artery disease, and recent coronary artery stent insertion. Certain vascular procedures may also require ongoing clopidogrel. As a general principle, CNB should not be performed in this circumstance. However, risk:benefit assessment may swing in favour of CNB, if the patient has other significant comorbidity.

Sepsis

Systemic or local infection represents a theoretical ↑ risk of epidural abscess formation or meningitis. Administration of antibiotics may reduce this risk but as this is a rare complication, no data is available regarding risk reduction. Again, risk:benefit analysis should be undertaken on an individual patient basis; this may warrant CNB in septic patients who are receiving antibiosis. Data from the 3rd National Audit Project suggest an incidence of 1:47,000 for epidural abscess formation following CNB, similar to the rate of spontaneous events in the population.

Impaired capacity to consent

CNB is invasive and warrants informed consent. Consent can only be valid if adequate information is supplied and the patient has the capacity to understand it and make a balanced decision, free from coercion. Adults have capacity to consent to a medical procedure if they are able to understand and remember the information given to them about the procedure, and to use that information in order to decide whether or not to undergo the treatment proposed. When capacity is impaired, invasive procedures may be undertaken when they demonstrate benefit or prevention of harm in the eyes of 2 practitioners. This commonly occurs in the setting of trauma, with elderly patients, Fracture of the neck of the femur, polytrauma victims, or those intubated on the ITU. Once an intervention is undertaken, if capacity returns to a patient it is important to attempt to gain retrospective consent. Even just touching a patient without consent may lead to a charge of battery.

Sterility and the teaching scenario

If a more senior practitioner takes over the performance of a procedure, very often the full aseptic precautions in place will be broken, in preference to speed of getting the procedure done. Regardless of who performs the procedure, aseptic precautions appropriate to the procedure must be maintained. For CNB, this includes mask, hat, gloves, and gown.

Side effects and complications

CNB is an invasive procedure with an established list of side effects and complications (see Table 47.1). A side effect is an anticipated effect of a procedure at a site or mechanism different to the intended; these are usually common and harmless. A complication is an unanticipated problem caused by a procedure; these are rare but generally more serious.

Outcome benefits

Outcome benefits any decision about performing CNB balances the perceived benefits and these complications. Results of a large randomized trial in 2002 did not demonstrate any significant reduction in mortality in high-risk patients undergoing major abdominal surgery with the use of epidural anaesthesia and analgesia. The same study, however, did demonstrate some reduction in respiratory failure, and improved analgesia during the first 3 postoperative days. Follow-up subgroup analysis failed to demonstrate any groups who benefited from a reduction in mortality. A similar trial within the New York Veterans group in 2001 demonstrated similar outcomes.

Other studies, looking at more restrictive patient groups, have found reductions in morbidity, particularly perioperative myocardial ischaemic events, respiratory performance, deep venous thrombosis, and infections. Other benefits established include reduced duration of stay, improved analgesia, ↑ satisfaction, and better early mobilization. Some of these benefits may also, however, have been influenced by advances in the overall quality of healthcare over time.

The decision to use CNB should be made with knowledge regarding the relevant pros and cons of the intended technique, with the input from an informed patient taking into account their wishes.

Table 47.1 List of side effect and complications of CNB and estimation of their incidence

Side effect/complication	Incidence
Hypotension	Common
Itching	Common (especially with opiates)
Shaking	Common
Incomplete epidural block	10%
Failed block	1–5%
Postdural puncture headache	1% (dependant on needle)
Temporary nerve damage	1 in 1,000
Permanent harm	4.2 in 100,000
Permanent nerve damage	1 in 5000–10,000
Infection	Very rare
Haematoma	Very rare
Paraplegia or death	1.8 in 100,000

Further reading

Auroy Y, Benhamou D, Bargues L, *et al*. (2002). Major complications of regional anesthesia in France. *Anesthesiology*, **97**(5),1274–80.

Broadbent CR, Maxwell WB, Ferrie R, *et al*. (2000). Ability of anaesthetists to identify a marked lumbar interspace. *Anaesthesia*, **55**(11), 1122–6.

Cook TM, Counsell D, Wildsmith JAW (2009). Major complications of central neuraxial block: report on the Third National Audit Project of the Royal College of Anaesthetists. *Br J Anaesth*, **102**(2), 179–90.

Horlocker TT, Wedel DJ, Benzon H, *et al*. (2003). Regional anesthesia in the anticoagulated patient: defining the risks (the second ASRA Consensus Conference on Neuraxial Anesthesia and Anticoagulation). *Reg Anesth Pain Med*, **28**(3), 172–97.

Park WY, Thompson JS, Lee KK. (2001). Effect of epidural anesthesia and analgesia on perioperative outcome; a randomized, controlled Veterans Affairs Cooperative Study. *Ann Surg*, **234**(4), 560–71.

Peyton PJ, Myles PS, Silbert BS, *et al*. (2003). Perioperative epidural analgesia and outcome after major abdominal surgery in high-risk patients. *Anesth Analg*, **96**(2), 548–54.

Reynolds F (2001). Damage to the conus medullaris following spinal anaesthesia. *Anaesthesia*, **56**(3), 238–47.

Rigg JR, Jamrozik K, Myles PS, *et al*. (2002). Epidural anaesthesia and analgesia and outcome of major surgery: a randomized trial. *Lancet*, **359**(9314), 1276–82.

Epidural anaesthesia and analgesia

Thoracic epidurals

Indications

- High (T1–T6):
    - pneumonectomy
    - oesophagectomy
    - sternotomy
    - mediastinotomy
    - major breast reconstruction/plastics flaps.
- Mid (T7–T9):
    - thoracotomy
    - oesophagectomy
    - major abdominal surgery (especially upper GI)
    - open nephrectomy
    - AAA repair.
- Low (T10–T12):
    - major abdominal surgery (especially lower GI)
    - major gynaecological surgery
    - abdominal-based leg revascularization procedures.

Anatomy

- The thoracic region consists of 12 vertebrae in a normal kyphosis. This can be marginally exacerbated by flexion.
- The thoracic spinal cord is sizeable.
- Spinous processes are long and angulated caudally with a slight curve. See Fig. 48.1.
- Intervertebral foramina are smaller than the lumbar or cervical regions.
- Transverse processes are long and articulate with ribs.
- Skin to epidural depth is shallow, often as little as 3cm.
- Blood supply to the spinal cord comes from 1 anterior and 2 posterior arteries. The anterior spinal artery arises from a branch of each vertebral artery; the 2 posterior spinal arteries usually arise from the posterior inferior cerebellar arteries on each side. The anterior artery acquires contributions from intercostal arteries, the main contribution being from the artery of Adamkiewicz. This is responsible for supplying blood to the anterior 2/3 of the cord in the mid-thoracic to lumber territory, and innervates the main motor tracts.

Clinical implications

- Spinal anaesthesia is essentially inappropriate at thoracic levels.
- Patient flexion may marginally improve access.
- Midline approach may prove difficult, particularly in shorter patients.
- Paramedian approach is easier and more reliable, especially in the mid-thoracic region.
- Lateral angulation may result in a paravertebral catheter and unilateral anaesthesia.
- Accidental dural puncture is possible at relatively low distances, and may results in cord damage.

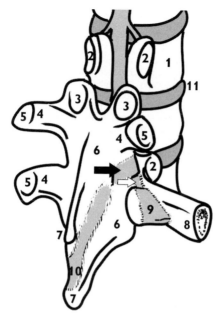

Fig. 48.1 Thoracic vertebrae. **1** vertebral body; **2** costal hemi-facet; **3** superior articular process; **4** transverse process; **5** facet for tubercle of rib; **6** lamina; **7** caudally angled spinous processes; **8** rib; **9** lateral costo-transverse ligament; **10** interspinous ligament; **11** intervertebral disc; White arrow, superior costo-transverse ligament; Black arrow, ligamentum flavum.

Approaches and technique

Common features

- Strict asepsis—mask, hat, gloves, gown.
- Chlorhexidine 0.5% in 70% alcohol skin prep; apply and leave to dry completely to achieve a true sterile field.
- Drapes should be applied to leave only the immediate area exposed.
- Local anaesthetic for skin/ligament anaesthesia; this should be applied subcutaneously initially, then inject 1–2mL lateral to the ligamentous structures. The nerve supply to the ligaments is variable, although generally sparse, and originates from the sympathetic chain and rami communicantes. This injection should block some of these branches.
- Equipment preparation. The epidural catheter and filter should be connected and flushed to ensure patency and connectability. As little as 1mL of air injected into the filter may obstruct it and prevent infusion, despite injection being possible.

Midline
- Can be very difficult between T5 and T8 and it may be best to use a paramedian approach at these levels; it can still be a challenging technique at other levels depending on patient. Familiarity with the paramedian approach is often required as a 'plan B'.
- Standard interlaminar approach; see Chapter 47.
- Acute cephalad angle required, accentuation of flexion may be needed to complete passage through ligamentum flavum.
- Loss of resistance to saline is now probably the technique of choice. Air may be used if experienced with this technique but the loss of resistance may be less obvious due to the compressibility of air, however CSF from an inadvertent dural puncture is more easily recognizable.
- Should have distinct moderate–low–high resistance feel.
- Distance from skin through to ligamentum flavum may be under 3cm.

Paramedian
- Often more reliable in majority of patients, especially between T5 and T8.
- Insertion point 1–2cm lateral to SPs.
- Infiltration vertically down onto lamina of vertebra; a small amount of LA onto periosteum may be needed.
- Withdrawal needle 1cm; redirect around 30° medial and 30° cephalad to enter the ligamentum flavum of chosen SP interspace.
- Loss of resistance to saline technique. Air may be used if experienced at this technique.
- There may be only a single high-resistance feel prior to encountering the epidural space.
- May occasionally need to angulate, either more caudal or more cephalad.

Passing and securing the catheter
Once the epidural space is identified, the catheter should pass freely. For slim patients, leave 3–4cm catheter in the epidural space. For larger patients, leave 5–6cm within the epidural space as an increase in subcutaneous tissue allows for more 'play' of the catheter, increasing the risk of displacement of the catheter, and infection hazard.

Securing the catheter into position may be achieved in many ways. Specially designed 'Lock-its' may improve security, although may provide pressure areas on the patient's back when rested on them for hours. A loop in the epidural catheter is traditionally employed to provide protection against pulling and displacement of the catheter. The whole area should be enclosed in a dressing through which the insertion site can be visualized.

Confirming the epidural position
Several strategies are commonly employed to exclude intravascular and intrathecal catheterization.

Meniscal drop
The negative pressure in the thoracic epidural region in a sitting patient results in a falling meniscus within the epidural catheter if held vertically above the patient's catheter insertion site. A rising meniscus may indicate intrathecal placement.

Aspiration
To seek CSF withdrawal. If fluid is aspirated it can be tested for warmth (LA should be cold, CSF warm), or glucose (if present = CSF, absent = LA). To seek venous catheter, gentle aspiration may demonstrate venous blood.

Test dose of LA
This aims to identify intrathecal catheterization, and may demonstrate motor block or hypotension within 2 minutes of injection.

Test dose of epinephrine-containing solution. If heart rate increases by >20% within 30 seconds of injection, the catheter may be IV.

Caution: none of these tests absolutely confirm epidural placement, nor exclude intravascular or intrathecal placement. Epidural catheters may also 'migrate' after insertion. Constant vigilance regarding these complications is required, particularly if administering a bolus dose.

How to test an epidural block
Anaesthesia requires a dense sensory and motor block; this can be demonstrated by loss of light touch sensation and absent motor power in the required dermatomes. The Bromage scale (see Table 48.1) has been traditionally used to grade level of motor block in the lower limb for obstetric anaesthesia.

For analgesia, the first assessment is to ask the patient about their pain. Adequate analgesia may be present with very little demonstrable block, particularly if opiates and other adjuncts have been used. The light touch and motor pathways may well show normal responses. As pain and temperature sensations travel in similar size nerves and spinal tracts, demonstration of altered temperature sensation in the desired dermatomes should be adequate. This can, however, be misleading, as loss of temperature sensation is progressive at the extremes of the block; i.e. the block becomes denser over sequential dermatomes. Documenting the transition range from normal to most abnormal may be useful.

Table 48.1 Bromage scale

Grade	Criteria	Degree of block
0	Free movement of legs and feet	Nil (0%)
1	Just able to flex knees with free movement of feet	Partial (33%)
2	Unable to flex knees, but with free movement of feet	Almost complete (66%)
3	Unable to move legs or feet	Complete (100%)

Troubleshooting an epidural
Epidural anaesthesia or analgesia may not be complete for several reasons.
See Table 48.2.

Drugs
Different LAs may be used to achieve desired actions. Adjunct solutions
have also been used. Try to differentiate between anaesthesia and analgesia.
See Table 48.3.

Table 48.2 Troubleshooting problematic epidurals

Problem	Findings	Action
Low block	Inadequate anaesthesia	Lie flatter
		Bolus of LA
High block	Low BP/bradycardia	Support BP with pressor/ fluid
	Digital tingling	Sit up (when BP allows)
		Turn down/off infusion
Hypotension	Nausea/presyncope	Support BP with pressor/ fluid
	Vasodilatation	Consider ondansetron
Missed segment	Single dermatomal absence of block	Roll patient so missed side is downwards
		Withdraw catheter leaving 3cm in space
Unilateral block	Absent block down 1 entire side	Further bolus of LA
		Consider fentanyl bolus (50–100 micrograms)
		If no success; resite
Patchy block	Variably spread and density of block throughout; possible subdural catheter.	**Do not use**
		Stop infusion;
		Remove catheter
		Consider resite at another level
Severe itching	Opiate-related	Consider:
		Ondansetron
		Chlorphenamine
		Naloxone
		Remove opiate

Table 48.3 Local anaesthetic solutions and additives

Desired effect	Drug	Concentration/dose	Comments
Anaesthesia	Lidocaine	2% 20mg/mL	Onset 5–10mins; 1hr anaesthesia
	Bupivacaine	0.5% 5mg/mL	Onset 20mins; 2–4hrs anaesthesia
	Levobupivacaine	0.5% 5mg/mL	
	Ropivacaine	0.75% 7.5mg/mL	Onset 10–15mins; 2–4hrs anaesthesia
Analgesia	Bupivacaine	0.05–0.125% 0.5–1.25mg/mL	Low concentration gives analgesia with minimal motor block
	Levobupivacaine	0.05–0.125% 0.5–1.25mg/mL	
	Ropivacaine	0.2% 2mg/mL	
	Emulsified isoflurane		Experimental
Adjuncts	Fentanyl	1–8 micrograms/mL	May improve spread; short duration of action; systemic absorption
	Diamorphine	2.5mg	Moderate onset; around 12hrs analgesia; moderate itching and nausea
	Morphine (preservative free)	1–2mg	Onset around 1hr; around 24hrs analgesia; severe itching /nausea
	Sodium bicarbonate	1mmol/10mL (1mL 8.4%)	May speed onset
	Epinephrine	5 micrograms/mL 1:200,000	May prolong block
	Clonidine	1–2 micrograms/kg 1–2 micrograms/mL for infusion	Increases duration of block; moderate sedation
	Ketamine (preservative free)	1–2mg/kg	May improve analgesia

Lumbar epidurals

Introduction

The lumbar epidural is a standard anaesthetic technique and is generally regularly performed by most anaesthetists. It has a well-established place in the role of labour and caesarean section, anaesthesia and analgesia of lower limb and lower trunk surgery, and may be extended to provide anaesthesia/analgesia for mid and upper trunk procedures if needed. Lumbar epidurals are usually performed with a standard midline (or paramedian) approach and are therefore not described further except for the following features worth highlighting. See Chapter 47.

Anatomy

- Normal lumbar lordosis may be countered by flexion.
- Spinous processes broad and almost perpendicular to skin.
- Broad transverse processes. See Fig. 48.2.
- Spinal cord ends at L1/L2 90%; L2/L3 10%.
- Distance to ligamentum flavum *rarely* <4cm.

Clinical notes

- Flexion increases likelihood of successful epidural.
- Passage through ligament may only need slight cephalad angulation.
- At low lumbar levels, the needle may need to be perpendicular or even slightly caudad.
- Midline approach standard.
- Paramedian technique require less cephalad angulation (15°) than the thoracic approach.
- Epidural space triangular and several mm deep.
- Safest approach to the epidural space at L3/L4 or below. No risk of needle damage to cord.

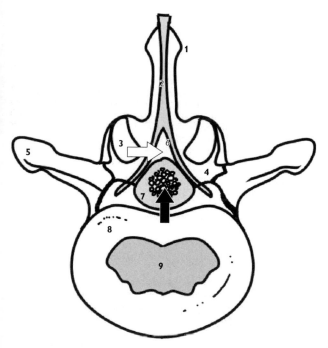

Fig. 48.2 Cross-section of lumbar vertebrae. 1 spinous process; 2 interspinous ligament; 3 superior articular process; 4 lamina; 5 broad transverse process; 6 ligamentum flavum; 7 CSF; 8 vertebral body; 9 nucleus pulposus; White arrow, epidural space; Black arrow, cauda equina.

Caudal epidural

Indications

Surgery below the umbilicus
- Hernia repair
- Hydrocoele repair
- Most urological procedures including TURP
- Lower limb surgery
- Ano-rectal procedures
- Vaginal repairs and surgery
- Chronic sacral pain
- Obstetric 2nd stage/instrumental delivery (rarely done now).

Introduction

The caudal is a technique most commonly performed in paediatric anaesthesia, where identification of the anatomy is clear and the caudal structures are not yet fully ossified. However, it can be of great use in the adult population, where anaesthesia and analgesia are required within the sacral dermatomes (e.g. vaginal repair).

Anatomy

- The epidural space extends through the sacrum to the sacrococcygeal membrane (SCM).
- Within the sacral canal, there is epidural fat, sacral epidural veins (usually ending at S4), the sacral canal containing the filum terminale and the sacral nerve roots.
- The SCM represents the failed fusion of the laminae of the 5th sacral vertebra. It may not be present in up to 20% of men or 5% of women.
- Distance to dural sac from SCM may be as short as 3.5cm.
- Volume of the epidural space is variable, from ~10mL up to >30mL, excluding dural sac and nerve roots.

Technique

- Lateral position, with hips flexed to 90°.
- Palpation of the sacral cornu marking the upper border of the SCM; the coccyx should be palpable marking the apex of the SCM triangle.
- A sterile technique should be used; most commonly this is performed using chlorhexidine skin preparation and a no-touch gloved technique.
- Use a short needle; ideally a short bevel. Remember in some patients 3.5cm may result in a dural puncture.
- Some practitioners prefer to cannulate the caudal epidural space using a 20G or 22G cannula.
- Insert the needle at 90° to the skin in the upper 1/3 portion of the SCM; feel the 'click' as you pass through SCM.
- Move the hub of the needle caudally by about 60°, then advance the needle/cannula by 1–2cm. See Fig. 48.3.
- Ensure no syringe is attached; watch for drainage of fluid/blood.
- Attach a syringe and ensure negative aspiration.
- Inject an appropriate volume of solution; 0.25% bupivacaine or similar.

- May require 20–25mL of LA for adults
- For paediatrics:
  - lumbarsacral: 0.5mL/kg
  - thoracolumbar: 1mL/kg
  - mid thoracic: 1.25mL/kg.
- Adjuncts such as clonidine, ketamine, and opiates can be used.

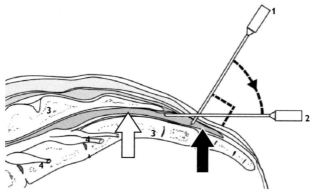

Fig. 48.3 Caudal epidural injection; showing re-angulation of needle after passing through SCM. **1** initial needle position; **2** re-angled needle after passing through the SCM; Black arrow, SCM; White arrow, epidural space; **3** sacrum; **4** nerve roots.

Further reading

Crighton IM, Barry BP, Hobbs GJ (1997). A study of the anatomy of the caudal space using magnetic resonance imaging *Br J Anaesth*, **78**(4), 391–5.

Spinal anaesthesia, combined spinal epidural, and continuous spinal anaesthesia

Spinal anaesthesia

Indications
- Surgery on the lower limbs or trunk
- LSCS
- Labour analgesia
- As analgesic adjunct for upper trunk/thoracic surgery
- Perineal/perianal surgery.

Introduction
Also known as subarachnoid block, this common technique involves the placement of a needle through the dura and arachnoid mater into cerebrospinal fluid, and the injection of medications, usually LA with or without adjuncts. The standard midline approach is described in Chapter 47 (see ⊃ Basic approach, p. 502). Paramedian approaches are often used and follow the same technique as for paramedian epidurals (see ⊃ Paramedian, p. 512), but obviously require the needle to be inserted slightly deeper to pass through the dura and arachnoid mater.

Equipment
The use of specific needles has reduced the incidence of complications related to puncturing the dura. There are 2 traditional needle designs in use, the bevelled needle tip (Quinke) and the pencil point (Whitacre and Sprotte) although there are newer hybrid versions appearing on the market. Beware of small gauge needles as the backflow of CSF can be slow, especially with pencil point needles. (See Fig. 49.1.)

Bevelled edge needles have a sharp long bevel which cuts effectively through ligament and dura. The stylet passes down to the distal hole, giving a reliable injection point. They are effective, and are less likely to deviate through the tissues they pass. However, they may 'cut' a hole in the dura, leading to an increased CSF leak and an ↑ risk of post dural puncture headache (PDPH).

Pencil-point needles have a cylindrical shaft formed to a point, with a more proximal hole, which the stylet passes down to. Available versions are the Sprotte and Whitacre needles, which differ according to location and size of the hole. They part ligament and tissues as they pass through, and are less likely to cut or tear dura, reducing PDPH risk. However, in order to aspirate CSF, the point and hole must be reliably through the dura. They are available in small diameters down to 29G; they also have a tendency to deviate as they pass through tissues.

Hybrid needles (e.g. Atraucan©) are a new development to try and maximize the benefits of both pencil-point and bevel spinal needles. The distal tip of the bevel is sharp, to make a small clean incision, with the remainder of the bevel designed to dilate the tissues. This should result in greater CSF flow per needle size, and a reduced likelihood of PDPH.

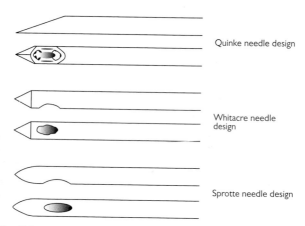

Quinke needle design

Whitacre needle design

Sprotte needle design

Fig. 49.1 Bevelled and pencil point needles.

Factors affecting spread of solution

Patient height influences length of spinal column and therefore the amount of drug required for effect.

The principal determinant of extent of spinal solution spread is the mass of drug injected; hence 2mL of 2.5mg/mL bupivacaine = 1mL 5mg/mL bupivacaine.

Baricity, and therefore patient positioning influences spread; 'Heavy' solutions, or drugs prepared with dense sugar formulations, will gravitate or 'sink'. Hypodense solutions, such as levobupivacaine, will 'float'.

Rapid injections may increase intrathecal spread; slow injections may localize injectate around injection site.

Factors which increase the volume of non-CSF components within the spinal canal may also increase the extent of block; i.e. the gravid uterus and morbid obesity increasing epidural venous volume. Spinal stenosis may increase spread of injectate by reducing the overall volume of the spinal canal.

Drugs

Principally LAs are injected intrathecally, with the most common being bupivacaine (with or without glucose). More recently both levobupivacaine and ropivacaine (with and without glucose) have been used without problem. Ropivacaine may have a shorter duration of action and less motor block. Lidocaine is rarely used in the UK due to persisting concerns over transient neurological symptoms (TNS). Prilocaine, for intrathecal use, and a resurgence of interest in chloroprocaine (currently unlicensed) may have benefits for day case spinal anaesthesia. Blocks are often supplemented with opiates and occasionally with clonidine or ketamine. It is imperative to use preservative free preparations of these drugs. See Table 49.1.

Modifications of spinal anaesthesia

Low-dose spinal anaesthesia

The combination of a small amount of LA with lateral positioning can provide anaesthesia in a small surgical field with minimal motor blockade and short duration of action, also minimizing the risk of urinary retention. A typical recipe consists of plain or heavy bupivacaine 5mg + fentanyl 10 micrograms to achieve a block suitable for knee arthroscopy in an outpatient setting. Each 1mg bupivacaine allows ~ 10 minutes of surgical anaesthesia. Patients will still retain motor function and may have skin sensation during surgery, particularly if aged below 50 years.

Unilateral spinal anaesthesia

Use of a hyperbaric solution injected with a patient in lateral position with desired block site downwards can achieve a degree of unilateral block. Usually the block is performed in the lateral position, with a very slow injection, and the patient remains lateral for 5–10 minutes afterwards. There is controversy over whether this remains truly unilateral; the blocks tend to start unilateral and subsequently spread bilaterally.

Saddle block

Use of small amounts of a hyperbaric solution with the patient in a sitting position can achieve a pure sensory block of the perineum, suitable for procedures such as haemorrhoidectomy, peri-anal abscess drainage, or fistulae exploration. A typical recipe would be 'Heavy' bupivacaine 5mg injected into a sitting patient very slowly.

Analgesic block

Use of opiate only intrathecal injections have been used for postoperative analgesia for major trunk and thorax procedures. Typically 200–300 micrograms diamorphine or 100–200 micrograms preservative-free morphine is used as a single preoperative injection. This will provide analgesia for ~ 12 and 24 hours respectively.

Complications specific to spinal anaesthesia

- Failed block
- PDPH
- Respiratory depression.

Table 49.1 Drugs used in spinal anaesthesia

	Drug	Dose	Properties	Duration
Local	Bupivacaine	5–15mg	Moderate onset. Slightly hypobaric	3–4hrs
	Heavy bupivacaine	5–15mg	Fast onset. Hyperbaric	3–4hrs
	Lidocaine		Not recommended due to concerns about TNS	
	Prilocaine	40–60mg (max 80mg)	Fast onset	1–2hrs
Opiates	Fentanyl	10–25 micrograms	Highly lipophilic. Rapid onset	1–2hrs
	Diamorphine	200–400 micrograms	Moderate lipophilic. Moderate onset	8–12hrs
	Morphine (preservative free)	100–200 micrograms	Hydrophilic. Slow onset	18–24hrs
Others	Clonidine	50–100 micrograms	Sedative analgesic. Prolongs block	Extra 25–50%
	Ketamine (preservative free)	0.1 mg/kg	Analgesic. ?reduces chronic pain. May reduce motor block	May reduce duration

Combined spinal epidural

A combination of neuraxial techniques can be performed on an individual patient. These can be performed at 2 distinct intervertebral spaces, or at a single space as a 'needle through needle' technique. This involves the location of the lumbar epidural space using a Tuohy needle as described in → Approaches and technique, p. 511, and the passage of a spinal needle through the Tuohy to penetrate the dura beyond the epidural space. Once intrathecal injection has occurred, the spinal needle is withdrawn, and the epidural catheter inserted as normal.

- Advantages:
  - needle through needle technique allows a single procedure where 2 were otherwise required
  - needle through needle technique may help localization of the spinal canal in the obese patient by ligament identification with a loss-of-resistance technique
  - lower volume of intrathecal injectate may minimize side effects
  - epidural volume expansion allows the elevation of a spinal block by epidural injection. 5mL of 0.9% NaCl is as effective as either 10mL of NaCl or LA solution, and will raise the block by ~ 2 segments
  - prolongation of anaesthesia possible using the epidural
  - an epidural catheter may provide postoperative analgesia.
- Disadvantages:
  - once intrathecal injection is complete, delay in threading and securing the epidural catheter may cause positional spinal spread (low block, unilateral block etc.)
  - passing the spinal needle through the Tuohy removes the secure 'grip' of the ligaments; this may allow repeated puncturing of the dura and increase risk of postdural puncture headache
  - using a needle through needle technique does not allow testing of the epidural catheter
  - a needle through needle technique may increase the risk of passing an intrathecal catheter, as dural perforation has already occurred
  - there is an ↑ risk of serious complications.

The CSE becomes particularly useful where regional anaesthesia is required but the duration of surgery has the potential to be prolonged; i.e. caesarean section following multiple previous lower abdominal operations, abdominal hysterectomy, lower limb revascularization procedures, endovascular aortic aneurysm stent insertion. Concerns regarding the increase in PDPH rate have led to development of CSE kits with fixators for attaching the spinal needle to the Tuohy needle to minimize multiple dural puncture.

Continuous spinal anaesthesia

Spinal anaesthesia provides profound, reliable anaesthesia but is limited by having a limited duration of action. Increasing the duration of action by increasing the dose of LA is associated with ↑ side effects especially in patients with significant comorbidities. Methods to allow repeated injections into the intrathecal space have been investigated for >100 years, and Tuohy investigated this in detail in the 1940s.

Achievement of CSA requires penetration of the dura, followed by passage of a catheter that remains within the subarachnoid space. Essentially this is achieved by techniques as for a lumbar epidural (see ➜ Approaches and technique, p. 511) but with deliberate penetration of the dura (as for a spinal).

Use of 20G needles to enter the intrathecal space led to concerns over the risk of PDPH, and smaller catheters (28G and 32G) were developed so that smaller needles could be used. These proved to be technically very difficult to use (10% unable to pass catheter; 15% failure) and were subsequently associated with incidents of cauda equina syndrome.

Cauda equina syndrome (CES) and continuous spinal anaesthesia (CSA)

CES consists of low back pain, sciatica, saddle sensory disturbances, bladder and/or bowel dysfunction, and variable lower extremity motor and/or sensory loss. It appeared to be caused by local pooling of toxic concentrations of LA. The small diameter of microcatheters meant that injection velocities were very low leading to pooling. If the catheters went caudally rather than cranially this tended to encourage the lack of spread leading to patchy block formation and encouraged repeated dosing of the LA. The use of a high concentration of drug (e.g. lidocaine 5%) led to neurotoxic concentrations pooled around unprotected nerves, and so to CES. In 1992 the FDA banned the use of catheters smaller than 24G. A recent evaluation of a series of 4000 CSA patients (using the 22G Spinocath©) showed no patients reporting neurology on discharge and no subsequent CES.

It is also of interest to note that the incidence of PDPH was no lower when microcatheters were used (possibly because of the technical difficulty in their use leading to multiple dural punctures).

CSA: operative anaesthesia

Present practice is to use either 20G catheters (PDPH incidence 3.7%, and <1% in patients over 67 years) or a 22G catheter placed over a 27G needle (Spinocath©).

CSA allows the use of smaller doses of LA with titration against effect. This is associated with reduced changes in MAP and HR (compared to single-shot spinal anaesthesia). Initial doses of 5mg of bupivacaine are used effectively particularly in the elderly. It is more consistent than continuous epidural anaesthesia and is associated with a lower need for conversion to GA.

CSA: postoperative analgesia

For postoperative analgesia CSA involves the use of low concentrations of LA and opioid mixtures. A practical formula is to use bupivacaine 300 micrograms/mL and diamorphine 100 micrograms/mL. This mixture is run as an infusion at 1–4mL/hour. Clearly it is important that there are policies in place to ensure that staff managing these patients understand the treatment being delivered and particularly how it differs from continuous epidural analgesia. The incidence of intrathecal infection appears to be extremely small in patients who have catheters in place for <60 hours and this duration can be recommended.

Further reading

Cook TM, Counsell D, Wildsmith JAW (2009). Major complications of central neuraxial block: report on the Third National Audit Project of the Royal College of Anaesthetists. *Br J Anaesth*, **102**(2), 179–90.

Denny NM, Selander DE (1998). Continuous spinal anaesthesia. *Br J Anaesth*, **81**(4), 590–7.

Nair GS, Abrishami A, Lermitte J, et al. (2009). Systematic review of spinal anaesthesia using bupivacaine for ambulatory knee arthroscopy. *Br J Anaesth*, **102**(3), 307–15.

Watson B, Allen J (2013). *Spinal Anaesthesia for Day Surgery Patients; A Practical Guide*. Norwich: British Association of Day Surgery. Available at: http://daysurgeryuk.net/en/shop/handbooks/spinal-anaesthesia-for-day-surgery-patients-a-practical-guide-3rd-edition.

Chapter 50

Ultrasound for central neuraxial blocks

Background

In 2008, NICE published guidelines on US-guided catheterization of the epidural space. Examining the limited evidence available at the time they came to the conclusion that 'it is safe and may be helpful in achieving correct placement'.

Like the use of US in peripheral regional anaesthesia, experts with many years of experience may not obtain as much benefit as novices or less experienced practitioners for the routine cases, but for everyone US can be particularly useful in those with problematic anatomy (e.g. obesity, scoliosis, previous back surgery, etc.) and/or prior history of difficulty in placement of neuraxial blockade.

The small gaps between adjacent vertebrae and the angulation of the spinous processes result in narrow acoustic windows into the intervertebral spaces. This is especially true in the mid-thoracic region. However, with a little practice, good information on the following can usually be obtained:

- More accurate determination of the vertebral level
- Location of the midline
- Identification of the optimal interspace
- Identification of the optimal angle of approach
- Evaluation of the depth to the epidural/spinal space.

This should result in ↓ technical difficulty and ↑ clinical efficacy.

Epidurals

Sacral (caudal epidural injection)

Imaging of the sacral hiatus and sacrococcygeal membrane can be achieved in most patients using a high-frequency linear array probe. Placed in a transverse orientation over the sacrum, the characteristic 'double hump' emerges as you slide over the sacral cornua. The hyperechoic line slung in between is the sacrococcygeal membrane with a deeper, parallel line corresponding to the anterior surface of the sacral canal (Fig. 50.1). If the probe is then carefully turned through 90°, a median sagittal view is obtained (Fig. 50.2). A cannula may then be introduced in plane and guided in real-time into the caudal epidural space.

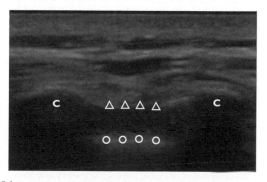

Fig. 50.1 Transverse view of the sacral hiatus. C, cornua; Triangles, sacrococcygeal membrane; Circles, anterior surface of the sacral canal.

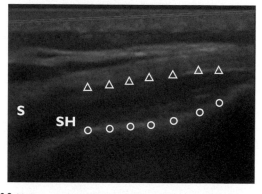

Fig. 50.2 Median sagittal view of the sacral hiatus. Triangles, sacrococcygeal membrane; Circles, anterior surface of the sacral canal; SH, sacral hiatus; S, sacrum.

Lumbar

In adults, a curvilinear, low-frequency (2–5MHz) probe is required to enable visualization of the deeper structures; however, this comes at the expense of resolution of the image obtained. Prior to scanning, the patient must adopt the same posture in which the block will be performed and the depth, focus and gain of the US machine should be optimized.

Although there are descriptions of real-time US-guided placement of epidurals in the literature, it often requires 2 experienced practitioners and is technically demanding. It is the author's opinion therefore, that more data is required before it can be recommended for routine use.

The use of US as a pre-procedural check of the relevant anatomy before proceeding with the traditional loss of resistance technique is relatively simple and potentially very useful. With a little practice it need not take any more time than using landmarks to guide your epidural placement, and in the more challenging patient it may indeed save time.

Pattern recognition is the key to success in this field, and only 2 views need to be mastered. These are the paramedian sagittal oblique and the transverse interspinous views.

Paramedian sagittal oblique (PSO) view

The probe is initially placed sagittally 2–3cm lateral to the midline and angled slightly medially to target the centre of the spinal cord (see Fig. 50.3). With additional small sliding and tilting movements a 'sawtooth' pattern can be seen (Fig. 50.4). The teeth of the saw correspond to the vertebral laminae, with the troughs in between formed by the hyperechoic ligamentum flavum and posterior dura. These are not commonly seen as separate entities. Another composite structure made up of the anterior dura, posterior longitudinal ligament and posterior surface of the vertebral body on the other side of the spinal canal is often seen as a further, deeper, single hyperechoic line parallel to the sawtooth pattern. See Fig. 50.5.

Once this image is obtained, sliding the probe caudally reveals the sacral bone as a flat hyperechoic line becoming more superficial the more caudal you scan. You can now visualize the L5 laminae as the first tooth of the saw, and hence mark off on the skin the L5/S1, L4/L5, L3/L4, and L2/L3 interspaces as each passes the centre of the image whilst moving the probe cranially. This is known as the 'counting up' method, but it is possible to 'count down' from the T12 lamina having first identified this vertebra by its attachment to the 12th rib laterally.

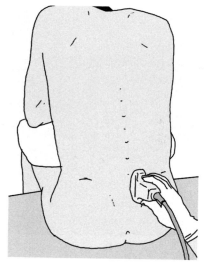

Fig. 50.3 Probe position for a paramedian sagittal oblique view of the lumbar spine.

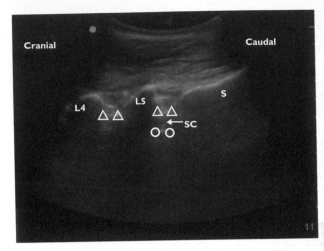

Fig. 50.4 Paramedian sagittal oblique view of the lumbar spine showing the 'sawtooth' pattern.

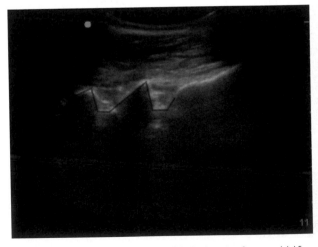

Fig. 50.5 Paramedian sagittal oblique view of the lumbar spine. S, sacrum; L4, L5, laminae; Triangles, ligamentum flavum/posterior dura complex; Circles, posterior surface of the vertebral body; SC, spinal canal.

Transverse interspinous view

If the probe is now turned 90° in a previously marked interspace (see Fig. 50.6), a 'flying bat' appearance will be revealed (Fig. 50.7 and Fig. 50.8). The head of the bat corresponds to the ligamentum flavum/posterior dura complex with the ears and wings formed by the shadows cast by the articular and transverse processes respectively. The posterior surface of the vertebral body (and related structures) on the other side of the spinal canal resembles the 'nose' of the bat. Some cephalad angulation of the probe may be required to improve this view.

Once the best picture is achieved, mark the skin at the middle of both the cranial and lateral surfaces of the probe. Later, these 2 marks can be extended with their intersect indicating the optimum puncture point. Prior to removal of the probe, a note should be made of the angle of the probe to the skin (best angle of approach to achieve a successful first pass) and then the image should be frozen allowing measurement of the depth to the epidural space with the in-built calipers.

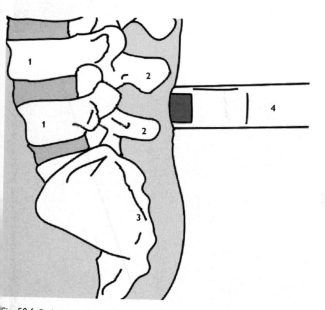

Fig. 50.6 Probe position for a transverse interspinous view of the lumbar spine.
1 vertebral bodies; 2 spinous processes; 3 sacrum; 4 ultrasound probe.

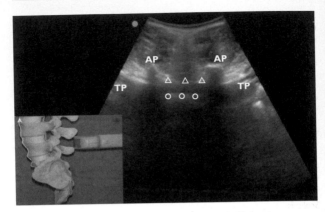

Fig. 50.7 Transverse interspinous view of the lumbar spine. AP, articular processes; TP, transverse processes; Triangles, ligamentum flavum/posterior dura complex; Circles, posterior surface of the vertebral body.

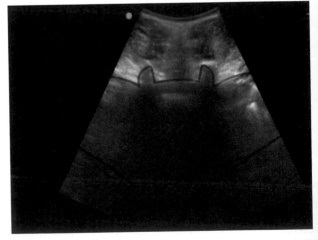

Fig. 50.8 Transverse interspinous view of the lumbar spine showing the 'flying bat' pattern.

Specific situations

Obese patients

- May have a significant amount of subcutaneous tissue between their skin and vertebral column.
- Avoid mistaking the erector spinae muscle shadows for the ears of the bat by starting with a larger depth of field (>15cm) before homing in on the flying bat pattern of the transverse view.
- Avoid significant underestimate of depth to epidural space by ensuring you release the pressure of the probe on the skin before freezing the image and taking measurements.
- Look for the ears and wings of the bat as the ligamentum may not be seen at the larger depths encountered in the obese. Just measure down to an imaginary line joining the base of the 2 flying bat's 'ears' in the transverse view (between the bases of adjacent 'sawteeth' in the PSO view).
- If you can only see the deeper, more hyperechoic vertebral body then there will be a clear passage to the epidural space.

Scoliosis

- This can be both rotational and lateral. Try to find an interspace with normal symmetrical sonoanatomy. Failing this, an asymmetrical image will allow you to estimate the angle off midline with which to aim. One may be able to achieve a more symmetrical image by angling the transversely orientated probe left or right. Again note the angle of the probe.

Elderly patients

- They tend to have more calcification or narrowing of the interspinous space with ossification of the interspinous ligaments and osteophytosis of the facet joints. If a 'flying bat' picture cannot be captured, the PSO orientation's 'sawtooth' pattern often saves the day.

Thoracic

The lower 4 thoracic vertebral interspaces can generally be viewed in the same manner as the lumbar region. However, between T5 and T8 the spinous processes project with a sharp inferior angle making the transverse interspinous view impossible. Even the laminae overlap making the PSO view more difficult with more horizontal 'sawteeth'. Even so, using the PSO orientation you can usually find a narrow acoustic window through to the epidural space. This can be marked off on the skin, and estimates of angle of approach and depth can still be made.

The upper thoracic (T1–4) interspaces again start to increase in size with their spinous processes becoming less severely angled. Again the sawtooth pattern of the PSO view can easily be observed.

Cervical

Cervical epidural injections can also be facilitated by US. With the interspaces again widened at the C6/C7, C7/T1 level it is certainly possible to get a transverse interspinous image, however the PSO view may be more clinically useful, especially if performing a paramedian approach to the epidural space. It is also possible to use US to guide a cervical medial branch nerve block for use in the diagnosis and treatment of cervical zygapophyseal joint pain.

Paediatric considerations

The distances involved in epidural placement in children (1–4cm) mean that a high-frequency linear array probe is effective. The added resolution provides relatively detailed images. In infants up to 6 months of age vertebrae have not yet ossified. The acoustic window is therefore limitless and the probe can be used in a median sagittal orientation. This, together with the 2 previously described views not only enables easy identification of the epidural space and dura, but also the neural structures within the spinal canal, and even the central canal of the spinal cord (Fig. 50.9 and Fig. 50.10).

Caudal injections can be performed as described earlier, but in neonates and preterm infants the distance to the epidural space can be as little as 0.5cm. Add to this the fact that the dural sac can extend to S4 means that US use is of great benefit to avoid dural puncture.

Confirmation of epidural placement can be made by injecting small doses of saline (0.1mL/kg) and observing the ventral movement of the posterior dura prior to injecting the LA. LA spread may also be monitored.

Correct epidural catheter tip placement can be confirmed either by direct visualization or inferred on monitoring spread of injectate. This allows less LA volume to be used and avoidance of opioids resulting in reduced risks of respiratory depression or poor analgesia.

Posterior (skin)

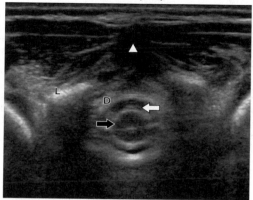

Anterior

Fig. 50.9 Transverse interspinous view of the paediatric spine. D, dura; L, lamina; White triangle, spinous process; White arrow, CSF; Black arrow, spinal cord (the central canal is also visible in the middle).

Posterior/superficial

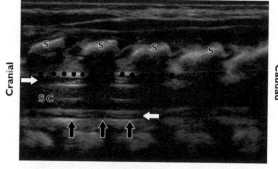

Anterior

Fig. 50.10 Paramedian sagittal oblique view of the paediatric lumbar spine. S, spinous process; SC, spinal cord; Black dots, posterior dura; White arrows, CSF; Black arrows, anterior dura.

Spinals

The spinal cord terminates most often at the level of L1, but can in certain individuals extend to L3. Add to this the fact that anaesthetists have been shown to only correctly identify an interspace 30% of the time lends more support to preprocedural US use. US is by no means perfect and still only manages to identify the correct level in 70%, but identification is misinterpreted by only 1 space compared to sometimes up to 4 spaces when relying solely on surface landmarks.

Again, preprocedural scanning using the techniques described in ➲ Epidurals, pp. 533–41 can be very useful in assessing patients with challenging anatomy (e.g. elderly trauma patients, the obese, etc.) and those with previous spinal surgery.

Single-operator real-time US guidance for performing spinal anaesthesia is much more feasible than for epidurals as the 2-handed counter-pressure technique is not required. This can be successfully achieved using the views described earlier in this chapter (➲ Epidurals, pp. 533–41). An alternative approach (a US enhancement of a technique first described in 1940 by an American anaesthetist Dr Taylor) is given here:

The L5/S1 interspace provides the largest access to the spinal canal. The curvilinear array probe is placed diagonally from lateral to medial between a point 1cm below and medial to the posterior inferior iliac spine, and the L5 lamina. The needle can then be introduced inferolaterally in-plane and followed into the spinal canal for 1st pass success (Fig. 50.11 and Fig. 50.12).

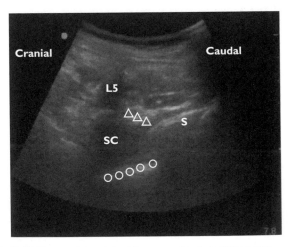

Fig. 50.11 Ultrasound view of the oblique approach to the L5/S1 interspace. 1 L5 vertebra; 2 Ilium; 3 sacrum.

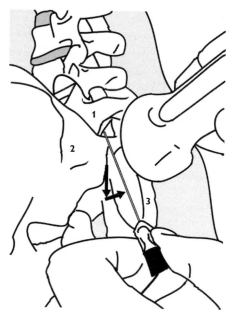

Fig. 50.12 Orientation of probe for an oblique approach to the L5/S1 interspace **1** L5 vertebra; **2** Ilium; **3** sacrum.

Further reading

Carvalho JCA (2008). Ultrasound-facilitated epidurals and spinals in obstetrics. *Anesthesiol Clinics*, **26**,(1) 145–58.
Chin KJ, Karmakar MK, Peng P (2011). Ultrasonography of the adult thoracic and lumbar spine for central neuraxial blockade. *Anesthesiology*, **114**(6), 1459–85.
Chen CPC, Tang SFT, Hsu T-C, et al. (2004). Ultrasound guidance in caudal epidural needle placement. *Anesthesiology*, **101**(1), 181–4.
Kim SH, Lee KH, Yoon KB, et al. (2008). Sonographic estimation of needle depth for cervical epidural blocks. *Anesth Analg*, **106**(5), 1542–7.
Roberts S, Syed SK (2010). Ultrasound for paediatric neuraxial blocks. *Int J Ultrasound Appl Techn Perioperat Care*, **1**(1), 1–8.

Index